Cancer and Aging
Progress in Research and Treatment

Terry V. Zenser, Ph.D.

Rodney M. Coe, Ph.D.

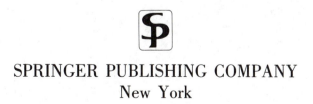

SPRINGER PUBLISHING COMPANY
New York

Springer Publishing Company, Inc.
536 Broadway
New York, NY 10012

88 89 90 / 5 4 3 2 1

Cancer and aging / Terry V. Zenser and Rodney M. Coe, editors.
   p.   cm.
     Includes bibliographies and index.
     ISBN 0-8261-6360-2
     1. Cancer—Age factors. 2.Geriatric oncology. I. Zenser, Terry
V. II. Coe, Rodney M.
RC281.A34C36 1988   88-31199
616.99'4071—dc19   CIP

Printed in the United States of America

*This volume is dedicated to Bernard B. Davis, M. D.,
physician, scientist, teacher, friend, and Director of the St.
Louis Geriatric Research, Education and Clinical Center since
its inception in 1976, for his dedication to excellence in
academics, science, and clinical medicine.*

Contents

PART III   Pharmacological Aspects of Cancer in the Elderly

PART IV   Special Issues in the Care of the Elderly Cancer Patient

Preface

The fact that chronological age is related to the development of cancer at different sites is no longer a matter of debate. It has been shown with increased frequency that advancing age is a major risk factor in carcinogenesis, and age-specific cancer incidence and mortality rates increase as a function of age (Crawford & Cohen, 1987). What is less certain is how aging is related to the development of cancers. Some view carcinogenesis as being age-related and largely due to extrinsic factors in the environment that result in malignant expression only after long-term exposure. Others see carcinogenesis as age-dependent and mostly intrinsic to basic genetic processes concerning fidelity in cell replication. Between these extremes are several variations of this theme such as viewing carcinogenesis as a product of stochastic environmental events during the individual's life that alter the processes controlling the fidelity of cell replication or as a product of natural processes of immunosenescence (Blumenthal, 1983).

The issue of age-relatedness versus age-dependence is still a matter of vigorous debate and ongoing research. The chapters in this volume do not resolve this issue, but they do provide some important insights to the relationship. Part I presents some general information on biological mechanisms common to aging and the development of cancers, e.g., the formation of radicals, lipid peroxidation, and changes in the genome. Major epidemiologic trends linking age with rates of morbidity and mortality from cancer at various sites are also presented. This section concludes with a discussion of types of cancers commonly seen in elderly patients and factors influencing treatment decisions.

New therapeutic interventions and diagnostic techniques made possible by rapid advances in molecular biology which have potential for treatment of older patients are described in Part II. Results are presented of human trials with biological response modifiers such as interleukin-2 (IL-2) and lymphokine-activated killer (LAK) cells, interferon and monoclonal antibodies. Also described in some detail is the treatment of solid tumors in humans by transplantation of autologous bone marrow.

Part III focuses on chemotherapy, including an initial statement concerning age-related changes in pharmacokinetics and pharmacodynamics. A related chapter considers the effects of the patient's age on specific anticancer drugs and concludes with a belief that the fact that the elderly do not tolerate cancer chemotherapy well often leads to treatment with suboptimal dosages. The mechanism by which human cancer cells can develop a resistance to some chemotherapeutic agents along with potential methods for preventing resistance are described. Finally, oncogenes are discussed along with experiments which show that their expression can be controlled by certain growth factors.

The final section, Part IV, addresses several issues concerning cancer and the elderly. One chapter reports the preventive practices of office-based physicians with respect to screening elderly patients for cancers. Another examines the application of surgical interventions in the treatment of cancer in the elderly. A third identifies common psychiatric symptoms in elderly cancer patients and describes ways to treat them. The final chapter outlines some basic standards for nursing care for older cancer patients. Despite apparent diversity, these papers have a common theme—stereotypes of the elderly are pervasive among health care providers and often find expression in practice (i.e., less comprehensive screening, reluctance to operate, comingling of age and disease in psychiatric symptoms, etc.). Fortunately, there is increasing recognition of the effects of stereotyping and more effective education to limit these effects and greater effort to enlist the older cancer patient in participation in his or her own health promotion and treatment.

This book is intended to be provocative rather than definitive in the hope of stimulating interest and further growth in cancer research and treatment.

REFERENCES

Blumenthal, H.T. (1983). The aging-disease connection in retrospect and prospect. In Blumenthal H.T. (Ed.), *Handbook of diseases of aging.* New York: Van Nostrand Reinhold.

Crawford, J., & Cohen, H.J. (1987). Relationship of cancer to aging. *Clinics in Geriatric Medicine, 3:*419–432.

Terry V. Zenser, Ph.D.
Rodney M. Coe, Ph.D.
St. Louis, Missouri 1988

Acknowledgments

The preparation of this edited volume was aided by many sources of support. The symposium at which the ideas expressed in these papers were presented was financially supported by grants from the Veterans Administration's Office of Geriatrics and Extended Care and the National Cancer Institute, R13 CA46754. Administrative support was also received from the VA South Central Regional Medical Education Center, St. Louis University School of Medicine, St. Louis University School of Nursing, the St. Louis College of Pharmacy, and the Missouri Division of the American Cancer Society. We are also indebted to Cheryl Mason, GRECC secretary and secretary of the symposium, for her exemplary handling of the myriad of details associated with the symposium and to Valerie Rincker, secretary in the Department of Community Medicine, for help with producing a manuscript. We also received helpful professional advice from Barbara Watkins of Springer Publishing Company. Finally, we thank the contributors of papers to this volume. They have done their work well, and any remaining errors or ambiguities are those of the editors and not the authors.

Contributors

Linda S. Birnbaum, Ph.D., DABT
Systemic Toxicology Branch
National Institute of Environmental Health
  Sciences
Research Triangle Park, North Carolina

David H. Boldt, M.D.
Divisions of Oncology and Hematology
University of Texas Health Science Center
San Antonio, Texas

James Carmichael, M.D.
Department of Medical Oncology
Newcastle Medical School
Newcastle-Upon-Tyne
England

David D. Celentáno, Sc.D.
Department of Behavioral Sciences and Health
  Education
School of Hygiene and Public Health
Johns Hopkins University
Baltimore, Maryland

Bruce A. Chabner, M.D.
Clinical Pharmacology Branch
National Cancer Institute
Bethesda, Maryland

Charles A. Coltman, Jr., M.D.
Divisions of Oncology and Hematology
University of Texas Health Science Center
San Antonio, Texas

Bernard B. Davis, M.D.
Geriatric Research, Education and
  Clinical Center
Veterans Administration Medical Center and
Department of Internal Medicine
St. Louis University School of Medicine
St. Louis, Missouri

Carlo DeAngelis, Pharm. D.
Toronto-Bayview Regional Cancer Centre and
Faculty of Pharmacy, University of Toronto
Toronto, Ontario

Jose A. Fernandez-Pol, M.D.
Veterans Administration Medical Center and
  Department of Internal Medicine
St. Louis University School of Medicine
St. Louis, Missouri

Robert L. Fine, M.D.
Hematology/Oncology Division
Duke University Medical Center
VA Hospital
Durham, North Carolina

Teresa A. Gilewski, M.D.
Department of Hematology/Oncology
University of Chicago Medical Center
Chicago, Illinois

Robin E. Goldman-Leikin, Ph.D.
Department of Hematology/Oncology
Northwestern University Medical School and
Veterans Administration, Lakeside Medical
  Center
Chicago, Illinois

Harvey M. Golomb, M.D.
Department of Hematology/Oncology
University of Chicago Medical Center
Chicago, Illinois

Jimmie C. Holland, M.D.
Department of Psychiatry
Cornell University Medical College and
  Memorial Sloan-Kettering Cancer Center
New York, New York

Edward H. Kaplan, M.D.
Department of Hematology/Oncology
Northwestern University Medical School and
Veterans Administration, Lakeside Medical
  Center
Chicago, Illinois

Ian G. Kerr, M.D.
Toronto-Bayview Regional Cancer Centre and
Faculty of Pharmacy, University of Toronto
Toronto, Ontario

William A. Knight, III, M.D.
Division of Oncology
St. Louis University School of Medicine and
  Veterans Administration Medical Center
St. Louis, Missouri

Vijaya M. Lakshmi, Ph.D.
Department of Biochemistry
St. Louis University School of Medicine
St. Louis, Missouri

Lynna M. Lesko, M.D., Ph.D.
Department of Psychiatry
Cornell University Medical College and
  Memorial Sloan-Kettering Cancer Center
New York, New York

Bernard S. Linn, M.D.
Department of Surgery
University of Miami School of Medicine and
  Veterans Administration Medical Center
Miami, Florida

Virgil Loeb, Jr., M.D.
President, American Cancer Society, 1987
Washington University
St. Louis, Missouri

Mary Jane Massie, M.D.
Department of Psychiatry
Cornell University Medical College and
  Memorial Sloan-Kettering Cancer Center
New York, New York

Michael B. Mattammal, Ph.D.
Geriatric Research, Education and
  Clinical Center
Veterans Administration Medical Center
St. Louis, Missouri

Jitendra Patel, Ph.D.
Biological Psychiatry Branch
National Institute of Mental Health
Bethesda, Maryland

James A. Radosevich, Ph.D.
Department of Hematology/Oncology
Northwestern University Medical School and
  Veterans Administration, Lakeside
  Medical Center
Chicago, Illinois

Lynn G. Ries, M.S.
Centers and Community Oncology
National Cancer Institute
Bethesda, Maryland

Steven T. Rosen, M.D.
Department of Hematology/Oncology
Northwestern University Medical School and
  Veterans Administration, Lakeside
  Medical Center
Chicago, Illinois

Geoffrey R. Weiss, M.D.
Divisions of Oncology and Hematology
University of Texas Health Science Center
San Antonio, Texas

**Deborah Welch-McCaffrey, R.N.,
  M.S.N., O.C.N.**
Good Samaritan Cancer Center
Phoenix, Arizona

Rosemary Yancik, Ph.D.
Office of Program Planning and Evaluation
Office of the Director
National Institutes of Health
Bethesda, Maryland

Jerome W. Yates, M.D., M.P.H.
Associate Director for Clinical Affairs
Roswell Park Memorial Institute
Buffalo, New York

Terry V. Zenser, Ph.D.
Geriatric Research, Education and
  Clinical Center
Veterans Administration Medical Center and
  Departments of Biochemistry and
  Internal Medicine
St. Louis University School of Medicine
St. Louis, Missouri

A. Michael Zimmer, Ph.D.
Department of Hematology/Oncology
Northwestern University Medical School and
  Veterans Administration, Lakeside
  Medical Center
Chicago, Illinois

Foreword

The term "cancer control" evokes many interpretations that extend from the emphasis on research sponsored by federal agencies to the more compassionate and personal concerns of the private health sector. The National Cancer Institute (NCI) has defined cancer control as "the reduction of cancer incidence, morbidity, and mortality through an orderly sequence from research on interventions and their impact in defined populations to the broad systematic application of the research results." The American Cancer Society (ACS) implements its cancer control mission by striving "to eliminate cancer as a human disease, to save more lives from cancer, and to diminish suffering from cancer through research, education, and service." Although expressed in clearly different terms, both statements refer essentially to the transfer of knowledge and technology from the laboratory to the individual for the benefit of the public health. Let us take a brief look at several of the areas of current emphasis and need.

CANCER PREVENTION AND DETECTION

It is clearly more efficient, more effective, and less costly to prevent rather than to treat cancer even if cure is a feasible outcome. How do we separate fact from fancy and how do we make use of whatever practical information is already available regarding cancer causation? Is it realistic to advocate and expect the elderly to adapt their lifestyles to take advantage of our best current information concerning the risk of developing cancer? One commonly hears today that 70% to 90% of all cancers are related to environmental factors and, therefore, according to one's orientation and perception, might be considered preventable. The nihilist will interpret these figures with futility and will question why one should stop smoking or alter his drinking and eating habits against such overwhelming odds. The realist, however, will recognize that the term "environment" is intended to refer not only to factors in air, food, and water over which the individual may have little control, but also to personal habits and to all voluntary exposures, i.e., everything other than heredity. As a consequence of our relatively meager knowledge concerning causation of specific cancers, current programs in prevention are virtually confined to stressing the importance of prudent health habits while giving recognition to the influence of socioeconomic and behavioral characteristics on specific population groups.

It has been found convenient to differentiate cancer prevention into two strategic subsets: primary prevention, wherein steps are taken to avoid those factors that might lead to development of cancer; and secondary prevention, referring to measures that might be taken to recognize malignant disease at its earliest detectable stage. Clearly, it is reasonable today to advocate primary prevention by abstaining from tobacco; by minimizing dietary fat, increasing dietary fiber, and avoiding obesity; by developing a respect for the dangers of overexposure to the sun; and by avoiding unnecessary contact with known carcinogens. At the same time such advice must be tempered realistically to recognize the specific needs and characteristics of the elderly and other population groups.

Although the term secondary prevention may evoke visions of mass public screening programs in the eyes of some individuals, the expression is really intended to emphasize the importance of detection and diagnosis of cancer at its earliest recognizable stage. This distinction between early detection and mass screening is an important issue. In the real world of medical practice, physicians recognize a major difference between early diagnosis or case finding in the doctor's office and screening of large populations as a public health measure. Nevertheless, the public tends to equate these two modalities. Why is it important to differentiate the two? Whereas reduction in mortality rate may represent the gold standard of the epidemiologist, the practicing physician as well as the public is understandably interested in measures that will have a positive impact upon such intermediate end points as morbidity and quality of life.

Fortunately, the health care delivery system and professional attitudes are changing. Health care providers appear ready to accept a larger role in cancer prevention activities. Primary care physicians and other health professionals have frequent contact with well individuals and should be among the prime educators in cancer prevention and early detection. The surveillance of healthy populations, all of whom are potential cancer patients, is delivered in a variety of settings including office practice, community hospitals, prepaid medical groups, clinics, emergency rooms, and health departments. Among barriers to the implementation of cancer prevention activities by primary care providers are costs, insurers' customary nonpayment for such interventions, lack of public knowledge, perceived inefficacy of the interventions, and the differences in current cancer prevention and detection guidelines issued by various health professional organizations. Only recently, for example, has there been convened an ecumenical council of concerned organizations charged with the responsibility of generating a common set of guidelines for early detection of cancer for the benefit of the public and the profession. This includes such general measures as screening mammography, Pap testing, and nutritional recommendations in addition to the identification of high-risk populations in need of individualized surveillance.

Is the elderly public interested in cancer prevention and early detection? Information derived from a recent focus group exploration of older persons' knowledge, attitudes, and practices regarding preventive health care is of considerable interest. The major finding that emerged was the participants' lack of understanding of the entire concept of preventive health care screenings or practices. Participants were unable to talk about the concept of preventive care without beginning a discussion of diagnostic tests, symptom-driven measures, or general nonmedical health promotion activities. In addition to this lack of understanding, participants were extremely reliant upon their physicians for both diagnosis and for initiation of preventive tests and screenings. This reliance served to further undermine participants' recognition that preventive health measures could and should be self-initiated. Clearly, it is essential that a conceptual framework for early detection of cancer can be provided, that an appropriate motivation be generated, and that relevant information be made available.

Optimal programs in cancer prevention and detection have among their goals a meaningful reduction in incidence of morbidity and mortality rates from cancer within defined populations. These programs should be efficient, self-sustained, and generalizable to other communities. They must be integrated into the usual health care system with degrees of penetration that may vary from pure research projects to temporary demonstration activities, from broadly based public health initiatives at the work site or at mass screening centers to individual counseling and early detection efforts in routine medical practice. Whereas the vast majority of medical care is given in the setting of general office practice, precious little time may be expended in promulgating those guidelines that represent the best of our current knowledge concerning cancer prevention and early detection. If the physician or nurse fails to suggest an intervention, we cannot blame the victim for his or her own indiscretion.

PUBLIC AND PROFESSIONAL EDUCATION

Public and professional education across the whole spectrum of cancer control activities must also be considered. How effective have efforts been to communicate with professional colleagues as well as with public constituents? How do we provide the motivation as well as the means for the public to become truly informed? Familiar concepts of education and learning are being replaced by new techniques in marketing and diffusion. One consequence is that information utilization has become essentially a passive phenomenon. Physicians claim to be too busy, too specialized, too insecure to serve as public health advocates; they are taught very little about this in medical school. Physicians need to expand their horizon so that health care actually means health service.

Local community groups, such as the ACS, regional health departments, hospitals, and cancer centers, may invest significant time and resources in pursuit of such cancer control priorities as prevention and early detection projects, screening clinics, and smoking cessation programs. There has been virtually no structured evaluation of the effectiveness of these activities as they exist in specific population groups. Our emphasis and directions must adapt to the societal as well as the biological differences in the characteristics of malignant disease in the young, the middle-aged, and the elderly. We need to coordinate wellness and preventive programs so that they encompass not only the cancer organizations but also those organizations concerned with heart disease, diabetes, stroke, *etc.* How many disease-oriented cookbooks does the public need in order to understand a prudent diet? Is it worth spending a lot of time with the hard-core smoker rather than educating youngsters as to the hazards of tobacco? How can we best carry the message to those who are not used to reading or speaking English; to those who are more concerned with day-to-day existence rather than long-term preventive measures; to those who have neither financial nor functional access to the health care system in any form?

What about management of the patient with cancer? How do we bring the fruits of our present knowledge regarding cancer treatment to the individual who may not even recognize his or her own problems and needs? We must ensure that the public is aware of available facilities and that these facilities are in fact accessible to everyone. It matters little if we create programs for the good of the public health if existing knowledge is not being applied or utilized. Why do we still see so many women presenting with advanced breast cancer or advanced cervical cancer or individuals with preventable lung cancer or with sun-induced melanoma? We need to encourage research into techniques of behavioral modification that will apply to all segments of the population, not just those who are easily studied. Management must be individualized to serve the needs of those constituents of society who are at greatest risk, not simply those who constitute the majority.

The tendency to let statistical significance take precedence over clinical significance in making treatment decisions has resulted in a preoccupation with the treatment of disease rather than with illness; less attention is being paid to the quality than to the duration of survival. At the same time, however, it is important for patients to be given the opportunity and the encouragement to participate in well-designed clinical trials; this should be the locus wherein the best of treatment strategies are available. Furthermore, we need to expand cancer control interventions within the community to include the reentry of cancer patients into the workplace, the school, and the family setting. We need to stimulate research on lifestyle factors and adaptations of individuals cured of cancer as well as those with stable or progressive disease.

COSTS AND FINANCING

What about the financial implications of all of these programs and services? There is undeniable evidence that cost factors are controlling health care today.

When patients will be treated, by whom, and for how long are no longer decisions left solely to the care providers. Institutional, state, and federal regulatory bodies have assumed increasing jurisdiction over these issues, and this influence will undoubtedly continue. Reimbursement programs tend to discriminate against chronic diseases such as cancer, whereas short-term, acute episodes in which patients improve or deteriorate rapidly fare far better in reimbursement. How can we convince those responsible for setting public policy that effective cancer control measures in prevention, early detection, and rehabilitation can offset many times over the massive costs of palliative care?

RESEARCH

Finally, let us look at some of the needs and opportunities for cancer control research. We should be examining how best to mobilize and utilize existing resources within the voluntary health agencies and the public health system. Programs need to be targeted specifically for the elderly, minorities, and the economically disadvantaged where cancer incidence is greatest independent of race or ethnic heritage. There is an overwhelming need to develop health promotion strategies that take into consideration the importance of behavioral modification, facilitation of communication, public awareness, and social interventions. We must take a hard look at the impact of societal and emotional factors on patterns of care and on the availability of state-of-the-art cancer detection and treatment facilities. Although the probability of developing cancer increases as one grows older, relatively little is known about how the problems of old age affect cancer patient workup, treatment, and care. Studies of cost-effectiveness are essential in order to transfer existing knowledge for the benefit of society. How do we reach the public and how do we convince the profession that we may be failing to exploit our current wisdom while waiting for something more dramatic to occur within the laboratory?

In summary, an attempt has been made to identify some opportunities as well as problems with current cancer control efforts, particularly as they interface with the elderly. Issues dealing with how best to expand and exploit growing knowledge of cancer prevention, diagnosis, and treatment are addressed in the pages that follow. Involvement of primary care professionals and allied health providers as intervening agents for cancer control programs must be encouraged. Knowledge such as that contained in the chapters in this volume will increase the ability of caregivers to apply the best of what is known for the benefit of everyone, but for the elderly in particular who cannot wait for the scourge of malignant disease to be eliminated.

Virgil Loeb, Jr., M.D.
President, American Cancer Society, 1987

PART I

Current Perspectives on Cancer and Aging

1

Biological Mechanisms of Cancer and Aging

Terry V. Zenser, Michael B. Mattammal, Vijaya M. Lakshmi, and Bernard B. Davis

Overlapping mechanisms pertinent to both cancer and aging will be the focus of this chapter. Aging consists of partly preprogrammed changes occurring during the lifetime of an organism which increase the risk of dying for all members of a species. Cancer is not one disease but a general term used in describing a class of diseases associated with malignant neoplasia. Cancer increases in incidence during the life of the organism and, like aging, is a multistep process. Aging may be complementary to and/or facilitate steps in the carcinogenic process.

AGING

During most of the 15,000 years that modern Homo sapiens have existed, the average human life expectancy was only about 20–40 years. As illustrated by the survival curves in Figure 1.1, there was little change in average life expectancy from 15,000 years to about 500 years ago (Cutler, 1984a). The similarity of the exponential-like decrease in percent survival implies that the probability of death was fairly constant and independent of chronologic age. Death was, for the most part, due to infectious diseases, malnutrition, accidents, and animal predators.

Supported by the Veterans Administration and by the USPHS Grant CA-28015 from the National Cancer Institute through the National Bladder Cancer Project.

The human's ability to control these environmental or external factors has resulted in an increase in average life expectancy. However, note that the maximum life span potential has not changed appreciably over this same period of time. For most of human history, the average life span has been made up of what might be considered today as young individuals. With a mean life span of 30 years, age-dependent declines in many processes had not yet occurred to a significant degree. From an evolutionary point of view, there was not a need to maintain good health past the age of 30 years. A large population of aging people is a relatively new problem for society.

CANCER

The essential feature that distinguishes a tumor cell from a normal cell is a heritable change that allows the tumor cell to undergo inappropriate cell proliferation with subsequent invasion and metastasis. Although aging occurs over a broad front in most cells, tumor cells are rare (relative to the 6×10^{13} cells in our body).

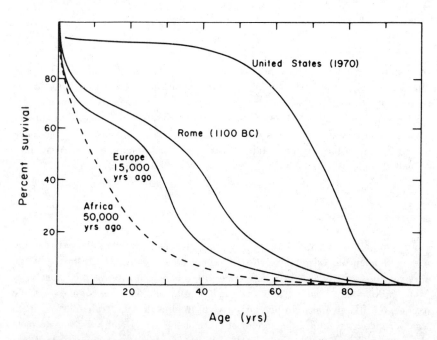

FIGURE 1.1. Percent survival curve for humans is depicted. Effect of different environmental hazard conditions is illustrated. Although the mean survival values are different, the maximum life span potential remains constant at about 100 years (from Cutler, 1984a).

The onset frequency of most cancers is found to be low until after age 30. Thereafter, risk of cancer increases with approximately the fourth power of age. At the end of the life span of a short-lived species (2–3 years), such as rodents, about 30% of the animals have cancer. Similarly, with long-lived species, such as humans, about 30% have cancer by 85 years. During the 60 million years of primate evolution, the increase in life span has been accompanied by a large decrease in cancer rates during early life (Ames et al., 1985).

Environmental factors were first recognized as causing cancer in the late 18th century. The English physician Pott noted that chimney sweeps had a high incidence of scrotal cancer. Many other occupational and environmental factors that enhance carcinogenesis are recognized today. About 60% to 90% of human cancers have important environmental factors in their etiologies (Higginson, 1969; Doll & Peto, 1981). Environmental factors that play a major role in the causation of human cancer include chemicals and ultraviolet and ionizing radiation. Such environmentally related cancers are thought to result from a multistep process in which a deleterious change in the genome becomes fixed and inherited. Because of increased longevity and industrial pollution, cancer is also a relatively new health problem.

MULTIPLE STEPS OF CARCINOGENESIS

Chemical carcinogenesis is a multistep process (Berenblum & Haran-Ghera, 1957; Foulds, 1965; Farber & Sarma, 1987). A procarcinogen is metabolically activated to the ultimate carcinogen that covalently binds to DNA. Some carcinogens are direct-acting and do not require activation to bind DNA. DNA adducts are subjected to excision repair and error-prone repair. Most adducts are properly repaired with no alterations occurring in the genome. Following replication alterations in DNA become fixed. This initiation step is not reversible. Expression of the neoplastic state depends upon promotion of the initiated cells. During promotion, growth of phenotypically altered cells occurs. Examples of these cells are nodules in liver, papillomas in the skin and urinary tract, and polyps in the colon. Promotion is reversible at first, but later becomes irreversible. During progression, promoted cells undergo a slow cellular evolution to a malignant neoplasm. Neoplasms become more prone to show invasion and then to metastasize.

COMPARISON OF CANCER AND AGING

A number of comparisons can be made between the processes of aging and cancer (Pitot, 1978). A few of these are delineated in Table 1.1. Both processes increase with longer survival time and involve alterations in the genome. Although cancer is well-characterized as consisting of multiple stages, stages in the aging process

TABLE 1.1. Comparison of the Processes of Aging and Cancer

Similarities
  Increases with longer survival time
  Alterations in the genome
  Multistage development
  Hormonal status modification
  Radicals and lipid peroxidation increase
  Antioxidants decrease
  Dietary restriction decreases or slows

Differences
  Life span of cells
  Proliferative capacity
  Size of cell population initiating process

have been described but are not as well-characterized (Finch, 1976). Both processes are influenced by hormonal status. Changes in hormonal status during aging are associated with the development of osteoporosis. Development of certain tumors is also influenced by hormonal status. Both processes are increased by radicals and lipid peroxidation, and accordingly are decreased by antioxidants. Dietary restriction decreases or slows both processes.

In addition to these similarities, there are some important differences between aging and cancer. Although the life span of normal cells is finite, as is their proliferative capacity, cancer cells are immortal and have a tremendous proliferative capacity. Aging appears to involve many or most cells of the organism, whereas cancer can be initiated by a single clonal population.

RADICALS AND LIPID PEROXIDATION

General

Radicals and lipid peroxidation are thought to be involved in both aging and carcinogenesis (Harman, 1986; Ames, 1983). A radical is an atom or group of atoms possessing an odd (unpaired) electron. In writing the symbol for a radical, a dot is included to represent the odd electron (i.e., $R^{\bullet}$). Radicals are reactive and form chemical bonds in a manner that will allow them to gain an electron. Radicals can cause cellular damage in several ways. Radicals can react with and alter critical cellular nucleophiles (nucleic acids and proteins). Radicals can cause a chain reaction that proliferates its deleterious effects. Radicals are natural by-products of cellular metabolism. Oxygen radicals are one example (Greenstock, 1986). Successive addition of electrons to oxygen results in the sequential formation of superoxide ($O_2^{\bullet}$), hydrogen peroxide (H_2O_2), and hydroxyl radicals ($^{\bullet}OH$).

$$O_2 \xrightarrow{\ e^- \ } O_2^{\bullet} \xrightarrow{\ e^-,2H^+ \ } H_2O_2 \xrightarrow{\ \ } {}^{\bullet}OH \xrightarrow{\ e^-,H^+ \ } H_2O \qquad [1]$$

Polyunsaturated fatty acids are a major component of membranous structures throughout the body. Polyunsaturated fatty acids are susceptible to radical mediated damage and the proliferation of that damage (Pryor, 1984). LH is an unsaturated lipid that loses its allylic hydrogen atom to form an allylic radical, L$^{\bullet}$ (equation 2).

$$\text{LH} \xrightarrow{\text{initiation}} \text{L}^{\bullet} \qquad [2]$$
$$\text{L}^{\bullet} + O_2 \rightarrow \text{LOO}^{\bullet} \qquad [3]$$
$$\text{LOO}^{\bullet} + \text{LH} \rightarrow \text{LOOH} + \text{L}^{\bullet} \qquad [4]$$

The allylic radical reacts with molecular oxygen to form a lipid peroxy radical, LOO$^{\bullet}$ (equation 3). The lipid peroxy radical can abstract a hydrogen atom from another polyunsaturated fatty acid (L$^{\bullet}$) continuing the process (equation 4). This is indicative of the chain reaction mechanism (equations 3 and 4) involved in lipid peroxidation that propagates the radical process. This chain reaction (rancidity) yields a variety of mutagens, promoters, and carcinogens. These include fatty acid hydroperoxides, epoxides, enals and aldehydes, and alkoxy and hydroperoxy radicals (Ames, 1983). The presence of numerous defense mechanisms within the cell to limit levels of radicals and lipid peroxidation and the damage induced by these processes emphasize the necessity for protection.

Aging

Aging is an extremely complex process. However, the maximum life span potential is relatively unaffected by different environmental conditions and is characteristic of each species. As such, Cutler (1985) has proposed that a common set of longevity genes may exist in all mammalian species. Functions of an organism that might contribute to aging are normal developmental and metabolic processes required for propagation and survival. Recognition of this fact was obtained by the correlation of specific metabolic rate versus maximum life span potential. Specific metabolic rate is a measure of the total energy used by an animal per unit body weight. For most nonprimate mammalian species, the relationship between specific metabolic rate and maximum life span potential is expressed by a common hyperbolic curve. Thus, the product of maximum life span potential and specific metabolic rate is nearly constant. This product is called life span energy potential, which represents the total energy used over a species' life span per unit body weight. For nonprimates and primates, the life span energy potential is about 220 kcal/g and 458 kcal/g, respectively. Humans have a significantly higher value (815 kcal/g). Thus, most species, regardless of their maximum life span potential, use up the same amount of energy on a per gram basis. The species' aging rate is proportional to its specific metabolic rate or amount of oxygen consumed. One important factor in longevity appears to be specific metabolic rate, which is much lower in humans than in rodents and markedly affects the levels of endogenous oxygen radicals.

Oxygen is used for metabolism because of its ability to yield a highly efficient energy output (as compared to anaerobic metabolism). Various by-products of oxygen metabolism include superoxide, hydroxyl radical, hydrogen peroxide, and products of lipid peroxidation. Toxic reactions caused by these by-products are thought to contribute to the aging process.

The role of lipid peroxidation in aging has been assessed. The age-related accumulation of an autofluorescent pigment in many postmitotic cell types appears to occur universally in animals. This pigment, termed lipofuscin, is thought to be the result of *in vivo* autoxidation of lipids (lipid peroxidation). Lipofuscin is proposed to be formed by malondialdehyde (a major product of lipid peroxidation and a mutagen and carcinogen) cross-linking protein and lipid. If the rate of lipid peroxidation is a major determinant of longevity, one would expect to find a correlation between a species' maximum life span potential and the rate of lipofuscin accumulation in their tissues. There is a linear increase with age in the amount of lipofuscin in the rat retinal pigment epithelium (Katz & Robison, 1986). In addition, short-lived mammalian species with high metabolic rates tend to accumulate lipofuscin at a faster rate than longer-lived species with lower metabolic rates. Consistent with these observations is the inverse correlation of serum lipid peroxide levels with life span energy potential in mammalian species (Cutler, 1985). Thus, lipid peroxidation, like the specific metabolic rate, appears to play an important role in the aging process. Lipid peroxidation is known to cause DNA damage (Inouye, 1984). Alterations in DNA bases have been shown to occur in old-aged animals (Randerath et al., 1986).

An antioxidant system functions to prevent deleterious effects of radicals and lipid peroxidation (Inouye, 1984). This system has enzymatic and nonenzymatic components. Enzymes involved include superoxide dismutases, catalases, and peroxidases. Superoxide dismutase concentrations in primate and rodent brain, liver, and heart were found to correlate with a species' life span energy potential (Cutler, 1985). The nonenzymatic defense system is comprised, for the most part, of small molecular weight compounds including beta carotene, vitamin A, vitamin E, glutathione, and urate. Plasma levels of beta carotene, vitamin E, and urate were found to correlate with species' life span energy potential (Cutler, 1984a; Cutler, 1985). Thus, the total amount of oxygen a species utilizes over its life span is directly proportional to the amount of protection provided by certain antioxidants against the toxic byproducts of oxygen metabolism. The synthetic antioxidant, ethoxyquin, has the capacity to extend the life span of rats (Comfort, 1971).

Antioxidant defense systems have evolved by changes occurring in genes and contribute to longevity.

Cancer

There is considerable evidence that radicals and the ensuing lipid peroxidation can affect carcinogenic processes. This may involve structural changes in the genome. Gene rearrangements or combined epigenetic–genetic mechanisms may be involved in initiation or modulation of the expression of genes related to tumor promotion and progression (Cerutti, 1985a).

Initiation. Oxidative damage to DNA can initiate carcinogenesis. For ionizing radiation, oxygen radicals (particularly hydroxyl radicals) are responsible for 60% to 70% of DNA strand breaks, chromosomal aberrations, mutations, and cell killing. A variety of chemicals can generate free radicals directly, such as *N*-hydroxy-2-naphthylamine and 4-hydroxy-aminoquinoline-*N*-oxide, or following metabolic activation, such as aromatic hydrocarbons and aminoazo dyes (Kaneko & Leadon, 1986). Thymine glycol (5,6-dihydroxydihydrothymine) and its nucleoside analogue, thymidine glycol, and 5-hydroxymethyluracil are oxidation products of thymine. These alterations in thymine could contribute to the formation of single-strand breaks or accelerate abnormal DNA replication and recombination. Specific enzymes can repair this damage with thymine oxidation products that are detectable in urine. This serves as a method for quantitating oxidative DNA damage. Assessing urinary excretion in humans, Ames and Saul (1986) estimated that an average of 1000 oxidized thymine residues per day per cell are formed (based on a total of 6×10^{13} cells in the body). This represents only three products of one oxidized base. It is likely that many thousands of additional DNA bases are altered per cell each day in humans but escape detection. Rats, which have a shorter life span and higher specific metabolic rate than humans, excrete about 15 times more thymine glycol and thymidine glycol per kilogram of body weight. In addition, *in vivo* and *in vitro* studies have demonstrated that *N*-hydroxy-2-naphthylamine elicits a dose-dependent increase in thymine glycol production. Thymine glycol production was significantly reduced or eliminated by either catalase or superoxide dismutase (Kaneko & Leadon, 1986).

Promotion. There appears to be a relationship between the generation of radicals, lipid peroxidation, and tumor promotion (Cerutti, 1985b). Tumor promoters induce a prooxidant state. This is characterized by the generation of radicals with structure–activity relationships that parallel the capacity of promoters to support tumorigenesis. In addition, agents that prevent promotion inhibit radical formation (Copeland, 1983). Benzoyl peroxide is widely used as a radical generating compound, primarily in the polymer industry as a polymerization initiator, curing agent, and cross-linking agent. It is effective in promoting skin papillomas and squamous cell carcinomas. Benzoyl peroxide, like the phorbol ester 12-*O*-tetradecanoylphorbol-13-acetate (TPA), induces epidermal hyperplasia and similar morphologic changes (e.g., dark keratinocytes) (Birnboim, 1981). TPA, in addition to other promoters, causes DNA damage (Slaga et al., 1982). In skin, antioxidants prevent DNA strand breaks and the promoting effects of TPA. DNA damage appears to be important in mouse skin tumor promotion. Thus, a "membrane-mediated chromosomal damage" model has been proposed to describe the actions of certain promoters (Copeland, 1983). According to this model, membrane active agents, such as TPA, stimulate release of certain unsaturated fatty acids such as arachidonic acid, elicit an oxidative burst, and disturb cellular membranes in a nonspecific way, thereby exposing phospholipids to autoxidation. An end result of this metabolic sequela is DNA damage. Promotion is frequently associated with inflammatory processes. Oxygen radicals and lipid peroxidation are thought to be the active participants in these inflammatory processes.

The biologic effects of certain carcinogens and promoters may overlap because they initiate common radical or lipid peroxidation reactions. Such carcinogens have been called complete carcinogens because they do not require promotion. Promoters such as TPA can facilitate peroxidase-mediated activation of carcinogens, i.e., aromatic amines, by supplying substrate in the form of hydrogen peroxide or lipid peroxide. In addition to prostaglandin H synthase, which has a hydroperoxidase activity, a variety of ubiquitous peroxidases exist in mammalian tissues (Zenser et al., 1983; Zenser & Davis, 1985). Furthermore, some chemical carcinogens are activated by radicals that are generated from unsaturated fatty acid hydroperoxides (Marnett, 1987). NADPH-dependent lipid peroxidation in rat liver microsomes has been shown to cause epoxidation of the carcinogen (+)-BP-7,8-diol.

INTERRELATIONSHIPS BETWEEN AGING AND CANCER

The involvement of radicals and lipid peroxidation in both aging and cancer suggests an overlap in mechanisms. Whether a radiation-induced hydroxyl radical is facilitating aging or cancer or both processes at any specific time is not possible to assess. Similarly, because lipid peroxides are known to cause DNA damage and mutations, it is not possible to determine whether a specific lipid peroxidation event is mediating aging and/or carcinogenic processes. DNA damage involved in aging versus carcinogenesis may be qualitatively different. The capacity of antioxidants to prevent both aging and cancer suggests radicals and lipid peroxidation are mediating events.

A summary of the role of radicals and lipid peroxidation in both aging and cancer is illustrated in a model by Greenstock (1986). Radicals can be formed by a variety of sources internal to the organism such as metabolism and autoxidation of lipids or external such as sunlight, ionizing radiation, and chemical carcinogens (Figure 1.2). Epoxides, peroxides, and other radical-derived products cause damage, resulting in DNA strand breakage and protein cross-linking. The ultimate biologic effects include cancer and aging along with other deleterious effects.

GENE STABILITY AND EXPRESSION

Chromatin may be considered a thread of duplex DNA coiled around a series of nucleosomes. Information in this mass of euchromatin must be accurately replicated and transcribed for the species to survive. The mechanism by which genetic material is directed to replicate or to be transcribed is only beginning to be understood. Many mechanisms appear plausible, and more than one may be

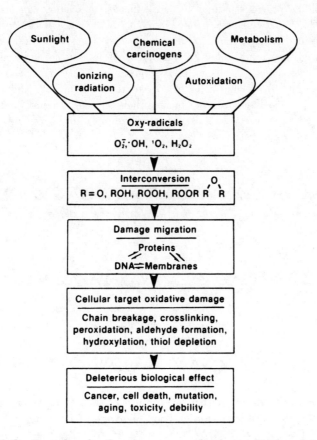

FIGURE 1.2. Postulated role of oxygen radicals in eliciting deleterious biologic effects including cancer and aging (from Greenstock, 1986).

functional. Methylation is one mechanism that appears to regulate the expression of certain genes (Lewin, 1985). An active gene may be described as under-methylated. Embryonic genes tend to have the best correlation with the under-methylated state. The state of methylation at specific sites is critical. Methylation modifies the structure of DNA such that its substrate characteristics for specific enzymes are altered. For example, certain unmethylated regions on DNA are hypersensitive to DNase I. Methylation can alter the recognition sites of restriction enzymes. Hpa II and Msp I are restriction enzymes that cleave the same DNA sequence (CCGG) but have a different response to the state of methylation (isoschizomers). This is illustrated in Figure 1.3. If the second C is methylated in the sequence (CC*GG), Hpa II no longer recognizes the sequence. However, Msp I still cleaves the site. If the sample DNA in Figure 1.3 were electrophoresed, bands corresponding to fragments 1, 3, 4, and 2 would appear following Msp I digestion. Hpa II digestion would yield only fragment 1 and new fragment 5. The drug 5-azacytidine provides indirect evidence that demethylation can result in gene expression. The drug is incorporated into DNA in the place of cytidine and cannot be methylated because the 5' position is blocked. The state of differentiation can be changed by 5-azacytidine. For example, muscle cells are induced to develop from nonmuscle cell precursors (Constantinides et al., 1977). A review by Riggs and Jones (1983) provides a list of 26 reports in which 5-azacytidine treatment activated previously silent genes (gene switching) and 40 reports indicating that CCGG sites in nonexpressing tissues or cell cultures are more highly methylated than in expressing tissues.

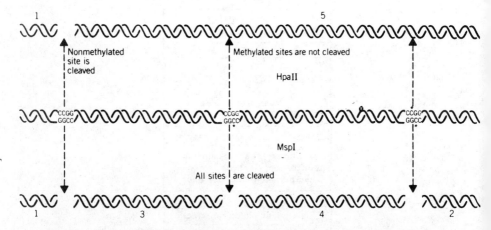

FIGURE 1.3. Schematic representation of the effect of methylation on gene expression. Restriction enzyme cleavage of DNA depends upon the degree of methylation. DNA fragments of differing length, represented numerically, may be expressed (from Lewin, 1985).

Aging

Age-related changes are often associated with DNA stability because of the central role DNA plays in the expression of cellular phenotype. Using a specific DNA probe, the intracisternal A particle gene was examined for age-related changes (Mays-Hoopes, 1985). A sequence in the probe contains one Msp I/Hpa II site. Genomic DNA was analyzed in livers from 6-, 12-, 18-, 24-, and 26-month-old mice. An increased sensitivity to both enzymes was observed with increasing age. A fivefold increase was observed during aging in the 0.5 kb fragment derived from Msp I digestion. A tendency toward smaller hybridizing fragments with increasing age from Hpa II digestion was also observed. As illustrated above in Figure 1.3, these effects may be due to demethylation of cytosine. In this regard, it is important to note that only approximately 6% of all methylable cytosines are assessable with this type of enzyme treatment. In addition to demethylation, there are other possible reasons for increased Msp I sensitivity, such as an increased number of copies of the intracisternal A particle gene.

Separate studies have shown that there is imperfect transmission of DNA methylation patterns from cell generation to generation in human diploid fibroblasts in and around endogenous gene loci (Shmookler Reis & Goldstein, 1982). A single treatment of cultured human fibroblasts with 5-azacytidine significantly shortens their life span (Holliday, 1985). In general, *in vitro* aging has been associated with a reduction in methylation. If DNA methylation is important in maintaining gene repression, then demethylation may lead to substantial expression of normally silent genes. Such activation may have progressively deleterious effects, with cell regulation no longer possible.

It is likely that other genomic changes, in addition to methylation, may contribute to senescence. Gene amplification and enhanced expression of cellular oncogenes have been observed for the proto-oncogene c-Ha-*ras*-1. Upon hybridization with a c-Ha-*ras*-1 DNA probe, a 6.6 kb band was observed that corresponds to the proto-oncogene (Srivastava et al., 1985). The intensity of this band increased twofold to fourfold during late passage (senescent) compared to early passage fibroblasts. When DNA was probed for other genes such as human chorionic gonadotropin and alpha- and gamma-globins, no changes in band intensity with increased passage were observed. The level of mRNA and protein product for c-Ha-*ras*-1 exhibited age-related increases of the same magnitude as observed with DNA. Proto-oncogenes confer normal growth-regulating effects on cells. Amplification of c-Ha-*ras*-1 may provide an advantage to late passage fibroblasts to traverse the G1 phase of the cell cycle. During late passage, an increasing number of fibroblasts are arrested in G1/S interphase, replicative senescence. Thus, selective pressure favoring oncogene amplification increases in late passage cells.

Changes in lymphocyte mRNA expression have also been observed during aging. The ability of mitogens to stimulate lymphocytes to proliferate declines with increasing age. Interleukin-2 is an intermediate in this proliferation process.

Following concanavalin A stimulation, lymphocyte interleukin-2 mRNA and polypeptide levels were 80% lower for lymphocytes from 29- compared to 6-month-old rats (Richardson et al., 1985). Alterations in the genome and subsequent gene expression are thought to contribute to the well-documented declines in immunologic function that occur with increasing age.

Cancer

Many human cancers are thought to be caused by the abnormal regulation of developmentally important genes. These genes are always present in the genome. According to this hypothesis, the new synthesis or increased synthesis of a developmental stage-specific gene product, which would normally be present in much smaller amounts, may result in cancer. Support for this hypothesis is provided by experiments that demonstrate that teratocarcinomas can be induced to differentiate and participate in normal development by being placed in an early embryo (Mintz & Illmensee, 1975). Methylation plays a fundamental role in governing gene expression during normal cell differentiation (Lewin, 1985). Therefore, irregularities in DNA methylation patterns may be responsible for some of the aberrant gene expression seen in cancer. The overall levels of cytosine methylation in transformed cells has been shown to be decreased. Primary hepatocarcinomas and transplantable mouse liver tumors contain decreased levels of 5-methylcytosine relative to normal liver (Lapeyre et al., 1981). Several carcinogens have been shown to inhibit the methylation of DNA. Most notable are the inhibitory effects of N-methyl-N'-nitro-N-nitrosoguanidine. This carcinogen directly alters DNA methyltransferase activity (Cox, 1980). Carcinogen adducts in the vicinity of methylation sites may alter recognition by methyltransferases resulting in demethylation (Wilson & Jones, 1983). The hepatocarcinogen, ethionine, substantially inhibits methylation in DNA shortly after or during carcinogen exposure. Ethionine is a competitive inhibitor of methylation after conversion to S-adenosylmethionine (Boehm & Drahovsky, 1979).

Methylation of DNA has been assessed during excision repair in human diploid fibroblasts (Kastan et al., 1982). DNA damage was induced by ultraviolet radiation, methyl-N-nitrosourea or acetylaminofluorene. In confluent, nondividing cells, methylation in repair patches induced by all three agents was slow and incomplete. In cells damaged during logarithmic phase, methylation of cytosine was much faster and reached an almost normal level in 10–24 hours. Hypomethylated repair patches in confluent cells became more methylated when the cells were stimulated to divide. However, the repair patch may not become fully methylated before cell division. Thus, DNA damage and repair induced by carcinogens may lead to a heritable loss of methylation in some sites. This may result in inappropriate gene expression and initiation of carcinogenesis.

Chromosomal rearrangement and demethylation have been shown, in certain instances, to be factors in the expression of oncogenes. There are many known examples of nonrandom and specific chromosome alterations in hemopoietic and lymphoid neoplasms (Rowley, 1984). Individual cases of leukemia have been subclassified on the basis of karyotype and different chromosomal abnormalities and correlated with clinical course. Many known oncogenes map to sites that are nonrandomly associated with chromosomal alterations. The C-*myc* oncogene is translocated to one of the immunoglobulin loci in many cases of Burkitt's lymphoma, a tumor of antibody-producing B cells. Hypomethylation has been demonstrated with cellular oncogenes H-*ras*, K-*ras*, and C-*myc*.

Interrelationships Between Aging and Cancer

Alterations in the integrity of the genome lead to a loss of genetic information required for cell regulation. Both aging and cancer are characterized by instability in the genome. Specific chromosomal alterations occur during aging and in many neoplasias. Normal cell differentiation involves subtle gene rearrangements that lead to the irreversible commitment of somatic cells to a given line of gene expression. As a result, the options for somatic cells become progressively fewer, making these cells more susceptible to random aberrant DNA alterations leading to aging. In a rare cell, abnormal DNA replication may lead to malignant transformation.

Specific protective genes may exist that maintain genomic stability. If such genes exist, they could function as suppressors of tumor growth and senescence. There are a considerable number of studies demonstrating tumor suppressor genes (Sager, 1986). Early studies fused pairs of cells, one normal and the other tumorigenic. Suppression of tumor formation was observed in hybrids. During late passage of hybrid cells, reexpression of tumor-forming ability was observed along with increasing chromosome loss. The loss of a specific chromosome was associated with tumorigenesis. Tumor suppressor genes were proposed to reside on the lost chromosome (Harris, 1971). Tumor suppression has been reported both in intraspecies and interspecies cell hybrids. Tumor lines used have been viral and oncogene-induced as well as spontaneously derived. These results suggest that the suppressor genes were highly conserved during evolution. These genes may be considered akin to the longevity genes referred to by Cutler (1984a,b). Genetic analysis of retinoblastoma patients has provided additional evidence for suppressor genes (Knudson, 1985; Sager, 1986). Formation of a tumor requires homozygosity of the inactive Rb gene. Homozygosity is attributed to nondisjunction of sister chromatids during mitosis. In all the diploid cells of these patients, the Rb gene located on chromosome 13 (13q14) is heterozygous. Survivors of the childhood disease often develop osteosarcomas, which also have a homozygous inactive Rb gene. Thus, differentiation controls the expression of the Rb locus. Rb may be classified as a dominant tumor suppressor, differentiation-related gene. Loss of Rb blocks terminal differentiation in committed cells and thereby permits further cell proliferation.

Because both aging and cancer are facilitated by instability in the genome, identification of antioncogenes will provide a means of better understanding and controlling both processes. One approach would be to apply methodology that has been used successfully to clone oncogenes (Shih & Weinberg, 1982). This would involve transfecting tumor cells with normal cellular DNA, then using a positive selection process, and selecting revertant nontumorigenic cells. DNA from nontumorigenic cells can then be cloned, sequenced, and the structure and function of the protein product determined. Molecular biology provides new insight into the mechanisms involved in aging and cancer and may provide a basis for therapeutic intervention.

REFERENCES

Ames, B.N. (1983). Dietary carcinogens and anticarcinogens. *Science, 221*:1256–1264.

Ames, B.N., Saul, R.L., Schwiers, E., Adelman, R., & Cathcart, R. (1985). Oxidative DNA damage as related to cancer and aging: Assay of thymine glycol, thymidine glycol, and hydroxymethyluracil in human and rat urine. In Sohal, R.S., Burnbaum, L.S., & Cutler, R.G. (Eds.), *Molecular biology of aging: Gene stability and gene expression* (pp. 137–154). New York: Raven Press.

Ames, B.N., & Saul, R.L. (1986). Oxidative DNA damage as related to cancer and aging. In C. Ramel, B. Lampert & J. Magnusson (Eds.), *Genetic toxicology of environmental chemicals, part A: Basic principles and mechanisms of action* (pp. 11–26). New York: Alan R. Liss.

Berenblum, I., & Haran-Ghera, N. (1957). A quantitative study of the systemic initiating action of urethane (ethylcarbamate) in mouse skin carcinogenesis. *British Journal of Cancer, 11*:77.

Birnboim, H.C. (1981). Skin tumor-promoting activity of benzoyl peroxide, a widely used free radical-generating compound. *Science, 213*:1023–1025.

Boehm, T.L.J., & Drahovsky, D. (1979). Effect of carcinogen ethionine on enzymatic methylation of DNA sequences with various degrees of repetitiveness. *European Journal of Cancer, 15*:1167–1173.

Cerutti, P.A. (1985a). Prooxidant states and tumor promotion. *Science, 227*:375–381.

Cerutti, P.A. (1985b). Active oxygen and promotion. In Fischer, S.M., & Slaga, T.J. (Eds.), *Arachidonic acid metabolism and tumor promotion* (pp. 131–168). Boston: Martinus Nijhoff.

Comfort, A. (1971). Effect of ethoxyquin on the longevity of C3H mice. *Nature, 229*:254–255.

Constantinides, P.G., Jones, P.A., & Gevers, W. (1977). Functional striated muscle cells from non-myoblast precursors following 5-azacytidine treatment. *Nature, 267*:364–366.

Copeland, E.S. (1983). A National Institutes of Health workshop report: Free radicals in promotion—a chemical pathology study section workshop. *Cancer Research, 43*:5631–5637.

Cox, R. (1980). DNA methylase inhibition in vitro by N-methyl-N'-nitro-N-nitrosoguanidine. *Cancer Research, 40*:61–63.

Cutler, R.G. (1984a). Free radicals and aging. In Roy, A.K., & Chatterjee, B. (Eds.), *Molecular basis of aging* (pp. 263–354). Orlando: Academic Press.

Cutler, R.G. (1984b). Antioxidants and longevity. In Armstrong, D., Sohal, R.S., Cutler,

R.G., & Slater, T.F. (Eds.), *Free radicals in molecular biology, aging, and disease* (pp. 235–266). New York: Raven Press.

Cutler, R.G. (1985). Antioxidants and longevity of mammalian species. In Woodhead, A.D., Blackett, A.D., & Hollaender, A. (Eds.), *Molecular biology of aging* (pp. 15–73). New York: Plenum Press.

Doll, R., & Peto, R. (1981). The causes of cancer: Quantitative estimates of avoidable risks of cancer in the United States today. *Journal of the National Cancer Institute, 66:*1192–1308.

Farber, E., & Sarma, D.S.R. (1987). Biology of disease. Hepatocarcinogenesis: A dynamic cellular perspective. *Laboratory Investigation, 56:*4–22.

Finch, C.E. (1976). The regulation of physiological changes during mammalian aging. *Quarterly Review of Biology, 51:*49.

Foulds, L. (1965). Multiple etiologic factors in neoplastic development. *Cancer Research, 25:*1339.

Greenstock, C.L. (1986). Radiation-induced aging and induction and promotion of biological damage. In Johnson, J.E., Jr., Walford, R., Harman, D., & Miquel, J. (Eds.), *Free radicals, aging, and degenerative diseases* (pp. 197–219). New York: Alan R. Liss.

Harman, D. (1986). Free radical theory of aging: Role of free radicals in the origination and evolution of life, aging, and disease processes. In Johnson, J.E., Jr., Walford, R., Harman, D., & Miquel, J. (Eds.), *Free radicals, aging, and degenerative diseases* (pp. 3–49). New York: Alan R. Liss.

Harris, H. (1971). Cell fusion and the analysis of malignancy. *Proceedings of the Royal Society of London. Series B: Biological Sciences, 179:*1–20.

Higginson, J. (1969). Present trends in cancer epidemiology. *Canadian Cancer Conference, 8:*40–75.

Holliday, R. (1985). The significance of DNA methylation in cellular aging. In Woodhead, A.D., Blackett, A.D., & Hollaender, A. (Eds.), *Molecular biology of aging* (pp. 269–283). New York: Plenum Press.

Inouye, S. (1984). Site-specific cleavage of double-stranded DNA by the hydroperoxide of linoleic acid. *FEBS Letters, 172:*231–234.

Kaneko, M., & Leadon, S.A. (1986). Production of thymine glycols in DNA by N-hydroxy-2-naphthylamine as detected by a monoclonal antibody. *Cancer Research, 46:*71–75.

Kastan, M.B., Gowans, B.J., & Lieberman, M.W. (1982). Methylation of deoxycytidine incorporated by excision–repair synthesis of DNA. *Cell, 30:*509–516.

Katz, M.L., & Robison, W.G., Jr. (1986). Nutritional influences on autoxidation, lipofuscin accumulation, and aging. In Johnson, J.E., Jr., Walford, R., Harman, D., & Miquel, J. (Eds.), *Free radicals, aging, and degenerative diseases* (pp. 221–259). New York: Alan R. Liss.

Knudson, A.G., Jr. (1985). Hereditary cancer, oncogenes, and antioncogenes. *Cancer Research, 45:*1437–1443.

Lapeyre, J.N., Walker, M.S., and Becker, F.F. (1981). DNA methylation and methylase levels in normal and malignant mouse hepatic tissues. *Carcinogenesis, 2:*873–878.

Lewin, B. (1985). The nature of active chromatin. In Lewin, B. (Ed.), *Genes* (pp. 489–512). New York: John Wiley & Sons.

Marnett, L.J. (1987). Peroxyl free radicals: Potential mediators of tumor initiation and promotion. *Carcinogenesis, 8:*1365–1373.

Mays-Hoopes, L.L. (1985). DNA methylation: A possible correlation between aging and cancer. In Sohal, R.S., Birnbaum, L.S., & Cutler, R.G. (Eds.), *Molecular biology of aging: gene stability and gene expression* (pp. 49–65). New York: Raven Press.

Mintz, B., & Illmensee, K. (1975). Normal genetically mosaic mice produced from malignant teratocarcinoma cells. *Proceedings of the National Academy of Sciences USA, 72:*3585–3589.

Pitot, H.C. (1978). Interactions in the natural history of aging and carcinogenesis. *Federation Proceedings, 37*:2841–2847.

Pryor, W.A. (1984). Free radicals in autoxidation and in aging. In Armstrong, D., Sohal, R.S., Cutler, R.G., & Slater, T.F. (Eds.), *Free radicals in molecular biology, aging, and disease* (pp. 13–41). New York: Raven Press.

Randerath, K., Reddy, M.V., & Disher, R.M. (1986). Age- and tissue-related DNA modifications in untreated rats: Detection by 32p-postlabeling assay and possible significance for spontaneous tumor induction and aging. *Carcinogenesis, 7*:1615–1617.

Richardson, A., Rutherford, M.S., Birchenall-Sparks, M.C., Roberts, M.S., Wu, W.T., & Cheung, H.T. (1985). Levels of specific messenger RNA species as a function of age. In Sohal, R.S., Birnbaum, L.S., & Cutler, R.G. (Eds.), *Molecular biology of aging: Gene stability and gene expression* (pp. 137–154). New York: Raven Press.

Riggs, A.D., & Jones, P.A. (1983). 5-Methylcytosine, gene regulation, and cancer. *Advances in Cancer Research, 40*:1–30.

Rowley, J.D. (1984). Biological implications of consistent chromosome rearrangements in leukemia and lymphoma. *Cancer Research 44*:3159–3168.

Sager, R. (1986). Genetic suppression of tumor formation: A new frontier in cancer research. *Cancer Research, 46*:1573–1580.

Shih, C., & Weinberg, R.A. (1982). Isolation of a transforming sequence from a human bladder carcinoma cell line. *Cell, 29*:161–169.

Shmookler Reis, R.J., & Goldstein, S. (1982). Variability of DNA methylation patterns during serial passage of human diploid fibroblasts. *Proceedings of the National Academy of Sciences USA, 79*:3949–3953.

Slaga, T.J., Klein-Szanto, A.J.P., Triplett, L.L., Yotti, L.P., & Trosko, J.E. (1982). DNA strand breakage in human leukocytes exposed to a tumor promoter, phorbol myristate acetate. *Science, 215*:1247–1249.

Srivastava, A., Norris, J.S., Shmookler Reis, R.J., & Goldstein, S. (1985). c-Ha-ras-1 Proto-oncogene amplification and overexpression during the limited replicative life span of normal human fibroblasts. *Journal of Biological Chemistry, 260*:6404–6409.

Wilson, V.L., & Jones, P.A. (1983). Inhibition of DNA methylation by chemical carcinogens in vitro. *Cell, 32*:239–246.

Zenser, T.V., Mattammal, M.B., Wise, R.W., Rice, J.R., & Davis, B.B. (1983). Prostaglandin H synthase-catalyzed activation of benzidine: A model to assess pharmacologic intervention of the initiation of chemical carcinogenesis. *Journal of Pharmacology and Experimental Therapeutics, 227*:545–550.

Zenser, T.V., & Davis, B.B. (1985). Peroxidatic activation of procarcinogens: A role for prostaglandin H synthase in initiation of chemical carcinogenesis. In Lands, W.E.M. (Ed.), *Biochemistry of arachidonic acid metabolism* (pp. 127–149). Boston: Martinus Nijhoff.

2

Epidemiological Features of Cancer in the Elderly

Rosemary Yancik and Lynn G. Ries

In this volume some authors address the clinical decision-making and techniques for assessment and surveillance of the elderly with respect to cancer prevention and treatment. Others focus on specific therapies, drug–drug and drug–age interactions, and caring for the elderly cancer patient. As a backdrop to the discussions on these issues, this chapter provides information that pertains to cancer in the elderly from the joined perspectives of cancer epidemiology and the epidemiology of aging. Drawing upon selected statistical data from each field, this cancer–aging epidemiology interface highlights selected aspects of cancer in the aged population.

Cancer prevention and treatment is truly a challenge for oncologists, geriatricians, and other health care professionals. This is attributed to the heterogeneity of cancer, the effects of aging as it affects the course of the malignancy, and the immense individual differences in the older-aged population.

Knowledge derived from the studies of the behavior, physical functioning, and characteristics of younger patients with cancer may not be generalizable to aged individuals because of any number of complicating age-related factors. Unfortunately, only limited data are available on the treatment and patterns of care for the aged cancer patient; the interaction of the normal and/or pathophysiologic processes of aging and cancer; the overlap of intercurrent diseases with cancer; and the interdisciplinary approaches for optimum cancer care for the elderly. Diagnosis and therapeutic interventions must be made with consideration of the full spectrum of pathologic conditions identified in the older-aged person afflicted with cancer.

THE CHANGING DEMOGRAPHY

The elderly, those aged 65 years or older, represent 12% of the U.S. population, or 26 million people. This age group is expanding in numbers faster than the rest of the population. The impact of the increase in the geriatric population is extremely relevant to this discussion on cancer in the elderly. When cancer statistics and health care utilization data are cast against the predicted expansion of the aged segment of the population for the next several decades, the sheer increases in the numbers of the aged alone will be a major burden for the U.S. health care system. The elderly require a disproportionate share of our nation's health care resources. This age group accounts for 31% of all health care expenditures: 75% of return office visits to physicians; 30% of hospital discharges; and 40% of hospital days of care received during a 1-year period (Waldo and Lazenby, 1984).

Let us contrast the recent phenomenal growth of the aging segment of the U.S. population and its expansion in future years with data from the U.S. Bureau of the Census (1984). Figure 2.1, compares the proportions of the aged in the U.S. since 1950 and provides estimates for selected years including the year 2030, the peak year for the rapid growth period.

If population projections of today hold true, in 2030 the older-aged segment of the United States will consist of about 64 million persons, constituting 20% or more of the population. One in every five Americans will be 65 years of age or more. Today every ninth American is in that age group, whereas in the 1950s every 12th American was 65 years or older.

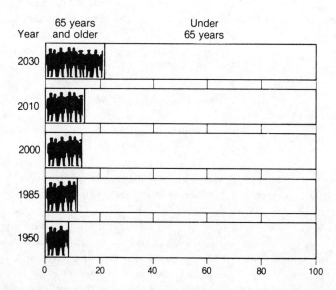

FIGURE 2.1. Percentage distribution of the U.S. population by age.

It is important to point out also that age shifts within the 65 years and older segment will bring about an expansion of the 75 years and older age group. The older population is getting older within the older-aged segment itself.

The elderly population as it currently exists already has many needs for health care and support systems. With the large expected expansion in this age segment during the next several decades, there is clearly an urgent need to emphasize prevention and other cancer control measures for the elderly.

CANCER INCIDENCE RATES IN THE ELDERLY

Old age is a high risk factor for vulnerability in developing cancers of the lung and bronchus, colon, rectum, stomach, pancreas, urinary bladder, prostate, and breast. Incidence data on approximately 700,000 cancer cases collected during 1973–82 by the Surveillance, Epidemiology, and End Results (SEER) Program, a population-based cancer registry system supported by the National Cancer Institute (NCI), indicate that 53% of all cancers occur in persons 65 years or older.

With the maturation of the NCI SEER Program, we now have the opportunity to bring the data from this unique cancer registry to bear upon specific age-related questions. The data reported here are from the SEER Program cancer registries in the states of Connecticut, Iowa, New Mexico, Utah, and Hawaii and the reporting regions of Detroit, Atlanta, San Francisco–Oakland, and Seattle–Puget Sound. This large population-based data system covers about 10% of the U.S. population. Details on SEER Program participants and a description of the program have been published in other documents (Horm et al., 1984; Young et al., 1981).

Demographic data, disease-specific information on primary site, histologic type, extent of disease, treatment, and follow-up are available for certain descriptive analyses. These registry data lend themselves to an exploration of the impact of age on cancer diagnosis, certain aspects of treatment, and survival to gain overall insights for clinical practice and to identify clinical research needs.

Incidence rates reflect the number of newly diagnosed cases occurring per 100,000 population during a specific time frame. As shown in Figure 2.2, which portrays the age of the SEER cohort in 5-year intervals, increased cancer incidence is strongly associated with advancing age. Cancer incidence rates begin to show a visible rise in the middle decades of life. Rates for persons aged 45 to 49 years are about 300 per 100,000 in this SEER cohort. For those a decade older, the rate is more than double: 750 per 100,000 persons aged 55 to 59 years. At the traditional old age demarcation of 65 years, the rates are almost doubled once again: at 1400 per 100,000 persons aged 65 to 69 years. The rates continue to increase even more dramatically, climbing to over 2000 per 100,000 cases for those 75 to 79 years of age. Rates culminate at more than 2300 per 100,000 cases for those 85 years or older.

Among older men and women, the men appear to be at greater risk for cancer.

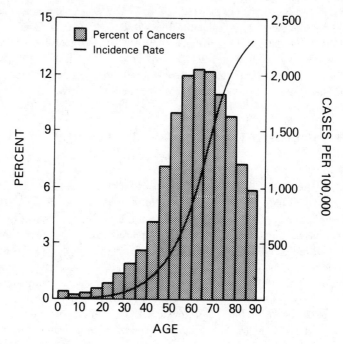

FIGURE 2.2. Incidence rates according to age.

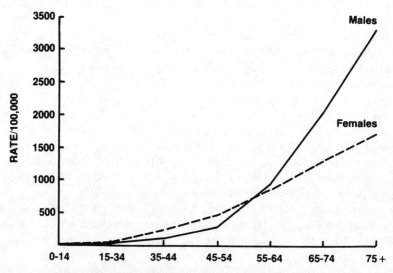

FIGURE 2.3. Incidence rates according to sex.

Contrasts are made in Figure 2.3 where the age groups are shown in 5-year intervals from 65 years according to sex. When compared with rates for females, cancer incidence rates for males are slightly lower under age 35 and quite a bit lower between the ages of 35 and 54 years. However, the rates for males rapidly escalate in the 55 to 64 years age group. They reach a point in the age segment 75 years and over where the rates are almost double those for females: 3365.0 per 100,000 as compared to 1735.0 per 100,000. These data reflect the different cancer types men and women tend to have. Males have much more lung cancer, a neoplasm with an extremely poor prognosis. Men have more colon, rectum, stomach, urinary bladder, and pancreas cancer. Prostate cancer also contributes to an extremely high sex differential.

Figure 2.4 presents a gender comparison by selected malignancy. The cancers with the highest incidence rates for the malignancies common to both sexes are lung and bronchus, colon, rectum, pancreas, urinary bladder, and stomach. All of these malignancies show higher rates for men than for women. For example, between 65 to 75 years, the incidence rates for lung and bronchus are about four times greater. After the age of 75 years the incidence rates are five times higher for men than for women. In the decade of 65 to 75 years, the incidence rates are about four times higher. Urinary bladder cancer rates are about four times greater for males than for females in every 5-year age segment. For stomach cancer men have twice the rates observed for women in every 5-year age segment.

Incidence rates are shown separately for breast and prostate cancers (Figure 2.5). Rates increase for both according to advancing age. Prostate cancer incidence rates increase by approximately 1.5-fold for each successive 5-year age group from 65 years on. Rates are over 1000 for males 80 years of age or older. Breast cancer incidence rates are over 300 for women 70 years or older, reaching a high of 378 per 100,000 for females 85 years and older.

CANCER MORTALITY RATES

Sixty percent of all cancer deaths are in the age group of persons 65 years or older. The median age for cancer deaths is 67.9 years (Young et al., 1981). The SEER Program has compiled cancer mortality statistics for selected years (Horm et al., 1984). A comparison of cancer mortality rates for the six cancers common to older-aged men and women by 5-year age groups is presented in Table 2.1. Breast cancer and prostate cancer mortality rates are also shown.

The severity of these major malignancies especially as they affect older-aged men is made quite apparent if one considers all cancer mortality rates over 200 per 100,000, an arbitrary selection. Ten of the 5-year age groups shown for males have mortality rates greater than this rate. Indeed, all of the rates for lung and bronchus cancer are over 350 per 100,000 population. For the oldest-old, prostate cancer

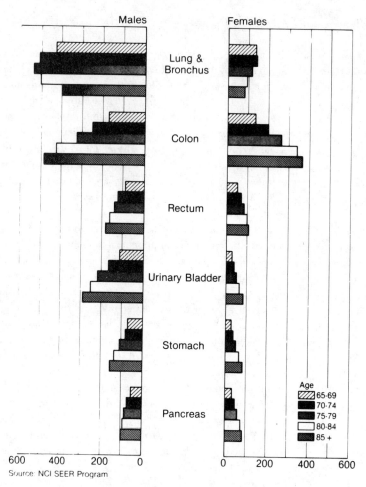

FIGURE 2.4. Average annual age-specific incidence rates per 100,000 population of common prominent cancer sites for males and females of all races, 1978–1981.

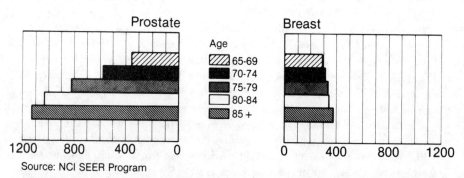

FIGURE 2.5. Average annual age-specific incidence rates per 100,000 population of prostate and breast cancer sites for all races, 1978–1981.

mortality rates soar to close to 600 per 100,000 population. Colon cancer for women in the 85 years and over age group is the only 5-year age segment that has rates over 200 per 100,000 population.

These contrasts mirror the cancer incidence data previously shown for the SEER cohort aged 65 years and older. All the prominent cancers affect the elderly disproportionately. However, older men are likely to get even more cancer than older women. The sex differences in the cancer statistics reflect the general mortality rates.

For all leading causes of death of persons aged 65 years and older, with the exception of diabetes, mortality rates are higher for men. Sex differences in life expectancy at birth and at the age of 65 years are shown in Table 2.2. Although both males and females experience greater longevity now than ever before, females can anticipate a greater advantage. On the average, women who are currently 65 years of age can expect to live approximately 5 years longer than men (Waldo and Lazenby, 1984). The quality of the lengthened life span for both men and women, however, is questionable (Verbrugge, 1984). Special problems of the aged such as living alone, being isolated, institutionalized, having functional limitations, restricted activity and bed disability, multiple chronic diseases, and low income status are noted in the health statistics and gerontologic literature. Inaccessibility of medical care and preventive health services contribute to these problems. As future generations age, there will be even greater numbers with social, economic, and health care needs.

SOME RESEARCH PRIORITIES

A number of research efforts from the broad cancer control spectrum of prevention, early detection and diagnosis, treatment, and continuing care efforts should be organized with a specific focus on the elderly. Some studies have been done in recent years, but there are still too few data available. Many of the more prominent areas of research urgently needing concentrated cancer control research efforts were described in the NCI announcements in 1983. Despite this pioneer program, major knowledge deficiencies still exist. We have just begun to address some of the multiple concerns about cancer in the elderly. The subsequent studies supported by the NCI and NIA raise issues for targeting future research.

Prevention

Studies are needed to evaluate the short- and long-term effects of cancer prevention programs for the aged. New knowledge has been developed on effective cancer prevention and early detection measures (e.g., smoking cessation, breast cancer

TABLE 2.1. Average Annual Age-specific Mortality Rates per 100,000 Population by Selected Cancer Sites for Elderly Males and Females, 1978–81

	Males					Females				
	65–69	70–74	75–79	80–84	85+	65–69	70–74	75–79	80–84	85+
Lung/Bronchus	359.4	444.4	478.5	467.0	361.3	95.5	97.3	92.1	86.4	82.5
Colon	87.6	132.2	181.8	245.7	305.1	63.7	93.8	133.3	185.7	239.6
Rectum	20.0	28.0	38.7	53.4	73.3	10.2	14.6	21.1	30.0	47.6
Urinary bladder	25.4	43.8	67.2	101.9	140.6	7.1	10.8	18.6	29.2	47.0
Stomach	35.0	49.6	68.7	91.2	111.0	14.8	22.8	31.8	46.6	63.8
Pancreas	48.5	67.4	83.5	99.4	102.5	31.3	42.8	56.6	70.9	79.5
Prostate (in males)/Breast (in females)	76.0	146.0	256.0	410.4	592.1	95.7	106.6	116.8	136.9	168.1

Source: NCI SEER Program, Horm et al., 1984.

TABLE 2.2 Life Expectancy at Birth and at 65 Years of Age, by Sex for Selected Years

Year	At birth		At 65 years	
	Male	Female	Male	Female
1900	46.3	48.3	11.5	12.2
1950	65.6	71.1	12.8	15.0
1975	68.8	76.6	13.8	18.1
1982	70.8	78.2	14.4	18.8
2005	73.6	81.2	16.0	21.0

Source: U.S. Bureau of the Census, Series P-25, No. 952, 1984.

screening). This body of information and the renewed emphasis on our national goals for health promotion and disease prevention should be incorporated into specific research strategies for the elderly.

Early Detection

Research should be conducted on variations in response to signs and symptoms of cancer by older-aged individuals. Improved cancer cures depend on early recognition and appreciation of signs and symptoms of the malignancy and prompt referral to treatment. The actions taken by older persons in response to the signs and symptoms of cancer will affect their ability to survive cancer, the number of complications, and morbid sequelae. Elderly persons are often directly or indirectly excluded from most early cancer detection efforts. Rarely are they singled out as a target group for early detection studies.

Treatment

Studies are also needed on the assessment of the effectiveness of different treatments relative to cancer, the stage of the disease, and significant features and characteristics of old age (e.g., poor repair mechanisms, functional loss, greater susceptibility to toxicity of treatment). We know very little about how physicians care for older-aged patients. There are few studies on the behavior of neoplasms and tumor characteristics as they are found in the elderly. However, the multiple clinical problems of the aged frequently require physicians to look for subtle or masked features of adverse conditions in addition to the presenting complaint. These special features of aging and symptoms of illness in old age influence the treatment and care of the elderly cancer patient and tend to complicate carrying out prescribed regimens for cancer therapy.

Increased clinical trials research is very much needed to develop a sound information base for cancer treatment of the elderly. Questions that address the problems concomitant with old age, i.e., effects of previous illnesses, concurrent illnesses, stage of disease at initial diagnosis, second primaries, recurrence, and level of physical functioning, should be answered to develop baseline data on cancer in the elderly.

Continuing Care

We know very little about how older-aged individuals cope with cancer, what family stress is invoked by cancer, and what the organization of care is under these trying circumstances. Various forms of social support diminish as a person grows older. The aged person may experience loss of friends, family, and spouse. Often the cancer patient must be cared for in the home by someone who is also in relatively poor health.

CONCLUSION

The challenge of understanding the multidimensional aspects of cancer in the elderly is before us. We have seen with the SEER Program population-based data that the aged are at very high risk for various types of malignancies. Indeed, even after age 65, we see that the risks tend to increase within this subset of the population. Furthermore, with advancing chronologic age, there are great variations in physiologic age and physical functioning as well.

Cancer, as multiple diseases, when coupled with the many concerns of the aging process creates unique interdisciplinary problems for professionals in oncology, gerontology, and geriatrics. Elderly Americans deserve an aggressive cancer control research agenda that at a minimum includes an exploration of the influence of old age on the array of current strategies being developed to prevent, treat, and manage cancer.

REFERENCES

Horm, J.W., Asire, A.J., Young, J.L., & Pollack, E.S. (Eds.), (1984). *SEER Program: Cancer incidence and mortality in the U. S., 1973–1981.* Bethesda, Maryland: Department of Health and Human Services: NIH Publication No. 85-1837.

U. S. Bureau of the Census, Current Population Reports, Series P-25, No. 952, (1984). *Projections of the population of the United States, by age, sex, and race: 1983 to 2080.* Washington, D.C.: U.S. Government Printing Office.

Verbrugge, L.M. (1984). Longer life but worsening health? Trends in health and mortality of middle-aged and older persons. *Milbank Memorial Fund Quarterly/Health and Society, 62:* 475–519.

Waldo, D.R., & Lazenby, H.C. (1984). Demographic characteristics and health care use and expenditures by the aged in the United States: 1977–1984. *Health Care Financing Review, 6:* 1–29.

Young, J.L., Percy, C.L., & Asire, A.J. (Eds.) (1981). *Incidence and mortality data: 1973–77.* National Cancer Institute Monograph 57, DHHS No. (NIH) 81-2330. Washington, D.C.: U.S. Government Printing Office.

3

Characteristics of Elderly Cancer Patients

Jerome W. Yates

EARLY DETECTION IN THE ELDERLY

The early dissemination of small asymptomatic primary cancer in the elderly makes them virtually impossible to cure. The cancers most amenable to surgical cure are those that grow slowly and metastasize late. The relatively early metastases from small primaries in lung, prostate, pancreas, and even breast diminish the possibility of cure without an effective systemic therapy. One report of age trends in lung cancer from the Comprehensive Cancer Center Registries suggests that more localized disease may occur in the elderly (O'Rourke et al., 1987). Understaging among the elderly and the differential referral of young patients with disseminated disease to cancer centers is a probable explanation for these proportional differences. Markers for premalignant disease and the identification of individuals at high risk of developing cancer could improve outcomes through earlier detection. With only palliative treatments for disseminated lung, prostate, and colorectal cancers, increasing survival in the elderly is not possible. Earlier detection may be enhanced in the future by using monoclonal antibodies or DNA probes to detect premalignant changes. Mammography for the early detection of breast cancer deserves more widespread utilization in the elderly.

The natural history of specific cancers provides some understanding of the biology of these cancers. Locally aggressive tumors occurring in critical anatomic areas such as soft tissue sarcomas or adult glioblastomas are virtually unresectable and as a result incurable. Slow-growing basal cell carcinomas may be followed for years and are almost always curable because they remain localized. A better understanding of the natural history of the common cancers in the elderly would facilitate the future design of improved detection and treatment methods.

The two major risk factors for cancer, age and a history of a previous cancer, make the elderly the largest and most easily identified high-risk population. This should strongly stimulate the planning for programs aimed at the early detection of cancer in the elderly. Recently, the National Cancer Institute (NCI) has accepted a new set of early detection guidelines that may give new impetus to those providers caring for the elderly (NCI, 1987). Special studies dedicated to identifying the appropriate workup and treatment specifically for the elderly are needed. Most of the treatment information is derived from reports of clinical trials conducted among younger patient populations with median ages for the study groups 5–10 years less than the general population (Begg et al., 1983; Brinker, 1985; Cohen & Bartolucci, 1985; Hunter et al., 1987). It is important that an appreciation of the critical need for more complete information and the existing limitations in the data available be stressed. Expanding our base of knowledge first followed by targeted efforts to improve cancer management for the elderly should be pursued.

ADVANCED CANCER IN THE ELDERLY

Possible explanations for the association of more advanced disease with selected cancers common in the elderly are as follows: (1) a longer prediagnostic delay on the part of the patients or their physicians, and (2) the cancers may be biologically more aggressive (Yancik et al., 1983; Ershler, 1987). Subsequent discussion will suggest that cancers are not biologically more aggressive in the elderly. Limitations in our existing cancer classification based on organ of origin, pathology, and other factors (e.g., receptor status) may obscure some age-related biologic differences. The onset of the first symptoms and signs of the cancers do not always lead to immediate discovery.

The elderly are known to tolerate symptoms better than their younger counterparts with similar conditions. This is probably related to a lifetime of symptomatic experience and also a multiplicity of confusing stimuli arising from the accrual of physical problems associated with normal aging. Bone pain or extremity swelling may be attributed to long-standing arthritis, blood in the stools may be thought to come from hemorrhoids, constipation can be expected as age-associated changes in dietary habits and bowel function occur, and repetitive bronchitis in heavy smokers is common and seldom thought to deserve medical attention. Elderly patients often have an array of co-morbid conditions that detract their attention from routine health needs. These co-morbid conditions may obscure the true source of the symptoms and delay the diagnosis of an early cancer. Patients with other conditions requiring medical follow-up may focus only on these specific problems. For example, women with moderate hypertension may forget to get a Pap smear aimed at the early detection of cervical cancer. Their physicians may forget or delay routine cancer examinations. Patients often defer the responsibility for their total care to their physicians when they concentrate only on immediate medical problems. Smokers with chronic lung disease are susceptible to head and neck and lung cancers, but hemoptysis is often ignored by those patients. The elderly become desensitized to the importance of fecal blood or constipation because they often have a long history of previous episodes not considered serious by their physicians. It is the combination of patient tolerance and physician inattention to peripheral medical problems that promotes delay and leads to late cancer detection for this population.

AGE, CO-MORBIDITY, AND CANCER

Many host factors may be accentuated with advancing age and deserve attention. The presence of co-morbid conditions, immunologic changes, and the increased risk of developing second cancers are all important. In addition, the normal reduction in function of the cardiovascular, respiratory, renal, hepatic, and mucocutaneous systems contribute to changes in both the course of the cancer and the feasibility of successful treatment.

It has been suggested that the biologic characteristics of the cancers in the elderly should actually favor survival and discovery at an early state (Colapinto, 1985). Animals have provided conflicting results depending on the model system studied. Some have demonstrated slower local tumor growth, a delayed growth of known metastatic lesions, and fewer metastases when compared with younger control animals. It is assumed that an assortment of factors play a role in these differences. Circulatory changes affecting local nutrition, oxygenation, and decreased angiogenesis in the area of the tumor may all inhibit the implantation and growth of metastases. Local tissue reaction such as desmoplasia and hormonal effects may slow progression, and there is a suggestion that retention of relatively larger numbers of natural killer lymphocytes may benefit older animals. The suggestion that the cancers are less aggressive locally and less likely to metastasize in the older animals has been anecdotally discussed. Clinicians more easily remember their treatment successes and forget their detection or treatment disasters. Selective referral patterns, aggressive diagnostic pursuits and the availability of a curative treatment all favorably influence outcomes for the younger age groups.

By examining human relative survival data in cohorts selected by age and stage at the time of diagnosis, aging appears to confer an additional disadvantage for survival in the older cohorts. Survival from cancer is dependent on four factors: (1) extent or stage of cancer; (2) cancer biology or aggressiveness; (3) host factors or resistance; and (4) available curative treatment. By looking at only a group of patients presenting with advanced cancer, for which there is only palliative treatment, an assessment of the influence of host factors on outcome is possible. Disseminated cancer implies the presence of a biologically aggressive disease. Survival differences for patients with advanced lung cancer grouped by age demonstrate an early age-related decrease in survival (Figure 3.1). These SEER data taken for patients (both sexes and all races) diagnosed from 1977 to 1982 show a decreased survival for each successive age cohort. Advanced lung cancer, in those older than 65 years reflect the greatest aged-related disadvantage. Because this information is population-based, selection biases resulting from referral patterns and systematic differences in supportive care do not play a role. Because this is advanced disease, lead time bias and the beneficial treatment effects are not factors.

MANAGEMENT INFORMATION

One of the major limitations in assessing clinical trials data is the paucity of information related to cancer management of the elderly. Coupled with this is the marked divergence of chronologic and physiologic age that occurs for those older than 60 years (Yancik, et al., 1983). Because it is possible to select elderly patients who are physiologically younger than their chronologic colleagues, the

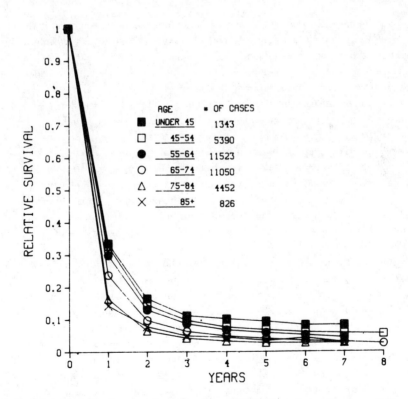

FIGURE 3.1. Relative survival data for all SEER patients diagnosed from 1977 to 1982 partitioned by age at diagnosis.

available clinical trials data are usually biased. Owing to co-morbidity and other factors that may influence the utilization of effective treatment, outcome comparisons among the elderly may be less interpretable than for younger populations with the same cancer. For example, co-morbidity such as lung disease or compromised renal function may alter the ability to deliver curative surgery in the elderly patient (Colapinto, 1985; Greenberg et al., 1982). Infectious or hemorrhagic complications may truncate aggressive curative efforts and result in the premature demise of the patient. Intracavitary reservoirs such as pleural and peritoneal effusions may influence the pharmacokinetics of drugs, and attenuated organ function may influence the pharmacodynamics. In summary, survival in the elderly cancer patient is related to the extent of disease, the biology of the cancer, a complex set of host factors, and the availability of effective treatment. For each elderly patient an appreciation of the specific host factors important to that individual is necessary to assure appropriate management.

DECISION PROCESS

When the decision process for early detection and treatment selection is reviewed there are important age-imposed considerations. These stages of information-gathering and assessment leading to prevention and treatment are outlined in Figure 3.2. The history taken from the patient must have a much broader scope than that commonly collected from their younger counterparts. Beyond the specific cancer-related medical history, the physician or his or her extender must explore issues such as co-morbidity, medications, risk factors (e.g., smoking, alcohol), and nutrition. Information related to physical performance status, strength, balance, appetite, sleep habits, pain history, social support, and other social factors including living arrangements may influence patient access, utilization, and compliance to treatment. The presence of co-morbid conditions can obscure the early suspicions of cancer for both the patient and the physician. As part of the physical examination, the patient's mental acuity, physical performance, and potential risk from other compromised organ systems (e.g., cardiorespiratory, hepatic, or renal function) must be considered.

Because the management of these patients has to be individualized to a greater extent than their younger counterparts, the diagnostic studies should be selected with attention given to probable treatment. If the treatment intent is curative, then it is critical that the patient be accurately staged before being subjected to curative attempts; the extension of disease may make only palliation the treatment of choice. Because the homeostasis of the aged may be precarious and their ability to withstand severe physical stress may be poor, it is critical that the probable treatment benefit be weighed against the potential harm. There are often ethical considerations that are peculiar to the elderly regarding treatment, supportive care, and extraordinary lifesaving interventions. These decisions are generally made ad

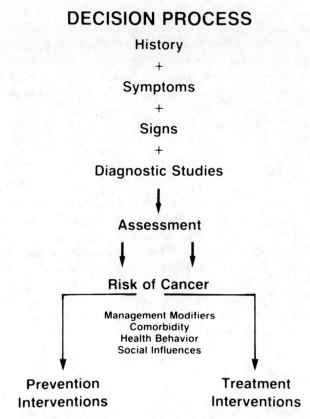

FIGURE 3.2. Information, assessment and selection of interventions in the prevention (primary and early detection) and treatment of cancer in the elderly.

hoc by the attending physician with variable input from the patients and their families.

Special problems peculiar to the elderly warrant further attention. Conditions that diminish patient awareness, access to, or utilization of treatment are often underestimated. The patients may be too timid to ask appropriate questions, they may have hearing difficulties, or they may be unable to comprehend or understand the treatment plans. Access to appropriate treatment may be impaired because of a lack of transportation, a proud avoidance of asking for help, and the presence of unanticipated economic barriers (e.g., lack of health insurance and/or excessive out-of-pocket costs).

When physicians select a specific treatment for an elderly patient, they should attempt to anticipate potential complications. Rehabilitation plans should be considered at the time of initial treatment. Their awareness of particular patient vulnerabilities may avoid complications. This is particularly true for episodes of bleeding, infection, and malnutrition. Prior to treatment the physician should try to optimize physical function, eliminate unnecessary medication, reduce obstructions to normal secretions, anticipate potential sources of infections, and adequately assess respiratory, cardiac, and renal reserve. A plan for maintaining mobility that includes an educational program for both the patient and family can improve effective outpatient and home care management.

FUTURE NEEDS

Increased interest and targeted attention from the oncologists toward the elderly and from the geriatricians toward cancer will be required if a multidisciplinary knowledge base is to develop. More descriptive studies to assess current cancer management is important. An increased emphasis on clinical trials involving the elderly could provide useful information. A set of guidelines aimed at improving early detection, treatment, and rehabilitation with particular emphasis on the elderly would be of great use to geriatricians. A greater understanding of some of the biologic issues and the opportunities and limitations to existing treatment should be a goal for all those caring for the elderly cancer patient.

REFERENCES

Begg, C.B., Zelen, M., Carbone, P.P., McFadden, E.T., Brodovsky, H., et al. (1983). Cooperative groups and community hospitals. *Cancer, 52*:1760–1767.

Brincker, H. (1985). Estimate of overall treatment results in acute nonlymphocytic leukemia based on age-specific rates of ancidence and of complete remission. *Cancer Treatment Reports, 69*:5–11.

Cohen, H.J., & Bartolucci, A. (1985). Age and the treatment of multiple myeloma. Southeastern Cancer Group Experience. *American Journal of Medicine, 79*:316–324.

Colapinto, N.D. (1985). Is age alone a contraindication to major cancer surgery? *Canadian Journal of Surgery, 28*:323–326.

Ershler, W.B. (1987). The change in aggressiveness of neoplasms with age. *Geriatrics, 42*:99–103.

Greenburg, A.G., Saik, R.P., Farris, J.M., & Peskin, G.W. (1982). Operative mortality in general surgery. *American Journal of Surgery, 144*:22–28.

Hunter, C.P., Frelick, R.W., Feldman, A.R., Bavier, A.R., Dunlop, W.H., Ford, L., et al. (1987). Selection factors in clinical trials: Results of the Community Clinical Oncology Program physician's patient log. *Cancer Treatment Reports, 71*:559–565.

National Cancer Institute. (1987). Minutes of the National Cancer Advisory Board. Bethesda, Maryland; September 28–30.

O'Rourke, M.A., Feussner, J.R., Feigl, P., & Laslo, J. (1987). Age trends of lung cancer stage at diagnosis. *Journal of the American Medical Association, 258*:921–926.

Yancik, R., Carbone, P.P., Patterson, W.B., Steel, K., & Terry, W.D. (Eds.) (1983). *Perspectives on prevention and treatment of cancer in the elderly.* New York: Raven Press.

PART II
Therapy by Biological Response Modifiers

4

Cancer Clinical Trials of Interleukin-2 and Lymphokine-Activated Killer Cells

Geoffrey R. Weiss, David H. Boldt, and Charles A. Coltman, Jr.

The past two decades have witnessed extraordinary advancements in molecular biology, which only recently have provided dividends in the management of human disease. Despite substantial progress in the understanding of mammalian and human immunology and its relation to malignant disease, the development of effective immunotherapies against cancer has been extremely elusive. Active immunotherapies utilizing nonspecific immunostimulants such as Bacillus Cal-mette-Guérin (BCG), Corynebacterium parvum and levamisole, among others, have not materialized into useful cancer treatments for patients with advanced malignancies. In contrast, recent developments in the adoptive immunotherapy of cancer, a form of passive immunotherapy wherein sensitized immunologic effector cells (e.g., lymphocytes or monocytes) are administered to the tumor-bearing host, have shown evidence of important and potentially useful clinical antitumor activity (Rosenberg, 1984).

Supported in part by contract CA32102 from the National Cancer Institute, Department of Health and Human Services, Bethesda, Maryland 20205, and by an American Cancer Society Clinical Oncology Career Development Award (Dr. Weiss).

Rosenberg and his colleagues at the National Cancer Institute (NCI) Surgery Branch have performed a series of experiments in mice bearing virus-induced lymphomas or transplantable sarcomas and melanomas, which have provided the model for the human clinical protocols of adoptive immunotherapy (Mazumder et al., 1984; Lafreniere & Rosenberg, 1985). Essential to the accomplishment of human clinical trials has been the recognition of theoretical concepts fundamental to successful adoptive immunotherapy and the ability to surmount a number of technical challenges inherent in the generation of effector cells for human administration. Among these challenges are the following: (1) defining a source of the effector cells; (2) recognizing the number of cells necessary to achieve clinical antitumor activity; (3) providing the agents in sufficient quantity necessary for sensitization of effector cells; and (4) synthesizing a treatment administration schedule that optimizes effector cell antitumor activity *in vivo*. Several principles have become central to the successful clinical use of adoptive immunotherapy for human cancer: (1) the effector lymphocyte becomes sensitized and reaches maximum antitumor activity after incubation with interleukin-2; (2) very large numbers of effector lymphocytes ($>10^8$) are necessary for mediation of antitumor activity in the host; (3) autologous effector cells appear to be most active; and (4) coadministration of interleukin-2 in very high dosage and the effector lymphocytes results in maximum effectiveness of this form of adoptive immunotherapy.

INTERLEUKIN-2

A fundamental requirement for the accomplishment of adoptive immunotherapy was the identification and isolation of the lymphokine, interleukin-2 (IL-2). Discovered by Morgan et al. (1976), IL-2 was first called T-cell growth factor (TCGF) and was considered necessary for the maintenance and proliferation of activated T-cells in long-term culture. It was learned that IL-2 possessed the capability of stimulating the *in vivo* clonal expansion of antigen- or mitogen-activated T-cells, and natural killer cell activity (Hefeneider et al., 1983; Wagner et al., 1980; Lotze et al., 1985). The sequence analysis of the cDNA coding for IL-2 and the molecular structure of the human protein were described by Taniguchi and his coworkers (1983). Recombinant human interleukin-2 (rIL-2) may now be produced in high quantity in very pure form by incorporation of the human IL-2 gene into an *Escherichia coli* plasmid. The resultant protein retains all of the properties of native IL-2 including sustained growth of activated human peripheral blood lymphocytes, stimulation of the generation of cytolytic lymphocytes in the presence of stimulator cells, and generation of lymphokine-activated killer (LAK) cells (Rosenberg et al., 1984). It is the production of LAK cells that is the property of rIL-2 exploited for adoptive immunotherapy.

LYMPHOKINE-ACTIVATED KILLER CELL

Although IL-2 may well possess anticancer activity and is being actively investigated for this attribute, the LAK cell's cytotoxic activity is examined in this review. The features of the LAK cell that render it unique among immunologic effector cells include its generation after incubation of murine or human peripheral blood lymphocytes with IL-2 alone and its ability to lyse fresh NK cell-resistant primary and metastatic tumor cells *in vitro* and *in vivo* (Rosenstein et al., 1984; Lotze et al., 1981). LAK cells begin to emerge after 1–2 days of IL-2 incubation and become maximal in 3–6 days. The LAK precursor cell is a null lymphocyte, expressing no T-cell surface markers or surface immunoglobulin. However, precursors may express CD16 cell surface antigens that correspond to the Fc-IgG receptor shared by NK cells and granulocytes (Phillips & Lanier, 1986). With acquisition of the LAK effector phenotype, CD16 and Leu-19 antigens are expressed on the surface of the cells, suggesting NK cell-like activation. Yet it appears that LAK activity also develops in a subset of CD3-positive T-cells.

The following clinical trials described herein reflect the development of technologies capable of generating LAK effector cells in large quantity (10^{10} cells) for the treatment of human malignancy.

CLINICAL TRIALS OF ADOPTIVE CELLULAR IMMUNOTHERAPY

The NCI Surgery Branch Experience

In 1985 Rosenberg and coworkers published the results of their initial clinical trials of autologous LAK and rIL-2 for the treatment of patients with metastatic cancer. Twenty-five patients with a variety of advanced cancers received intravenous rIL-2 every 8 hours in dosages of 10,000, 30,000, or 100,000 units per kg body weight. Treatment was accomplished in three components: an induction phase of rIL-2 treatment for 5 days; five daily lymphocytaphereses to harvest LAK precursor cells for 3–4 days of rIL-2 incubation and LAK activation; and transfusion of LAK cells into the patient accompanied by 4–5 additional days of high-dose intravenous rIL-2. Eleven objective antitumor responses were observed among the treated patients: three partial responses in three renal cancer patients, three partial responses and one complete response in seven melanoma patients, three partial responses in seven colorectal cancer patients, and one partial response in a lung adenocarcinoma patient. Although the results were quite dramatic in this group of previously treated cancer patients, the therapy came at substantial cost in toxicity. Treated patients experienced marked fluid retention and weight gain, pulmonary edema and dyspnea (requiring endotracheal intubation in two patients), oliguria, fever, chills, malaise, skin rash, nausea, vomiting, diarrhea, glossitis, nasal congestion, and mental confusion. Laboratory abnormalities included creatinine elevation, hyperbilirubinemia, eosinophilia, anemia requiring transfusion, and thrombocytopenia. Although all patients required treatment in the intensive care unit (ICU), most of the toxicities were rapidly reversible with discontinuation of rIL-2 and were therefore largely attributed to rIL-2 administration alone and not to LAK cell administration. LAK cell transfusion may be accompanied by fever and chills.

A progress report on the NCI Surgery Branch experience was published in 1987 (Rosenberg et al., 1987). In a larger group of 106 patients (including the original 25 patients) receiving LAK cells and IL-2 on a schedule similar to that reported in the initial trial, 8 complete responses (4 renal cancer, 2 melanoma, 1 colorectal cancer, and 1 non-Hodgkin's lymphoma) and 15 partial responses (8 renal cancer, 4 melanoma, 2 colorectal cancer, and 1 non-Hodgkin's lymphoma) were observed. The overall response rate was 22%, yet substantial and durable responses were still observed in renal cell carcinoma and melanoma after only one course of treatment. It is noteworthy that those patients treated with rIL-2 alone experienced fewer objective responses (13%), an observation suggesting that LAK cells contributed to the antitumor activity of the therapy.

The Biological Therapy Institute Experience

West and his coworkers at the Biological Therapy Institute in Memphis, Tennessee conducted an investigation of an aggressive regimen of rIL-2 and LAK cells in 40 evaluable patients with advanced refractory cancer (1987). Patients received all rIL-2 by continuous intravenous infusion and underwent a 5-day course of rIL-2 alone (days 1–5), 4 days of leukapheresis (days 7–10), 5 days of rIL-2 and LAK cells (days 10–15), and, in some cases, another 4 days of leukapheresis (days 17–20) and 5 additional days of rIL-2/LAK (days 20–25). Doses of rIL-2 ranged from 1×10^6 to 7×10^6 units/m^2/day by intravenous continuous infusion. Responses were noted in 13 of 40 treated patients (overall response 32.5%; 5 of 10 melanoma patients, 3 of 6 renal cancer patients, 1 of 5 lung cancer patients, 1 of 2 parotid cancer patients, and 1 each of ovarian cancer, Hodgkin's disease and nodular lymphoma patients). The toxicity of this therapy permitted treatment outside the ICU in the majority of cases (only six patients required ICU care), yet the dominant toxicities remained fever, anemia requiring transfusion, fatigue, diarrhea, azotemia, oliguria, hypotension, and glossitis. One treatment-related death occurred.

The authors proposed that anticancer responses appeared to correlate best with administration of high doses of rIL-2 during the priming phase, with the magnitude of postpriming lymphocytosis (≥ 6000/mm^3), with low pretreatment performance status, and with high pretreatment peripheral blood lymphocyte count (≥ 1400/mm^3).

The NCI Extramural IL-2/LAK Working Group Experience

The results of the NCI Surgery Branch clinical trials of rIL-2 and LAK cells stimulated the rapid establishment of a clinical trials resource with the capability of generating LAK cells in high volume. Six cancer centers (Loyola University School of Medicine, Chicago; Tufts-New England Medical Center, Boston; Einstein-Montefiore Medical Center, New York; University of Texas Health Science Center, San Antonio; City of Hope Medical Center, Duarte, California; University of California, San Francisco) were awarded contracts to conduct phase II trials of LAK/rIL-2 based upon the NCI Surgery Branch protocol. The protocol schema is illustrated in Figure 4.1.

The extramural program was open to patients with metastatic malignant melanoma, colorectal cancer, or renal cell carcinoma. Patients received a 5-day priming course of rIL-2 followed by five daily 4-hr leukaphereses to harvest LAK precursors. Harvested cells were incubated *in vitro* with rIL-2 for 3–4 days, then were transfused back into the patients while additional intravenous rIL-2 was administered. Patients were followed monthly after conclusion of therapy with appropriate examinations or studies to evaluate response. Repeat courses of treatment were initiated at 3-month intervals if evidence of antitumor activity was observed.

Toxicities of the therapy in the hands of the extramural investigators were quite similar to those induced in patients in the NCI Surgery Branch trials; one treat-

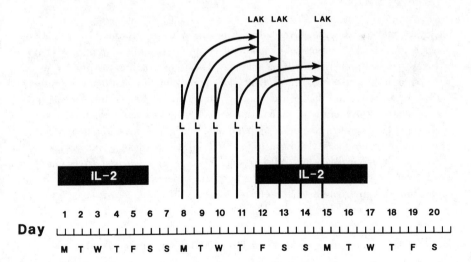

FIGURE 4.1. Schema for the protocol utilized by the NCI Extramural LAK/IL-2 Working Group. L, leukapheresis; IL-2, 100,000 u/kg iv q 8 hr; LAK, infusion of LAK cells iv.

ment-related death occurred among 83 patients and all patients required management in the ICU. An unexpected, but self-limited toxicity in the extramural trials was the occurrence of hepatitis A in 22 patients. Evidence strongly suggested that virus-contaminated human sera used in the preparation of LAK cell growth media were responsible for transmission of the infection.

Antitumor responses have been observed in patients of each category of disease treated on the extramural clinical trials. By December 1986, 85 evaluable patients had been treated by the extramural centers. Response data are shown in Table 4.1 (Fisher et al., 1987; Dutcher et al., 1987).

Variables that do not seem to correlate with response are the number of LAK cells administered, amount of rIL-2 administered, and *in vitro* cytolytic activity of LAK cells. Evidence suggests that the magnitude of tumor burden correlates negatively with response. At all extramural sites, generation of LAK activity assayed by *in vitro* ^{51}Cr release from the K562 NK-sensitive cell line, the Daudi NK-resistant cell line, and fresh tumor has been uniformly demonstrated.

The initial goals of the NCI extramural trials have been met and included the transfer of LAK generation technology beyond the NCI Surgery Branch, the safe management of rIL-2 induced toxicity by the extramural centers, and the demonstration of anticancer activity for the rIL-2/LAK preparation.

CONCLUSION

Clinical trials of rIL-2 and LAK cells are ongoing and will certainly be expanded in scope with the FDA approval of modified group C guidelines for pursuit of this therapy at comprehensive cancer centers. The issues of highest priority to be explored in future trials are methods for increasing the antitumor activity of rIL-2/LAK, reduction of the toxicity of treatment, reduction of the expense and complexity of the therapy by automating some LAK generation procedures, utilizing safe LAK growth medium preparations, etc., and identification of other responsive tumor types. Adjuvant trials of rIL-2/LAK in sensitive tumor types are in progress and will undoubtedly expand in scope. The current trials must be regarded as exploratory because the requisites necessary for the delivery of optimum therapy remain to be defined.

TABLE 4.1 Response Data from NCI Extramural Trials

Disease	Evaluable	CR	PR	%CR + PR	Duration (mo)
Renal	32	2	3	16	6+,7,9+,9+,10+
Melanoma	32	1	5	19	2,4,6,7,8+,9+
Colon	21	1	2	14	2,4,7+

REFERENCES

Dutcher, J.P., Creekmore, S., Weiss, G.R., et al. (1987). Phase II study of high dose interleukin-2 (IL-2) and lymphokine activated killer (LAK) cells in patients (pts) with melanoma. *Proceedings of the American Society of Clinical Oncology, 6*:246.

Fisher, R.I., Coltman, C.A., Doroshow, J.H., et al. (1987). Phase II clinical trial of interleukin II plus lymphokine activated killer cells (IL-2/LAK) in metastatic renal cancer. *Proceedings of the American Society of Clinical Oncology, 6*:244.

Hefeneider, S.H., Conlon, P.J., Henney, C.S., & Gillis, S. (1983). *In vivo* interleukin-2 administration augments the generation of alloreactive cytolytic T-lymphocytes and resident natural killer cells. *Journal of Immunology, 130*:222–227.

Lafreniere, R., & Rosenberg, S.A. (1985). Successful immunotherapy of murine experimental hepatic metastases with lymphokine-activated killer cells and recombinant interleukin-2. *Cancer Research, 45*:3735–3741.

Lotze, M.T., Grimm, E.A., Mazumider, A., Strausser, J.L., & Rosenberg, S.A. (1981). Lysis of fresh and cultured autologous tumor by human lymphocytes cultured in T-cell growth factor. *Cancer Research, 41*:4420–4425.

Lotze, M.T., Matory, E.L., Ettinghausen, S.E., et al. (1985). *In vivo* administration of purified human interleukin-2. II. Half-life, immunologic effects, and expansion of peripheral lymphoid cells *in vivo* with recombinant IL-2. *Journal of Immunology, 135*:2865–2875.

Mazumder, A., & Rosenberg, S.A. (1984). Successful immunotherapy of natural killer-resistant established pulmonary melanoma metastases by the intravenous adoptive transfer of syngeneic lymphocytes activated *in vitro* by interleukin-2. *Journal of Experimental Medicine, 159*:495–507.

Morgan, D.A., Ruscetti, F.W., & Gallo, R.C. (1976). Selective *in vitro* growth of T-lymphocytes from normal bone marrows. *Science, 193*:1007–1008.

Phillips, J.H., & Lanier, L.L. (1986). Dissection of the lymphokine-activated killer phenomenon. Relative contribution of peripheral blood natural killer cells and T-lymphocytes to cytolysis. *Journal of Experimental Medicine, 164*:814–825.

Rosenberg, S.A. (1984). Adoptive immunotherapy of cancer: Accomplishments and prospects. *Cancer Treatment Reports, 68*:233–255.

Rosenberg, S.A., Grimm, E.A., McGrogan, M., et al. (1984). Biological activity of recombinant human interleukin-2 produced in *Escherichia coli*. *Science, 223*:1412–1415.

Rosenberg, S.A., Lotze, M.T., Muul, L.M., et al. (1985). Observations on the systemic administration of autologous lymphokine-activated killer cells and recombinant interleukin-2 to patients with metastatic cancer. *New England Journal of Medicine, 313*:1485–1492.

Rosenberg, S.A., Lotze, M.T., Muul, L.M., et al. (1987). A progress report on the treatment of 157 patients with advanced cancer using lymphokine-activated killer cells and interleukin-2 or high-dose interleukin-2 alone. *New England Journal of Medicine, 316*:889–897.

Rosenstein, M., Yron, I., Kaufmann, Y., & Rosenberg, S.A. (1984). Lymphokine activated killer cells: Lysis of fresh syngeneic natural killer-resistant murine tumor cells by lymphocytes cultured in interleukin-2. *Cancer Research, 44*:1946–1953.

Taniguchi, T., Matsui, H., Fujita, T., et al. (1983). Structure and expression of a cloned cDNA for human interleukin-2. *Nature, 302*:305–310.

Wagner, H., Hardt, C., Heeg, K., et al. (1980). T-cell-derived helper factor allows *in vivo* induction of cytotoxic T-cells in *nu/nu* mice. *Nature, 284*:278–280.

West, W.H., Tauer, K.W., Yannelli, J.R., et al. (1987). Constant-infusion recombinant interleukin-2 in adoptive immunotherapy of advanced cancer. *New England Journal of Medicine, 316*:898–905.

5

Interferon in the Treatment of Malignant Disease

Teresa A. Gilewski and Harvey M. Golomb

During the past 15 years, a new class of agents has emerged for the treatment of human disease. This promising group is frequently referred to as biologic response modifiers (BRM) and constitutes a form of therapy known as biological therapy. The basis of this treatment, as noted by Smalley and Oldham (1984), "involves the modulation or utilization of the individual's own biological responses." Substances specifically included in this group are: immunomodulating agents, lymphokines (products produced specifically by lymphocytes) and other cytokines (i.e., growth factors, interferons), tumor antigens, antitumor cells, and antibodies directed against either the host or tumor. The studies performed with interferons have been particularly exciting because results have indicated a definite role for interferons in the treatment of human malignancy and possibly viral-induced infections. Recent technologic advances, specifically in molecular biology, have made it possible to produce significant amounts of highly purified interferon. This allows for a more controlled and standardized use of interferon in clinical trials.

INTERFERONS

Interferons comprise a group of biologically active, naturally occurring polypeptides, produced by eukaryotic cells in response to stimulation by inducing agents, such as viruses, mitogens, antigens, tumor cells, and other nonviral inducers (Strander, 1986). Isaacs and Lindenmann (1957) defined the term interferon in reference to their antiviral activity. Subsequently, Gresser (1961) documented the production of interferon by human leukocytes, and in the ensuing years much research was devoted to the development and purification of interferon. Initial clinical trials were hindered by impurities, lack of standardization, and small quantities of interferon (Spiegel, 1987).

There are three basic types of interferons: alpha(α), beta(β), and gamma(γ), which have been well documented (Pestka, 1983). The presence of a fourth type of interferon has been alluded to, although not proven (Wilkinson & Morris, 1983). Alpha and beta interferons are Type 1 interferons owing to their stability at a pH of 2, whereas gamma interferon is labile at pH of 2 and therefore is considered a Type II interferon (Clark & Longo, 1987). There are at least 20 subtypes of alpha interferon, and it has been noted that up to 40 subtypes may actually exist (Borecky, 1986; Collins, 1986). The presence of multiple subtypes in beta and gamma interferons has not been clearly established. Alpha interferons are produced by leukocytes, whereas beta interferons are derived from fibroblasts, yet they demonstrate an approximately 30% to 50% homology between their amino acid sequences (Taniguchi et al., 1980; Borecky, 1986). Gamma interferons are produced primarily by T lymphocytes, and differ in amino acid composition, with approximately 20 fewer amino acids than the other two types (Palacios et al., 1983). It has been suggested that chromosome 9 is the location of the alpha and beta genes, whereas the gamma gene is located on chromosome 12 (Sagar et al., 1981; D'Eustachio & Ruddle, 1983; Shows et al., 1982). However, the sensitivity of a cell to interferon may also be influenced by genes on chromosomes 16 and 21 (Tan et al., 1974; Borecky, 1986). The actual mechanisms involved in the synthesis and release of interferons have not yet been clearly established. Cell receptors for alpha and beta interferon (Type I) differ from gamma interferon receptors (Branca & Baglioni, 1981). However, chromosome 21 appears to contain the gene coding for both the alpha and gamma receptors (Weil et al., 1983). It has been suggested that the number of cell receptors may correspond to the sensitivity of the cell to interferon (Baglioni et al., 1982), although conflicting data have been presented (Tovey et al., 1983; Faltynek et al., 1986). In addition, it has been suggested that interferon receptors may contain two separate binding sites for activation of the antiviral mechanism in the cell and for binding of the interferon molecule to the cell (Borecky, 1986).

Following the discovery that human leukocytes could produce alpha interferon, extensive research was conducted to obtain a highly purified substance. A widely used method of purification was developed by Cantell, although this was expensive, time consuming, and yielded impure products (Cantell & Hirvonen, 1978). Subsequently, interferon derived from stimulation of human lymphoblastoid cell lines, (specifically the Namalwa cell line) with Sendai virus, was developed and yields an approximately 90% pure preparation of both alpha (90%) and beta (10%) interferon (Krown, 1986). In addition, monoclonal antibodies have played an important role in the purification of alpha interferon (Secher & Burke, 1980). However, since the development of recombinant alpha interferon (Goeddel et al., 1980), which has greater than 95% purity, limitations of natural interferon, i.e., differences in preparations, impurities, and possible viral contaminations have been markedly reduced (Wadell, 1977). There are two types of recombinant alpha interferon currently used in clinical trials. They differ only by one amino acid at position 23, and are identified as alpha 2a (Hoffman-La Roche) and alpha 2b (Schering) interferon. Natural beta and gamma interferon have also been used in clinical trials, although current studies frequently use the highly pure recombinant forms. Human beta interferon was cloned in 1979 (Taniguchi et al., 1982), followed by recombinant gamma interferon in 1982 (Gray et al., 1982). Current studies are evaluating any possible differences between the natural and recombinant products.

MECHANISMS OF ACTION

The actions of interferon encompass a wide array of changes, affecting not only the biochemical, but structural aspects of the cell as well . As previously documented in the literature, interferon has demonstrated a role as an antitumor agent, yet the exact mechanisms by which it exerts this effect currently remain unclear. Nevertheless, research thus far has indicated several major effects that may be related to its use in the treatment of malignancy. These specifically include antiproliferation, cell differentiation, antiviral, and immunomodulatory aspects.

Antiproliferative

The antiproliferative effects of interferon were first noted by Paucker et al. (1962) and affect both malignant and normal cells (Strander, 1986). Several studies have indicated a possible antagonism between growth factors and interferon, yet this has not been definitely established (Inglot, 1983; Taylor-Papadimitriou & Rozengurt, 1982). Resting tumor cells (those in G0, G1, or G2 phases) appear more sensitive to growth inhibition than those that are synthesizing or dividing (Horoszewicz et al., 1979; Creasey et al., 1981; Taylor et al. 1984). Balkwill and Taylor-Papadimitriou (1978) noted a delay in the progression of cells in the G1/G0 phase to further stages in the cell cycle after treatment with interferon. Some controversy exists regarding correlation of serum concentration and antigrowth effects. Kading et al. (1978) noted an association between serum concentration of the medium and tumor growth in a mouse cell line, whereas Ratner et al. (1980) found no correlation. The latter study suggested that interferon itself may be responsible for the antiproliferative effects, as opposed to other factors in the serum. Human cell lines have also demonstrated different sensitivities to the antiproliferative effects of the various interferons (Borden et al., 1982b). In addition, the same type of tumor from different patients has differed in response to the antigrowth effects of interferon (Ernberg et al., 1981). Interestingly, Ito and Buffet (1981) have documented human tumor cell lines that have distinct and separate susceptibilities to either the antiproliferative, antiviral, or cytocidal action of interferon.

The antigrowth effect may be influenced by temperature, as noted by Heron and Berg (1978) and Fleischmann et al. (1986), who have demonstrated an enhancement of antiproliferative activity with an increase in temperature. Whether antipyretic agents, which are frequently used clinically, affect the sensitivity of the cells to interferon is not known. The antiproliferative effects tend to be dose-related and are frequently reversible after interferon is removed (Salmon et al., 1983; Blalock et al., 1980). However, gamma interferon *in vitro* has been associated with direct cytotoxicity of cells and may therefore cause irreversible changes (Rubin & Gupta, 1980). In addition, there have been reports of stimulation of tumor growth after treatment with interferon *in vitro* (Ludwig et al., 1983; Bradley & Ruscetti, 1981). Whether this phenomenon occurs *in vivo* is not known.

Gresser (1985) has developed a very interesting experimental model using Friend erythroleukemia cells injected intraperitoneally in mice and subsequently treated with intraperitoneal mouse interferon (alpha/beta). His results revealed a greater than 99% tumor cell loss in 3–4 days. He concluded that the interferon caused a host-mediated tumor cell destruction, as opposed to a direct effect on the tumor, caused by inhibition of cell multiplication or antiviral effect. Possible mechanisms included the following: (1) production of toxic oxygen intermediates by interferon-induced peritoneal leukocytes or macrophages; (2) production of cytotoxic factors by interferon-induced lymphocytes or macrophages; (3) interferon-induced cell differentiation of tumor cells; (4) effect of interferon on normal surrounding tissues (i.e., vascular/stromal tissues), which deprives the tumor of a vital nutrient; (5) the enhancement of an already operative host response (possibly endogenous interferon); and (6) the interferon receptor acts as a contact growth factor which is inhibited by interferon (Lindenmann, 1985). The fourth and fifth mechanisms were advocated by Gresser (1985) as the most likely etiologies of the antiproliferative effects of interferon in this specific model. Others have also suggested that factors probably involved in the antiviral mechanism (i.e., protein/RNA/DNA synthesis inhibitors) may also contribute to the antiproliferative effect (Clark & Longo, 1987). Therefore, as previously demonstrated, the details surrounding the antiproliferative effect of interferon are complex and not clearly defined.

Cell Differentiation

Interferon can either induce or repress cellular differentiation (Rossi, 1985). For example, human alpha interferon can inhibit granulocyte differentiation (Verma et al., 1981), whereas gamma interferon can stimulate monocytic differentiation in myeloid cells (Perussia et al., 1983) and enhance B lymphocyte differentiation

(Sidman et al., 1984). Part of this mechanism may be secondary to its effect on specific genes involved in differentiation (Lotem & Sachs, 1978). The dose of and timing of interferon administration may also determine the effect on differentiation. For example, in DMSO-stimulated Friend leukemia cells, low doses of interferon have increased differentiation (Belardelli et al., 1980), whereas higher doses reversibly inhibited growth and differentiation (Rossi et al., 1977). However, the specific underlying mechanism of action has not been determined thus far.

Antiviral

The antiviral action of interferon, in addition to other factors, may involve its effect on viral adsorption, RNA synthesis, protein synthesis, and virus maturation and release. Perhaps the most well-documented effect includes its interaction with $2'-5'$ oligoadenylate synthetase (2-5A), and protein kinase (McMahon & Kerr, 1983). Specifically, interferon may induce the cleavage of RNA via a 2-5A-activated endoribonuclease, in addition to the activation of a protein kinase, followed by phosphorylation of initiation factor II (Taylor et al., 1984). A recent trial comparing the antiviral activity of natural and recombinant alpha, beta, and gamma interferons on vesicular stomatitis virus revealed no significant difference with various combinations (Stebbing & May, 1982). However, further studies are needed to determine the exact mechanism of action and the responses obtained with various interferons.

Immunomodulating Effects

The effects of interferon on the immune system are complex and not completely understood. Interferon induces changes on cell surface receptors and antigens, B lymphocytes, T lymphocytes, macrophages, and natural killer (NK) cells. Heron et al. (1978) reported an increase in beta 2 microglobulin and HLA antigen expression of human peripheral mononuclear cells after treatment with human interferon. Interferon has also increased shedding of tumor-associated and HLA antigens (Giacomini et al., 1984). Further studies noted that increased HLA synthesis occurred secondary to an increase in HLA mRNA (Burrone & Milstein, 1982). Gamma interferon has a greater stimulatory effect in this respect than does alpha or beta interferon (Dolei et al., 1983). In addition, interferons, especially gamma interferon, can increase the number of Fc receptors in human cell lines and normal monocytes (Guyre et al., 1983).

B Lymphocytes

The interaction between B lymphocytes and interferon can result in the augmentation or suppression of antibody formation. Both the dose and time of administration of interferon in relationship to the presentation of antigen can affect the outcome (Zarling, 1984; Sonnenfeld, 1984). However, interferon may not induce a change in antibody production, and its ultimate role in this particular area has not been clearly established.

Proliferative Responses of B and T Lymphocytes

Interferons primarily suppress the proliferative responses of human B and T cells to antigens and mitogens, although the effect on T cells is greater (Zarling, 1984). However, Miorner et al. (1978) have also noted an increase in the proliferative response after treatment with interferon. Gamma interferon may also augment the proliferation of B cells, alone and after stimulation with interleukin II (Romagnani et al., 1986). Again, the effect of interferon may be related to the dose and timing of interferon exposure.

T Lymphocytes

In contrast, although T cell cytotoxicity can be suppressed by interferon, it is usually enhanced and is also dependent upon dose and timing of interferon administration (Heron et al., 1976). The mechanism of cytotoxicity may also be related to the degree of suppressor cell function (Heron & Berg, 1979). Mittelman et al. (1983) have demonstrated an initial *in vivo* decrease in the helper/suppressor T cell ratio in humans after interferon therapy. However, the mechanism by which interferon may induce changes in T cell cytotoxicity remains unclear.

Macrophages

The phagocytic, cytolytic, and tumoricidal activity of macrophages is usually enhanced by interferons (Huang et al., 1971; Zarling, 1984). However, suppression of differentiation of peripheral blood monocytes to macrophages has also been documented (Lee & Epstein, 1980). The effect on macrophages may also be related to the dose and duration of exposure of interferon (Borden & Ball, 1981).

Natural Killer Cells

The effect of interferon on natural killer (NK) cells is probably the most extensively researched area of interferon-mediated immune modulation. In 1978, reports of enhanced NK cell activity and target cell resistance to cell-mediated lysis after exposure to interferon were published (Trinchieri & Santoli, 1978; Einhorn et al., 1978). Since then, numerous studies have demonstrated that both natural and recombinant human interferons usually cause increased NK cell activity and increased antibody-dependent cell cytotoxicity (ADCC) *in vitro* (Zarling et al., 1979; Masucci et al., 1980). Studies conducted in humans, *in vivo*, have resulted in various responses including an initial decline in NK cell activity and ADCC followed by an increase in activity (Koren et al., 1983), no significant change in NK cell activity, and depressed NK cell activity (Maluish et al., 1983). The response to interferon may also be related to the dose and timing of administration (Koren et al., 1983; Edwards et al., 1985; Ng et al., 1983). Lotzova et al. (1982) divided cancer patients and normal individuals into groups based on the peripheral blood NK cell activity. They noted that those with higher activity were primarily the normal donors, whereas cancer patients comprised more of the low responders. After treatment with interferon, the NK cell activity was enhanced in the low responder group, whereas it was essentially unchanged in the high responders. In a later trial, they detected no association between serum interferon levels and NK cell cytotoxicity (Lotzova et al., 1983). In addition, to date there has been no definite association between NK cell activity and clinical responses (Einhorn et al., 1982). The mechanism of enhanced NK cell activity may be related to an increased proportion of active NK cells as opposed to an increase in the number of target binding cells (Targan & Dorey, 1980). Therefore, the changes in NK cell activity after treatment with interferon are varied and inconsistent.

Other Actions

Numerous cellular changes have been associated with exposure to interferon (Taylor et al., 1984). Structural alterations include development of abnormal microtubules/lupus inclusions (Rich, 1981), decreased cellular motility (Tamm et al., 1981; Pfeffer et al., 1980a), altered expression of cell membrane receptors, i.e., concanavalin A and estrogen receptors (Pfeffer et al., 1980b; Dimitrov et al., 1984), and changes in cell membrane composition (Chandrabose & Cuatrecasas, 1981). Alterations in protein synthesis include increased expression of beta 2 microglobulin (Heron et al., 1978) and carcinoembryonic antigen (Attallah et al., 1979), while other biochemical changes such as depression of hepatic cytochrome P-450 system (Renton & Mannering, 1976) and increased prostaglandin synthesis (Yaron et al., 1977; Fuse et al., 1982) have also been reported. Additional effects include interference with oncogene expression (Clemens, 1985), suppression of the leukocyte migration inhibitory factor (Szigeti et al., 1980), and numerous other functions (Taylor-Papadimitriou, 1984).

Finally, it should be stressed that gamma interferon seems to be the most active of the interferons in respect to immune modulation. It is a strong monocyte activator, increases expression of histocompatibility antigens, enhances interleukin II receptor expression on T cells (Johnson & Farrar, 1983), and participates in generation of lymphokine activated killer cells (Itoh et al., 1985). As previously mentioned, the timing, dose, and route of interferon administration may exert a significant role in the ultimate effects of interferon on the patient.

PHARMACOKINETICS

In order to determine better the pharmacokinetics of the various interferons, both bioassays and immunoassays have been developed. The majority of pharmacologic data is from studies using various types of alpha interferon. Although numerous routes of administration have been used, including rectal, topical (eye drops, intranasal, skin), intradermal, intralesional, intravenous (IV), intramuscular (IM), subcutaneous (SQ), and intrathecal applications, most clinical trials have used either IV, IM, or SQ routes (Scott, 1982). After IM or SQ administration of either natural or recombinant alpha interferon, peak levels occur approximately 4–8 hr after injection and are minimally detectable at 24 hr. However, IV injection results in a peak level in 15–30 min with minimal serum levels obtainable at 4 hr (Gutterman et al., 1980, 1982; Kirkwood et al., 1985a; Spiegel, 1985). Data from beta interferon administration is not as vast, although IM injections produce inconsistent and low levels (Hawkins et al., 1984). IV infusions produce peak levels almost immediately with minimal levels detected after 12 hr (Rinehart et al., 1986). A phase I trial of natural gamma interferon resulted in rapid serum clearance after IV bolus, whereas IM injections yielded no detectable levels (Gutterman et al., 1984). Recombinant gamma interferon injected intramuscularly yielded a half-life of 3.5–7.5 hr (Kurzrock et al., 1986b). However, during or after IV administration at doses of 2×10^6 U/m^2/day, gamma interferon levels were not detected. At doses of 10×10^6 U/m^2/day and greater, peak levels were noted at 4–6 hr during a 6-hr infusion, with no detectable activity present 2 hr after the infusion (Vadhan-Raj et al., 1986; Brown et al., 1987). This again suggests a rapid plasma clearance. Alpha and beta interferon are primarily metabolized in the kidney with less than 5% excreted in the urine (Bino et al., 1982; Bocci et al., 1982). Pharmacokinetics of leukocyte interferon, however, have not been altered in chronic renal failure patients receiving dialysis, although further investigation is needed (Hirsch et al., 1983).

TOXICITIES

The toxicities of alpha, beta, and gamma interferon are basically similar, although most of the clinical trials have used alpha interferon and, therefore, unknown toxicities of beta and gamma interferon may exist. It was initially suggested that some of the toxicities of the natural interferons would be eliminated with the more purified and recombinant forms (Krown, 1986). Unfortunately, this has not occurred, and subsequently both the natural and highly purified interferons share similar toxicities (Scott et al., 1981). Toxicities can affect numerous organ systems as illustrated below.

Constitutional Symptoms

The majority of patients, upon initial exposure to interferon, will experience fever, myalgias, tachycardia, headaches, and chills (i.e., flu-like symptoms). The severity of these symptoms are related to the type of interferon, dose, schedule, route of administration, and the age of the patient (Quesada et al., 1986a). The fever usually begins within 6 hr of exposure and resolves within 24 hr. If interferon is administered on a daily schedule, the fever tends to diminish after 7–10 days, whereas patients treated with intermittent doses develop fevers after each dose. Fever can be well-controlled with acetaminophen; the mechanism is unclear, although it may be related to elevated prostaglandins in the hypothalamus (Dinarello et al., 1984). Another very common symptom is fatigue, which tends to be more pronounced in older patients, in those receiving high doses of interferon, and with chronic daily administration. This is a major dose-limiting toxicity, but it can be improved with dose reduction, intermittent administration, and evening injections (Abrams et al., 1985). Another frequent complaint is anorexia, which can be associated with weight loss, especially at high doses.

Hematopoietic System

Hematologic toxicity is also fairly common and can be dose-limiting. A leukopenia with decrease in both granulocyte and lymphocyte counts frequently occurs within several hours after interferon exposure, and reaches bottom within 1 week. However, counts normalize rapidly after discontinuation of the interferon. The mechanism may be related to a reversible inhibition of release of cells from the bone marrow (Ernstoff & Kirkwood, 1984) and possible inhibition of myeloid differentiation (Verma et al., 1981). However, there has been no definite increase of infections in patients with normal pretreatment counts (Quesada et al., 1986a). Occasionally, a mild thrombocytopenia will develop after a few weeks of therapy. In addition, a normochromic/normocytic anemia can also occur, usually with chronic therapy, but normalization of counts may not develop until a few months after discontinuation of interferon (Ingimarsson et al., 1980). These hematologic toxicities appear to be more severe in patients with hematologic malignancies (Quesada et al., 1984a). Immune thrombocytopenias, anemias, and coagulopathies have been reported (McLaughlin et al., 1985; Mirro et al., 1985).

Nervous System

Neurotoxicity is primarily manifested by central nervous system abnormalities, although peripheral neurotoxicity including parasthenias and muscle atrophy have been noted (Mattson et al., 1983; Bernsen et al., 1985). At high doses, confusion, somnolence, psychosis, and hallucinations may occur. Electroencephalogram evaluations have revealed a diffuse encephalopathy, although there has been no association between these changes and interferon levels in the cerebrospinal fluid (Rohatiner et al., 1983b). The complaint of fatigue may be a manifestation of frontal lobe dysfunction, possibly secondary to a direct effect of interferon or to a disruption of normal neurotransmitter activity (Adams et al., 1984). In addition, headaches and seizures have been reported (Kirkwood et al., 1985a).

Cardiovascular System

Few reports of cardiovascular toxicity have been documented, although episodes of congestive heart failure, myocardial infarction, pericardial effusions, and arrythmias have occurred during interferon treatment (Quesada et al., 1986a). More frequently, physical findings of tachycardia, hypotension, and diaphoresis can be attributed to fever. Nevertheless, interferon should be administered with caution to those with evidence of cardiovascular disease (Oldham, 1982).

Other System Effects

Gastrointestinal System. Gastrointestinal symptoms have generally been limited to nausea, vomiting, diarrhea, and altered taste. These symptoms seem to increase in intensity with dose escalation. Approximately 25% of patients will also develop transient elevations in hepatic transaminase levels that are dose-related, and less often experience increases in lactic dehydrogenase and alkaline phosphatase levels (Quesada et al., 1986a). Acute hepatic necrosis has been noted in mice, but thus far not in humans (Gresser et al., 1975).

Genitourinary System. Proteinuria (usually less than 1 g/day) develops in approximately 15% to 20% of patients (Quesada et al., 1986a). Reports of interstitial nephritis and minimal-change nephropathy have also been associated with acute renal toxicity and the nephrotic syndrome (Averbuch et al., 1984).

Musculoskeletal System. Musculoskeletal toxicities have consisted primarily of diffuse transient myalgias and arthralgias. However, chronic myelogenous leukemia patients treated with interferon have occasionally developed weakness and severe myalgias (Talpaz et al., 1987).

Mucocutaneous. Mucocutaneous symptoms have included alopecia, rashes, urticaria, increased eyelash growth, and worsening of psoriasis, although alopecia is the most common of these and occurs primarily with chronic therapy (Foon & Dougher, 1984; Quesada et al., 1986a). Interferon has also been documented in fluid from psoriatic lesions (Bjerke et al., 1983).

Miscellaneous. Significant laboratory abnormalities have included increased 11-hydroxycorticosteroids, hypercalcemia/hypocalcemia, hyperkalemia, hypothyroidism/hyperthyroidism, decreased circulating progesterone/estrogen levels, elevated antidiuretic hormone, acute tumor lysis syndrome, and vasculitis (Bottomley & Toy, 1985; Fer et al., 1984; Clark and Longo, 1987). Initial reports suggested a significant effect of alpha interferon on testicular function (Davidson et al., 1985). However, subsequent analysis failed to demonstrate a definite correlation between interferon and testicular dysfunction, noting that gonadal toxicity owing to interferon is probably uncommon (Schilsky et al., 1987). Phenobarbital toxicity, possibly due to interference of drug metabolism has also been noted (Krown et al., 1987).

Toxicities owing to beta interferon are similar to those produced by alpha interferon although possibly milder (Sarna et al., 1986; Liberati et al., 1985). Gamma interferon also has similar toxicities to alpha interferon, although dose-limiting toxicities in several Phase I trials have included neurotoxicity, hypotension, fever, and cardiovascular toxicity (Vadhan-Raj et al., 1986; Brown et al., 1987). Tachyphylaxis to fever may not occur as frequently with gamma interferon as with alpha interferon. The etiology of the fever with gamma interferon may be related to release of interleukin I, as opposed to hypothalamic alterations (Quesada et al., 1986a). Hypertriglyceridemia (Kurzrock et al., 1986a) has also been reported. This is in contrast somewhat to the hematologic and constitutional abnormalities that are more frequently noted with alpha interferon.

HEMATOLOGIC MALIGNANCIES

Hairy Cell Leukemia

Thus far the disease that has benefited most from the clinical use of interferon is hairy cell leukemia (HCL). Bouroncle et al. (1958) described a distinct clinical entity, termed leukemic reticuloendotheliosis; Schrek and Donnelly (1966) later used the term "hairy" cell to describe the peculiar cytoplasmic projections that typify the characteristic cell found in this disease. HCL accounts for approximately 2% of all leukemias (Bouroncle, 1979) and occurs primarily in males with age of onset usually in the sixth decade (Golomb et al., 1978). Clinical features frequently include complaints of fatigue, bleeding, abdominal pain, and infections, and physical examination often reveals splenomegaly, mild hepatomegaly, and rare lymphadenopathy (Jansen et al., 1981; Flandrin et al., 1984). Laboratory data reveal a pancytopenia in approximately 66% of untreated patients, with up to 20% presenting in the leukemic phase (Golomb, 1983). The diagnosis can be confirmed by bone marrow biopsy, which reveals a characteristic mononuclear cell infiltrate (Burke, 1978) and the hairy cells are frequently (90% to 95% of patients) tartrate-resistant acid phosphatase (TRAP) positive, although this factor alone does not confirm the diagnosis (Yam et al., 1971). HCL is a lymphoproliferative disorder of primarily B cell lineage, although a T cell variant has been reported (Rieber et al., 1979; Jansen et al., 1982; Saxon et al., 1978). Indications for treatment include anemia (hct < 25%), granulocytopenia (ANC < 500/μL), thrombocytopenia (platelet count $< 50,000/\mu L$), bone involvement, frequent infections, symptoms secondary to splenomegaly, and bulky retroperitoneal disease (Golomb, 1987).

Approximately 90% of patients will require treatment at some point. Androgens (Magee et al., 1981), leukapheresis (Yam et al., 1984), lithium (Blum, 1980), bone marrow transplantation (Cheever et al., 1984), chlorambucil (Golomb et al., 1984), and combination chemotherapy (Calvo et al., 1985) have all been reported to achieve responses. Several of these responses, however, have been anecdotal or in the case of chemotherapeutic agents, frought with infectious complications and death. Radiation therapy has been used primarily for local control (Lembersky et al., 1985). However, splenectomy has been considered the treatment of choice because all patients have an initial improvement in their peripheral blood counts (Mintz & Golomb, 1979), although recent data indicate that almost 50% of splenectomized patients will require further treatment. The interval from splenectomy to treatment ranges from 1–164 months with a median of 8.3 months (Golomb et al., 1986a).

Quesada et al. (1984b) reported a 100% response rate in seven patients with HCL treated with IM injections of partially purified alpha interferon (three complete responses, four partial responses). Within 12 weeks all patients had improvement in one or more of the peripheral blood counts and six patients demonstrated $\leq 5\%$ hairy cells in the bone marrow. Since then, several clinical trials have been conducted using primarily recombinant alpha interferon, and occasionally highly purified lymphoblastoid interferon (Golomb et al., 1987; Quesada et al., 1986c; Foon et al., 1986b; Golomb et al., 1986b; Worman et al., 1985). The overall response rate is approximately 90%. Many patients achieve a response within 6 months, although occasionally responses will occur later. Most trials have treated patients for a period of 12 months, using IM or SQ injections daily or three times per week, with doses ranging primarily from 3–4 million units per day. However, although the overall response rate to interferon is high, the complete response rate and subsequent chance of cure is low. The duration of response to interferon therapy is currently being evaluated. Twenty-four patients evaluated by Ratain et al. (1987) at a median of 8.5 months following interferon therapy, revealed only one patient requiring further treatment. However, most of the patients' bone marrow samples demonstrated a marked decrease in normal elements and a relative increase in the percentage of hairy cells, although peripheral counts remained stable. Further long-term follow-up is necessary to determine the duration of response to interferon and the need for maintenance therapy. However, it appears that peripheral blood counts do not rapidly decrease after completion of therapy. A current randomized multicenter trial is evaluating the benefit of an additional 6 months of interferon therapy compared to observation alone. Preliminary data demonstrated 18% of patients (observation alone) relapsed, compared to only 7% in the treatment group (Golomb et al., 1987). However, further investigation is necessary prior to any definite conclusion.

Hematologic parameters in interferon-treated patients frequently reveal a normalization of platelet count after 2 months of therapy, increase of hemoglobin within 4 months, and improvement of granulocyte count within 5 months (Golomb et al., 1986b). The number of serious infections and transfusion requirements has also decreased dramatically. Review of bone marrow biopsies 3 months after commencement of interferon has revealed a decrease in the cellularity and percentage of hairy cells, persistence of increased reticulin, and conversion of many TRAP positive hairy cells to TRAP-negative (Naeim & Jacobs, 1985). Further evaluation of bone marrow samples during 6–12 months of interferon therapy have demonstrated a reduction in the hairy cell index (bone marrow cellularity × percentage of hairy cells/10,000), although a complete absence of hairy cells did not occur (Bardawil et al., 1986). The majority of HCL patients treated with interferon develop a transient myelosuppression during the first month of treatment, with a nadir neutrophil and platelet count occurring at a median of 1 week after initiation of therapy (Ratain et al., 1986). However, as previously noted, the platelet count frequently normalizes within 2 months of treatment, whereas the hemoglobin and neutrophil count normalize later, usually after 4 months of therapy (Golomb et al., 1987).

The exact mechanism of action of interferon in the treatment of HCL is unclear. Although patients with HCL have decreased NK cell activity (Ruco et al., 1983), which can increase after treatment with interferon (Foon et al., 1986b), there is no definite evidence to attribute the clinical response to this factor. Other possible mechanisms include an antiproliferative (Paganelli et al., 1986), differentiating (Dolei et al., 1986), or protein synthesis effect (Samuels et al., 1987). A decrease in the number of alpha interferon receptors on the hairy cell surface after treatment with interferon has also been noted (Billard et al., 1986).

In summary, the use of interferon is recommended as initial therapy in those patients with a nonpalpable spleen and diffuse marrow involvement associated with decreased peripheral counts (Golomb & Ratain, 1987). Interferon can also be used in splenectomized patients who relapse, with an excellent response rate. The use of pentostatin (2-deoxycoformycin), an adenosine deaminase inhibitor, can result in high response rates, with a greater number of complete responses, compared to interferon (Spiers et al., 1984; Johnston et al., 1986; Kraut et al., 1986). However, further information on remission duration and toxicities are required prior to its use as initial therapy. Currently, its use is confined to clinical trials. Interferon, however, has been approved by the Food and Drug Administration for general use in the treatment of HCL.

Chronic Myelogenous Leukemia

The use of interferon in the treament of chronic myelogenous leukemia (CML) also appears promising. Human leukocyte and fibroblast interferons have been shown to exert inhibitory effects on normal and CML granulocytic progenitor cells (Oladipupo-Williams et al., 1981). Talpaz et al., (1983b) reported that a hematologic remission (normalization in peripheral WBC and platelet count) occurred in 5 of 7 patients treated with partially purified human alpha interferon. A decrease in serum B12 levels, lactic dehydrogenase levels, and splenomegaly was also noted. Induction doses ranged from 3 to 9×10^6 units, administered daily *via* IM injection. In 1987 Talpaz et al., (1987) updated their data on Philadelphia (Ph) chromosome-positive CML patients treated with human alpha interferon. Of the 51 patients treated, 71% achieved a complete hematologic response (CR) and 10% a partial response (PR). Improvement was noted in the peripheral blood, spleen, and bone marrow. A complete hematologic remission was noted at a median of 14 weeks into therapy, while a median of 9 months was required for Ph chromosome suppression. The median duration of disease control was 33+ months for those in CR (78% of these patients continued on maintenance therapy) and 9 months for those in PR, with a projected median 3-year survival of 76%. In addition, lymphoid or undifferentiated elements were frequently noted in those who developed a blast crisis. Recombinant alpha interferon has also been used with success in chronic phase CML (Niederle et al., 1987; Talpaz et al., 1986).

Talpaz et al. (1983a) have also used human leukocyte interferon for control of severe symptomatic thrombocytosis in patients with refractory CML with a 100% response rate. The exact mechanism of *in vivo* sensitivity and resistance to interferon in CML remains unclear. Down-regulation of IFN receptors during interferon therapy has been reported in both responders and nonresponders (Maxwell et al., 1985). Other studies have suggested that resistance may involve other factors besides interferon binding, such as a lack of increased 2,5-oligoadenylate synthetase activity (Rosenblum et al., 1986). This enzyme is frequently elevated in CML patients who respond to interferon therapy. It is too early to determine whether the use of interferon will prolong the chronic phase and increase survival. Its use in the blast phase has been limited, although anecdotal reports indicate a short-term benefit (Hill et al., 1982; Talpaz et al., 1985). Future use of interferon in CML may involve combination regimens with chemotherapeutic agents. For example, Bergsagel et al. (1986) have treated five patients in a busulfan-induced remission of chronic phase CML with alpha 2b interferon. A decrease in leukocyte doubling time and increased remission duration was noted in 4 of the 5 patients. However, further studies are needed to evaluate the value of combination therapy. The role of beta and gamma interferon is also being evaluated in clinical trials.

Acute Nonlymphocytic/Lymphocytic Leukemia

The response to interferon in other leukemias such as acute myelogenous leukemia (Mirro et al., 1986; Rohatiner et al., 1983a) and acute lymphocytic leukemia (Bratt et al., 1984) has been minimal, although the number of patients treated has been small. However, *in vitro* studies do suggest a possible future role for interferon in these diseases. For example, Hemmi and Breitman (1987) recently reported that retinoic acid in combination with either recombinant gamma or alpha interferon is synergistic in stimulating monocytic differentiation of the HL60 (human pro-myelocytic leukemia) cell line.

Chronic Lymphocytic Leukemia

The role of interferon in the treatment of chronic lymphocytic leukemia is unclear. Some studies have reported partial responses of approximately 25% with natural (Gutterman et al., 1980) and recombinant (O'Connell et al., 1986) alpha interferon. However, other recent trials using natural (Horning et al., 1985) and recombinant (Foon et al., 1985) interferon have revealed poor results. In the latter trial (Foon et al., 1985) only two of 18 patients obtained a brief partial response. Five patients had an acceleration of their disease during therapy. As of September, 1986, of the 57 patients reported in the literature, there were only eight PR and no CR (Foon et al., 1986a). Further trials using gamma interferon may be more promising, as *in vitro* studies reveal a phenotypic alteration toward a more differentiated cell in chronic lymphocytic leukemia cells after interferon treatment (Al-Katib et al., 1984).

Multiple Myeloma

Interferon was first used in the treatment of multiple myeloma by Idestrom et al. (1979). Since then, numerous studies have been conducted using alpha and beta interferon, although differences in doses, types of interferon, and response criteria necessitate careful interpretation of these reports. In a review by Wagstaff et al. (1985) of nine trials performed between 1979 and 1985, the overall response rate (CR + PR) was 18%. Most of these patients had been refractory to therapy or had relapsed. Ahre et al. (1984) conducted a randomized trial comparing leukocyte interferon to intermittent high-dose melphalan–prednisone in previously untreated patients. There was an overall response rate of 14% in the interferon-treated group compared to 44% in the chemotherapy-treated group. This difference was primarily due to a poor response of the interferon-treated IgG myelomas. Median duration of response was 23 months in the former group as opposed to 35 months in the latter group, although the overall survival did not differ significantly. Costanzi et al. (1985) reported an 18% response rate (one CR and six PR) in refractory or relapsed patients treated with alpha 2b interferon. There was a lower response rate (10.5%) in initially refractory patients compared to those who had relapsed after previous responses (26%). The duration of response ranged from 12 to 104+ weeks, with responses occurring from 7 to 14 weeks after initiation of treatment. Quesada et al. (1986b) noted a 50% response rate in previously untreated patients and a 15% response rate in all others after treatment with recombinant alpha interferon. Median duration of response ranged from 6 to 20 months. A normalization of subnormal serum immunoglobulin levels was noted in all responders.

Cooper et al. (1986) reported a 75% overall response rate (all PR) in previously untreated patients in a trial using a combination of alpha 2b interferon, prednisone, and melphalan. This response compared favorably with that expected from chemotherapy alone. Interferon followed by reinstitution of chemotherapy has also been successful in inducing responses (Costanzi & Pollard, 1987). Cooper has also reviewed the use of interferon in multiple myelomas (1986). Further trials are necessary to determine the role of interferon as a single agent or as part of a chemotherapeutic regimen in multiple myeloma. However, it appears that interferon is effective in treating both relapsed and previously untreated patients, with response durations of up to 2+ years (Cooper & Welander, 1986).

Non-Hodgkin's Lymphoma

The use of interferon in the treatment of non-Hodgkin's lymphoma appears limited to those with indolent, low-grade lymphomas. Patients with intermediate and high-grade lymphomas generally have poor responses to either natural or recombinant interferon; in a review of several trials only five of 36 reported cases obtained a response (Foon et al., 1986a). However, results in low-grade lymphomas have been more encouraging. Of 105 patients treated with either natural or recombinant alpha interferon, 11 CR and 34 PR were documented (Foon et al., 1986a). One of the earliest trials using human leukocyte interferon was reported by Merigan et al. (1978) and later updated by Louie et al. (1981). Four of seven evaluable patients with nodular lymphoma attained an objective response (1 CR + 3 PR) with response duration of 5–12 months. Subsequent studies using leukocyte interferon yielded similar results (Gutterman et al., 1980; Horning et al., 1985). In addition, Gams et al. (1984) reported an objective response rate of approximately 25% after treatment with lymphoblastoid interferon. The use of recombinant alpha interferon has also been studied in several trials, in both previously treated and untreated patients (Quesada et al., 1984a; Foon et al., 1984; Wagstaff et al., 1985; O'Connell et al., 1986; Leavitt et al., 1987).

Overall response rates are approximately 40%, although some studies indicate response rates of up to 60%. Median response durations are approximately 6 to 8 months, but remissions of 24+ months have been reported. Nodular poorly differentiated and nodular mixed lymphomas appear more responsive (Urba & Longo, 1986). There is no definite evidence to suggest that previously untreated patients are more responsive than those who have been treated; however, there is some suggestion that interferon responders relapse with more aggressive histology (Clark & Longo, 1987). Further studies are also needed to determine the difference in responses to high- and low-dose interferon. In addition, combinations of chemotherapy and interferon may prove to be beneficial (Hawkins et al., 1985). Beta interferon has also been used with minimal success (Siegert et al., 1982).

Hodgkin's Disease

The response to interferon in Hodgkin's disease has been minimal, although large trials have not been conducted (Blomgren et al., 1976; Horning et al., 1985; Leavitt et al., 1987).

Cutaneous T Cell Lymphoma

Recombinant alpha interferon has been used in the treatment of advanced cutaneous T cell lymphomas (Bunn et al., 1984; Foon & Bunn, 1986; Bunn & Foon, 1985). Of the 20 evaluated patients, there were two CR and seven PR for an objective response rate of 45%. All responses were noted within 1 month of treatment and ranged in duration from 3 to 36+ months (median, 5 months), with both cutaneous and extracutaneous improvement. The response may be partially dose-related because several patients improved further after dose escalations. The mechanism of action of interferon in this disease is unknown.

Kaposi's Sarcoma

A previously rare, indolent tumor, Kaposi's sarcoma, has dramatically increased in frequency and developed a more aggressive course in its association with the acquired immunodeficiency syndrome (AIDS) (Volberding, 1986). Interferon was initially used in this disease by Krown et al. (1983), and in a recent update of 75 patients treated with either high- or low-dose recombinant alpha 2a interferon, the response rate (CR + PR) was 38% for the high dose, 3% for the low dose, and 17% for patients escalated to high doses after initial low-dose treatment (Real et al., 1986). Median duration of response (from initiation of therapy) in the high-dose group was 18 months (4–31 months) and 10 months for those treated at lower doses. Responses were lower in those with a previous history of opportunistic infections, although responders later developed fewer infections with an apparent increase in survival (Krown et al. 1986b). Groopman et al. (1984) also reported a similar response rate of 30% after treatment with recombinant alpha interferon. Lymphoblastoid interferon has also been used with an objective response rate (CR + PR) of 13% (Gelmann et al., 1985). No responses to gamma interferon have been noted (Abrams & Volberding, 1986). Trials with combinations of interferon and chemotherapeutic agents have thus far not yielded better results compared to interferon alone, and may increase toxicity (Krown et al., 1986a; Lonberg et al., 1985). Immunologic changes do not correlate with responses, and the mechanism of action of interferon in this disease is unclear. (Abrams & Volberding, 1987).

Solid Tumors

The use of interferon in the treatment of renal cell carcinoma was first reported by Quesada et al. (1983). They noted a 26% response rate (all partial responses) with a median response duration of 6 months in patients receiving partially purified alpha interferon. Since then numerous trials have been conducted using leukocyte interferon (Kirkwood et al., 1985b), lymphoblastoid interferon (Vugrin et al., 1985; Neidhart et al., 1984; Trump et al., 1987), and recombinant alpha interferon (Quesada et al., 1985; Muss et al., 1987) with various doses, schedules, and routes of administration. Response rates (CR + PR) have ranged from 5% to 31%, with an overall major response rate of approximately 15% (Krown, 1985). Several studies have noted prolonged periods of time prior to response of 2–4 months and even up to 13 months (Muss, 1987). Most response durations are less than 1 year, but a response duration of 31+ months has been reported (Muss et al., 1987). Kirkwood et al. (1985b) noted a possible dose–response relationship, and Krown (1985) has suggested that intermediate doses may yield the best results. Other studies have suggested better responses in patients with small amounts of metastatic disease (Vugrin et al., 1985), in those treated previously with nephrectomy and without a history of bone metastases (Muss et al., 1987), or in those with lung metastases (Quesada et al., 1985), although these factors are not consistent findings. A few studies have been conducted using chemotherapeutic agents [i.e., vinblastine (Figlin et al., 1985) and doxorubicin (Muss et al., 1985)] in combination with interferon. Most of these studies have not resulted in an increased response rate, but greater toxicity has been a complicating factor. Although the benefit of interferon in regard to survival needs to be evaluated further, treatment with this agent is a reasonable option because response rates are frequently equal to or greater than those achieved with conventional chemotherapy. Current clinical trials are evaluating the efficacy of gamma interferon in the treatment of this disease.

Melanoma

Advanced melanoma has been very difficult to treat, with chemotherapeutic regimens resulting in response rates of approximately 20% with minimal impact on survival (Mastrangelo et al., 1985). Several studies have indicated immune alterations in patients with melanoma, i.e., the presence of cytotoxic T lymphocytes that react with autologous tumor cells (DeVries and Spits, 1984) and decreased expression of class I MHC antigens with progressive disease (Fossati et al., 1986). Therefore, the possibility of immunomodulation by interferons leading to positive clinical results has been suggested. Initial trials with either natural or lymphoblastoid alpha interferon have frequently resulted in response rates of less than 10% (Retsas et al., 1983; Krown et al., 1984; Goldberg et al., 1985). However, results for recombinant alpha interferon have been better, with response rates of up to 25% (Kirkwood et al., 1985a; Creagan et al., 1986). This may be related to differences in doses and patient selectivity. Overall, the response rate is approximately 18% (Goldstein & Laszlo, 1986), with median response duration of usually 4–6 months, although response durations of 25–36+ months have been reported

(Kirkwood & Ernstoff, 1985, 1986). Median time to response may be 3 months or longer. One study indicated that a combination of cimetidine (which inhibits suppressor T cell function) and interferon may be beneficial (Borgstrom et al., 1982), although subsequent trials have not revealed a significant advantage to this combination *versus* interferon alone (Ernstoff et al., 1984; Creagan et al., 1985). In a review of 96 patients by Creagan et al. (1986), a higher response rate was noted in patients with nonvisceral dominant disease and a definite dose–response relationship was not documented, although this has been previously suggested and will require further investigation. Combinations of interferon and chemotherapy (i.e., dacarbazine and nitrosureas) may also prove beneficial (Kirkwood & Ernstoff, 1986). Various combinations of alpha, beta, gamma interferons, monoclonal antibodies, and chemotherapeutic agents will, it is hoped, improve response rates (Legha, 1986; Abdi et al., 1985). Interferons may have a role not only in advanced melanoma but possibly as adjuvant therapy as well.

Gliomas

Several studies have documented systemic alterations in the immune system of patients with primary intracranial tumors; in addition, immune changes in the local environment of gliomas has been suggested (Mahaley et al., 1977; Bullard et al., 1986). For example, Fontana et al. (1984) have noted inhibition of interleukin II mediated effects and production of an interleukin-I–like factor by glioblastoma cells *in vitro*. Therefore, the use of immunomodulating properties of interferons, in addition to their antiproliferative and differentiating effects, may explain the responses noted after treatment. Thus far, trials have investigated the use of leukocyte, lymphoblastoid, and recombinant alpha interferon, in addition to beta interferon. The response rates range from 20% to 40%, with a median response rate of 24% (Goldstein & Laszlo, 1986). Median duration of response of 9+ months has been reported, with neurotoxicity as a significant dose-limiting factor (Mahaley et al., 1985). Interferon has been administered intravenously, intramuscularly, intratumorally and intrathecally. Further trials using gamma interferon and other combinations of biologic response modifiers are needed to determine their roles in unresectable disease or as an adjuvant therapy.

Ovarian Carcinoma

Several studies have used alpha interferon in ovarian carcinoma, either intravenously, intramuscularly, subcutaneously, or intraperitoneally with response rates ranging from 0% to 33%, with a median response rate of 14% (Goldstein & Laszlo, 1986). The highest response rate was noted by Berek et al. (1986) in patients with minimal residual disease, treated intraperitoneally with recombinant alpha interferon. Peritoneal fluid revealed an initial increase in NK cell activity, although this did not correlate with clinical response. Peritoneal fluid interferon levels were 30 to 1000 times those of blood levels. A recent trial of IV recombinant gamma interferon resulted in one CR and three PR in seven patients with recurrent disease (Welander et al., 1986). Because it has been suggested that the antitumor effects of gamma interferon may be mediated by tumor-associated macrophages, the use of interferon in this tumor may be beneficial not only systemically, but especially for local peritoneal disease (Saito et al., 1986).

Cervical Carcinoma

Interferon therapy in cervical carcinoma, has been used successfully in carcinoma in situ. Seto et al. (1984) reported a 100% response rate after intralesional application of alpha or beta interferon. Systemic treatment for recurrent or metastatic disease has been limited and has thus far yielded poor results (Einhorn et al., 1986).

Bladder Carcinoma

Intratumoral and intramuscular administration of natural alpha interferon was first used for treatment of malignant papillomatosis of the bladder by Ikic et al. (1981a) with remissions of up to approximately 24 months duration. A randomized trial of patients with superficial bladder cancer, using polyinosinic acid and polycytidylic acid (Poly I:C), an interferon inducer, versus observation post-transurethral resection, resulted in prolonged survival in the former group (Kemeny et al., 1981). Torti and Lum (1986) noted a 50% CR in patients with carcinoma *in situ* after administration of intravesical alpha 2b interferon. Some reports suggest immune alterations in patients with bladder carcinoma; therefore, further trials are needed to determine the role of interferon as first-line and/or adjuvant therapy (Lum & Torti, 1985).

Carcinoid

Oberg et al. (1986) have reported long-term results of 36 patients treated with natural alpha interferon for malignant carcinoid. A 47% objective response was noted with decreased urinary 5-hydroxyindolacetic acid and serum HCG levels, although minimal decrease in tumor size occurred. Those with midgut and pulmonary carcinoid responded, and combination therapy with chemotherapeutic agents was suggested for future trials.

Endocrine Pancreatic Tumors

Natural alpha interferon has also been used in the treatment of malignant endocrine pancreatic tumors by Eriksson et al. (1987). They reported an objective response rate of 83% with median response duration of 11 months (range, 2–36+ months). This was associated with a marked decrease in symptoms and peripheral hormonal levels, which may be secondary to inhibition of hormonal secretion by interferon. Anderson & Bloom (1987) have used recombinant alpha interferon with significant toxicities.

Head and Neck Carcinoma

Leukocyte interferon has been injected intratumorally with good response for various head and neck cancers (Ikic et al., 1981a). Connors et al. (1985) treated patients with nasopharyngeal carcinoma with IM leukocyte interferon, and noted two of 12 PR. Further studies are needed to determine the role of interferon in the treatment of head and neck cancer.

Sarcoma

Natural beta interferon and recombinant gamma interferon have been used in patients with nonosseous sarcomas with response rates of 5% and 0%, respectively (Harris et al., 1986; Edmonson et al., 1987). Response rates in osteosarcoma have thus far not indicated any definite benefit from therapy with natural alpha interferon or beta interferon, although further investigation is needed (Strander, 1986). Transient tumor reduction in pulmonary metastases has been reported (Ito et al., 1980).

Prostate Carcinoma

Experience with interferon therapy in prostate carcinoma has been limited and thus far has yielded minimal responses (Gutterman & Quesada, 1981–82).

Breast Carcinoma

Although initial trials with leukocyte interferon resulted in response rates (CR + PR) of 35% (Gutterman et al., 1980) and 22% (Borden et al., 1982a, 1982b, 1983), subsequent studies using lymphoblastoid, recombinant alpha, and beta interferon have yielded a median response rate of 0% (Goldstein & Laszlo, 1986). Although *in vitro* studies suggest a possible role for interferon, further investigation is needed, including studies using combinations of interferon and chemotherapy. There does not appear to be a role for interferon as a single-agent treatment, and at this time the use of interferon in breast carcinoma should be limited to clinical trials (Borden & Balkwill, 1984).

Colon Carcinoma

Response rates in colorectal cancer using natural, lymphoblastoid, and recombinant alpha interferon as single-agent therapy have been negligible (Goldstein &

Laszlo, 1986; Spiegel, 1986). However, despite lack of antitumor activity, immune alterations have occurred in patients after treatment (Krown et al., 1987). Combinations with other interferons or drugs may prove to have some efficacy.

Lung Carcinoma

Since 1980, a median response rate of 0% has been reported in both small cell and non-small cell lung carcinoma after alpha interferon therapy (recombinant/leukocyte/lymphoblastoid) (Goldstein & Laszlo, 1986; Strander, 1986).

Gastric Carcinoma

Experience with interferon therapy in gastric carcinoma has been limited, although one study using lymphoblastoid interferon reported no response in 14 patients (Strander, 1986).

Liver Carcinoma

Beta interferon has been used intravenously and intra-arterially, in addition to alpha interferon (intra-arterially) in the treatment of primary and metastatic liver carcinoma with essentially no response (Strander, 1986).

Antibodies

The development of neutralizing antibodies to human beta interferon was first noted by Vallbracht et al. (1981). Trown et al. (1983) then reported the presence of IgG antibodies after treatment with alpha interferon. Subsequently, neutralizing antibodies to recombinant alpha 2a interferon were documented in 153 of 559 (27.4%) patients during therapy (Jones & Itri, 1986), whereas only ten of 423 (2.4%) patients treated with systemic recombinant alpha 2b interferon developed antibodies (Spiegel et al., 1986). Nonneutralizing antibodies to recombinant beta interferon have also been reported (Pertcheck et al., 1985; Krown, 1986), whereas antibodies to gamma interferon have not been noted thus far (Quesada et al., 1986a). Renal cell carcinoma and Kaposi's sarcoma patients tend to develop antibodies (especially to alpha 2a) more frequently than in other malignancies (Spiegel, 1986). Some studies have documented a decrease in serum interferon levels and tumor progression with antibody development (Quesada et al., 1985), although this is not a consistent finding (Figlin et al., 1986). In addition, others have noted a decrease in toxicities owing to interferon antibodies, although there have been no side effects (i.e., increased viral infections or allergic reactions) associated with these antibodies. Antibodies to leukocyte interferon have also been noted in patients without prior interferon therapy (Krown, 1986).

Combination Therapy

Current research indicates a probable role for interferon, not only as a single agent, but also in combination with other factors such as chemotherapeutic drugs, radiation therapy, and other biologic response modifiers (Bonnem, 1987). Several *in vitro* and *in vivo* models have indicated an additive or synergistic effect of cytotoxic drugs and various interferons. Chemotherapeutic agents that have been used in clinical trials include doxorubicin (Green et al., 1985; Sarosy et al., 1986; Von Hoff et al., 1986), cyclophosphamide (Durie et al., 1986), cisplatin, chlorambucil, melphalan/prednisone, 5-fluorouracil, vinblastine, VP-16, and nitrosoureas (Bonnem, 1987; Green et al., 1985). The majority of these studies have been Phase I trials, attempting to determine safe doses of these agents and their toxicities when used in combination. Therefore, further Phase II trials are needed to reveal any significant efficacy clinically. Generally, no definite improvement in response has been achieved with combination therapy thus far. Several preclinical studies have indicated an additive or synergistic effect of interferons plus radiotherapy, with some suggestion that the interferon may act as a radiosensitizer (Namba et al., 1984). Torrisi et al. (1986) documented severe toxicity in a trial using recombinant alpha interferon and radiotherapy. Discontinuation of interferon was necessary in some patients. Again, further Phase II trials will determine any increased clinical benefit.

Interferons have also been used in combination with other biologic response modifiers. *In vitro* studies have demonstrated potentiation of the antiviral, antiproliferative, and immunomodulating effects of interferon therapy with various combinations of interferons (Bonnem, 1987; Schiller et al., 1986). Kurzrock et al., (1986c) noted a synergism between recombinant alpha and gamma interferon with respect to certain toxicities. Interferons, particularly gamma interferon, have also produced increased binding of tumor necrosis factor to cellular receptors, probably secondary to an increase in the number of receptors (Tsujimoto et al., 1986). Trials using interferons in combination with monoclonal antibodies (Murray et al., 1986) and with interleukin-II (Krigel et al. 1986) have also been conducted, although it is too early to determine any significant clinical benefit.

SUMMARY

There is a definite role for interferon in the treatment of human malignancy. However, it certainly is not the "cure-all" that it once was thought to be. Interferons have antiviral, antiproliferative, cell differentiating, immunomodulating, and other additional effects on cells. The mechanisms of action have not yet been clearly established. The majority of clinical trials have used alpha interferon, with smaller numbers using beta and gamma interferons. With recent advances in molecular biology, the availability of highly purified forms of recombinant interferons has markedly increased and allowed for better comparisons of clinical trials. The toxicities of interferons affect almost every organ system, but the most common of these include constitutional symptoms and myelosuppression. HCL has benefited most from the clinical use of interferon, with overall response rates of approximately 90%. Other hematologic malignancies, such as CML, cutaneous T cell lymphoma, Kaposi's sarcoma, and indolent non-Hodgkin's lymphomas have also responded to interferon therapy. The use of interferon in the treatment of solid tumors has unfortunately yielded poor response rates, especially in common tumors such as breast, lung, and colon cancer. Renal cell carcinoma and melanoma have obtained the best results, with response rates of 15% and 18%, respectively. The development of combination therapy, using chemotherapeutic agents, radiotherapy, and other biologic response modifiers, has only recently been used in clinical trials, although it should prove to be very interesting and promising research.

REFERENCES

Abdi, E.A., Kamitomo, V.J, Paterson, A.H., & McPherson, T.A. (1985). Combination Hu IFN β, DTIC, and cimetidine for advanced malignant melanoma. *Proceedings of the American Society of Clinical Oncology, 4*:134.

Abrams, D.I., & Volberding, P.A. (1986). Alpha interferon therapy of AIDS-associated Kaposi's sarcoma. *Seminars in Oncology, 13*(Suppl. 2):43–47.

Abrams, D.I., & Volberding, P.A. (1987). Alpha interferon therapy of AIDS-associated Kaposi's sarcoma. *Seminars in Oncology, 14*(Suppl. 2):43–47.

Abrams, P.G., McClamrock, E., & Foon, K. (1985). Evening administration of alpha interferon. *New England Journal of Medicine, 312*:443–444.

Adams, F., Quesada, J.R., & Gutterman, J.U. (1984). Neuropsychiatric manifestations of human leukocyte interferon therapy in patients with cancer. *Journal of the American Medical Association, 252*:938–941.

Ahre, A., Bjorkholm, M., Mellstedt, H., Brenning, G., et al. (1984). Human leukocyte interferon and intermittent high-dose Melphalan–Prednisone administration in the treatment of multiple myeloma: A randomized clinical trial from the multiple myeloma group of central Sweden. *Cancer Treatment Reports, 68*:1331–1338.

Al-Katib, A., Wang, C., & Koziner, B. (1984). Gamma interferon (IFN-γ)-induced phenotypic changes of chronic lymphocytic leukemia (CLL) and non-Hodgkin's lymphoma (NHL) cells. *Proceedings of the American Association of Cancer Research, 25*:235.

Anderson, J.V., & Bloom, S.R. (1987). Treatment of malignant endocrine pancreatic tumors with human leucocyte interferon. *Lancet, 1*:97.

Attallah, A.M., Needy, C.F., Noguchi, P.D., & Elisberg, B.L. (1979). Enhancement of carcinoembryonic antigen expression by interferon. *International Journal of Cancer, 24*:49–52.

Averbuch, S.D., Austin, H.A., Sherwin, S.A., Antonovych, T., Bunn, P.A., & Longo, D.L. (1984). Acute interstitial nephritis with the nephrotic syndrome following recombinant leukocyte A interferon therapy for mycosis fungoides. *New England Journal of Medicine, 310*:32–35.

Baglioni, C., Branca, A., D'Alessandro, S., Hossenlopp, D., & Chadha, K. (1982). Low interferon binding activity of two human cell lines which respond poorly to the antiviral and antiproliferative activity of interferon. *Virology, 122*:202–206.

Balkwill, F., & Taylor-Papadimitriou, J. (1978). Interferon affects both G1 and S + G2 in cells stimulated from quiescence to growth. *Nature, 274*:798–800.

Bardawil, R.G., Groves, C., Ratain, M.J., Golomb, H.M., & Vardiman, J.W. (1986). Changes in peripheral blood and bone marrow specimens following therapy with recombinant alpha 2 interferon for hairy cell leukemia. *American Journal of Clinical Pathology, 85*:194–201.

Belardelli, F., Ausiello, C., Tomasi, M., & Rossi, G.B. (1980). Cholera toxin and its B subunit inhibit interferon effects on virus production and erythroid differentiation of friend leukemia cells. *Virology, 107*:109–120.

Berek, J.S., Hacker, N.F., Lichtenstein, A., Jung T, et al. (1986). Intraperitoneal recombinant α interferon for "salvage" immunotherapy in stage III epithelial ovarian cancer: A gynecologic oncology group study. *Seminars in Oncology, 13*(Suppl. 2):61–71.

Bergsagel, D.E., Haas, R.H., & Messner, H.A. (1986). Interferon alpha-2b in the treatment of chronic granulocytic leukemia. *Seminars in Oncology, 13*(Suppl. 2):29–34.

Bernsen, P.L., Wong-Chung, R.E., & Janssen J.T. (1985). Neurologic amyotrophy and polyradiculopathy during interferon therapy. *Lancet, 1*:50.

Billard, C., Sigaux, F., Castaigne, S., Valensi, F., Flandrin, G., et al. (1986). Treatment of hairy cell leukemia with recombinant alpha interferon: II. In vivo down-regulation of alpha interferon receptors on tumor cells. *Blood, 67*:821–826.

Bino, T., Edery, H., Gertler, A., & Rosenberg, H. (1982). Involvement of the kidney in catabolism of human leukocyte interferon. *Journal of General Virology, 59*:39–45.

Bjerke, J.R., Livden, J.K., Degre, M., & Matre, R. (1983). Inteferon in suction blister fluid from psoriatic lesions. *British Journal of Dermatology, 108*:295–299.

Blalock, J.E., Georgiades, J.A., Langford, M.P., & Johnson, H.M. (1980). Purified human immune interferon has more potent anticellular activity than fibroblast or leukocyte interferon. *Cellular Immunology, 49*:390–394.

Blomgren, H., Cantell, K., Johansson, B., Lagergren, C., Ringborg, U., & Strander, H. (1976). Interferon therapy in Hodgkin's disease. *Acta Medica Scandinavica, 199*:527–532.

Blum, S.F. (1980). Lithium in hairy cell leukemia. *New England Journal of Medicine, 303*:464–465.

Bocci, V., Pacini, A., Muscettola, M., Pessina, G.P., Paulesu, L., & Bandinelli, L. (1982). The kidney is the main site of interferon catabolism. *Journal of Interferon Research, 2*:309–314.

Bonnem, E.M. (1987). Alfa interferon: Combinations with other antineoplastic modalities. *Seminars in Oncology, 14*(Suppl. 2):48–60.

Borden, E.C., & Balkwill, F.R. (1984). Preclinical and clinical studies of interferons and interferon inducers in breast cancer. *Cancer, 53*:783–789.

Borden, E., & Ball, L. (1981). Interferons: Biochemical, cell growth inhibitory and immunological effects. *Progress in Hematology, 12*:299–339.

Borden, E.C., Gutterman, J.U., Holland, J.F., & Dao, T.L. (1983). In Sikora, K. (Ed.), *Interferons and Cancer* (pp. 103–112). New York: Plenum Press.

Borden, E.C., Hogan, T.F., & Voelkel, J.G. (1982a). Comparative antiproliferative activity in vitro of natural interferons α and β for diploid and transformed human cells. *Cancer Research, 42*:4948–4953.

Borden, E.C., Holland, J.F., Dao, T.L., Gutterman, J.U., et al. (1982b). Leukocyte-derived interferon (Alpha) in human breast carcinoma—American Cancer Society phase II trial. *Annals of Internal Medicine, 97*:1–6.

Borecky, L. (1986). Current view on the perspectives of interferon therapy. *Acta Virologica, 30*:161–169.

Borgstrom, S., vonEyben, F.F., Flodgren, P., et al. (1982). Human leukocyte interferon and cimetidine for metastatic melanoma. *New England Journal of Medicine,* *307*:1080–1081.

Bottomley, J.M., & Toy, J.L. (1985). Clinical side effects and toxicities of interferon. In Finter, N.B., & Oldham, R.K. (Eds.), *Interferon: In vivo and clinical studies,* pp. 155–180. Amsterdam: Elsevier.

Bouroncle, B.A., Wiseman, B.K., & Doan, C.A. (1958). Leukemic reticuloendotheliosis. *Blood, 13*:609–630.

Bouroncle, B.A. (1979). Leukemic reticuloendotheliosis (hairy cell leukemia). *Blood, 53*:412–433.

Bradley, E.C., & Ruscetti, F.W. (1981). Effects of fibroblast, lymphoid, and myeloid interferons on human tumor colony formation in vitro. *Cancer Research, 41*:244–249.

Branca, A.A., & Baglioni, C. (1981). Evidence that types I and II interferons have different receptors. *Nature, 294*:768–770.

Bratt, G., Einhorn, S., Blomgren, H., Gahrton, G., Paul, C., & Strander, H. (1984). Interferon α treatment of a patient with acute lymphoblastic leukemia and Down's syndrome. *Scandinavian Journal of Haematology, 32*:49–54.

Brown, T.D., Koeller, J., Beougher, K., Golando, J., Bonnem, E.M., Spiegel, R.J., & VonHoff, D.D., (1987). A phase I clinical trial of recombinant DNA gamma interferon. *Journal of Clinical Oncology, 5*:790–798.

Bullard, D.E., Gillespie, G.Y., Mahaley, M.S., & Bigner, D.D. (1986). Immunobiology of human gliomas. *Seminars in Oncology, 13*:94–109.

Bunn, P.A., & Foon, K.A. (1985). Therapeutic options in advanced cutaneous T cell lymphomas: A role for interferon alpha-2a (Roferon-A). *Seminars in Oncology, 12*(Suppl. 5):18–24.

Bunn, P.A., Foon, K.A., Ihde, D.C., Longo, D.C., Eddy, J., et al. (1984). Recombinant leukocyte A interferon: An active agent in advanced cutaneous T-cell lymphomas. *Annals of Internal Medicine, 101*:484–487.

Burke, J. (1978). The value of the bone-marrow biopsy in the diagnosis of hairy cell leukemia. *American Journal of Clinical Pathology, 70*:876–884.

Burrone, O.R., & Milstein, C. (1982). The effect of interferon on the expression of human cell–surface antigens. *Philosophical Transactions of the Royal Society of London Series B: Biological Sciences, 299*:133–135.

Calvo, F., Castaigne, S., Sigaux, F., Marty, M., Degos, L., Boiron, M., & Flandrin, G. (1985). Intensive chemotherapy of hairy cell leukemia in patients with aggressive disease. *Blood, 65*:115–119.

Cantell, K., & Hirvonen, S. (1978). Large scale production of human leukocyte interferon containing 10^8 units per ml. *Journal of General Virology, 39*:541–543.

Chandrabose, K., & Cuatrecasas, P. (1981). Changes in fatty acyl chains of phospholipids induced by interferon in mouse sarcoma S-180 cells. *Biochemistry and Biophysical Research Communications, 98*:661–668.

Cheever, M.A., Fefer, A., Greenberg, P.D., Appelbaum, F.R., et al. (1984). Identical twin bone marrow transplantation for hairy cell leukemia. *Seminars in Oncology, 11*(Suppl. 2):511–513.

Clark, J.W., & Longo, D.L. (1987). Interferons in cancer therapy. In DeVita, V., Hellman, S., & Rosenberg, S.A., (Eds.), *Updates of cancer: Principles and practice of oncology,* (pp. 1–16). Philadelphia: J.B. Lippincott.

Clemens, M. (1985). Interferons and oncogens. *Nature, 313*:531–532.

Collins J. (1986). Personal communication. In Strander, H. Interferon treatment of human neoplagia. *Advances in Cancer Research, 46*:2.

Connors, J.M., Andiman, W.A., Howarth, L.B., Liu, E., et al. (1985). Treatment of nasopharyngeal cancer with human leukocyte interferon. *Journal of Clinical Oncology,* *3*:813–817.

Cooper, M.R. (1986). Interferon in the treatment of multiple myeloma. *Seminars in Oncology,* *13*(Suppl. 2):13–20.

Cooper, M.R., Fefer, A., Thompson, J., Case, D.C., Kempf, R., et al. (1986). Alpha-2 interferon/Melphalan/prednisone in previously untreated patients with multiple myeloma: A phase I–II trial. *Cancer Treatment Reports, 70*:473–476.

Cooper, M.R., & Welander, C.E. (1986). Interferon in the treatment of multiple myeloma. *Seminars in Oncology, 13*:334–340.

Costanzi, J.J., Cooper, M.R., Scarffe, J.H., Ozer, H., et al. (1985). Phase II study of recombinant alpha-2 interferon in resistant multiple myeloma. *Journal of Clinical Oncology, 3*:654–659.

Costanzi, J.J., & Pollard, R.B. (1987). The use of interferon in the treatment of multiple myeloma. *Seminars in Oncology, 14*(Suppl. 2):24–28.

Creagan, E.T., Ahmann, D.L., Frytak, S., Long, H. J., Chang, M.N., & Itri, L.M. (1986). Phase II trials of recombinant leukocyte A interferon in disseminated malignant melanoma: Results in 96 patients. *Cancer Treatment Reports, 70*:619–624.

Creagan, E.T., Ahmann, D.L., Green, S.J., et al. (1985). Phase II study of recombinant leukocyte A interferon (IFN-rA) plus cimetidine in disseminated malignant melanoma. *Journal of Clinical Oncology, 3*:977–981.

Creasey, A.A., Bartholomew, J.C., & Merigan, T.C. (1981). The importance of GO in the site of action of interferon in the cell cycle. *Experimental Cell Research, 134*:155–160.

Davidson, H.S., Schilsky, R.L., & Golomb, H.M. (1985). Gonadal and sexual function following treatment of hairy cell leukemia with recombinant alpha 2 interferon. *Proceedings of the American Society of Clinical Oncology, 4*:232.

D'Eustachio, P., & Ruddle, F.H. (1983). Somatic cell genetics and gene families. *Science, 220*:919–924.

DeVries, J.E., & Spits, H. (1984). Cloned human cytotoxic T lymphocytes (CTL) lines reactive with autologous melanoma cells. *Journal of Immunology, 132*:510–519.

Dimitrov, N.V., Meyer, C.J., Strander, H., Einhorn, S., & Cantell, K. (1984). Interferon as a modifier of estrogen receptors. *Annals of Clinical and Laboratory Science, 14*:32–39.

Dinarello, C.A., Bernheim, H.A., Duff, G.W., Le, H.V., Nagabhushan, T.L., Hamilton, N.C., & Coceani, F. (1984). Mechanisms of fever induced by recombinant human interferon. *Journal of Clinical Investigation, 74*:906–913.

Dolei, A., Capobianchi, M., & Ameglio, F. (1983). Human interferon-γ enhances the expression of class I and class II major histocompatibility complex products in neoplastic cells more effectively than interferon-α and interferon-β. *Infection and Immunity, 40*:172–176.

Dolei, A., Fattorossi, A., Pizzolo, J., Cafolla, A., Annino, L., & Dianzani, F. (1986). Alpha 2 (r)-interferon mediated differentiation of hairy cells in culture. *Journal of Interferon Research, 6*(Suppl. 1):45.

Durie, B.G., Clouse, L., Braich, T., Grimm, M., & Robertone, A.B. (1986). Interferon α-2b-cylclophosphamide combination studies: In vitro and phase I–II clinical results. *Seminars in Oncology, 13*(Suppl. 2):84–88.

Edmonson, J.H., Long, H.J., Creagan, E.T., Frytak, S., et al. (1987). Phase II study of recombinant gamma-interferon in patients with advanced nonosseous sarcomas. *Cancer Treatment Reports, 71*:211–213.

Edwards, B.S., Merritt, J.A., Fuhlbrigge, R.C., & Borden, E.C. (1985). Low doses of interferon alpha result in more effective clinical natural killer cell activation. *Journal of Clinical Investigation, 75*:1908–1913.

Einhorn, S., Ahre, A., Blomgren, H., Johansson, B., Mellstedt, H., & Strander, H. (1982). Interferon and natural killer activity in multiple myeloma. A lack of correlation between interferon-induced enhancement of natural killer activity and clinical response to human interferon-α. *International Journal of Cancer 30*:167–172.

Einhorn, N., Bertelsen, K., Bjorkholm, E., Davy, M., et al. (1986). In Strander H. Interferon treatment of human neoplasia. *Advances in Cancer Research, 46*:178. Vienna, Abstract.

Einhorn, S., Blomgren, H., & Strander, H. (1978). Interferon and spontaneous cytotoxicity in man. *Acta Medica Scandinavica, 204*:477–483.

Eriksson, B., Oberg, K., Alm, G., Karlsson, A., et al. (1987). Treatment of malignant endocrine pancreatic tumors with human leukocyte interferon. *Cancer Treatment Reports, 71*:31–37.

Ernberg, I., Einhorn, S., Strander, H., & Klein, G. (1981). Proliferation inhibitory effect of human α interferon on primary explants of Burkitts lymphoma: Inverse relationship to patient survival. *Biomedicine, 35*:190–193.

Ernstoff, M.S., Davis, C.A., & Kirkwood, J.M. (1984). Cimetidine plus interferon alpha-2 (IFN) does not remit metastatic melanoma which has failed IFN alone. *Proceedings of the American Society of Clinical Oncology, 3*:62.

Ernstoff, M.S., & Kirkwood, J.M. (1984). Changes in the bone marrow of cancer patients treated with recombinant interferon alpha-2. *American Journal of Medicine, 76*:593–596.

Faltynek, C.R., Princler, G.L., Rossio, J.L., Ruscetti, F.W., Maluish, A.E., Abrams, P.G., & Foon, K.A. (1986). Relationship of clinical response and binding of recombinant interferon alpha in patients with lymphoproliferative diseases. *Blood, 67*:1077–1082.

Fer, M.F., Bottino, G.C., Sherwin, S.A., Hainsworth, J.D., Abrams, P.G., Foon, K.A., & Oldham, R.K. (1984). Atypical tumor lysis syndrome in a patient with T cell lymphoma treated with recombinant leukocyte interferon. *American Journal of Medicine, 77*:953–956.

Figlin, R.A., deKernion, J.B., Maldazys, J. & Sarna, G. (1985). Treatment of renal cell carcinoma with α (human leukocyte) interferon and vinblastine in combination: A phase I–II trial. *Cancer Treatment Reports, 69*:263–267.

Figlin, R.A., deKernion, J.B., Mukamel, E., Schnipper, E.F., et al. (1986). Recombinant leukocyte A interferon (rIFN-αA) antibody development in advanced renal cell cancer. *Proceedings of the American Society of Clinical Oncology, 5*:222.

Flandrin, G., Sigaux, F., Sebahoun, G., & Bouffette, P. (1984). Hairy cell leukemia: Clinical presentation and follow-up of 211 patients. *Seminars in Oncology, 11*:458–471.

Fleischmann, W.R., Fleischmann, C.M., & Gindhart, T.D. (1986). Effect of hyperthermia on the antiproliferative activities of murine α, β, and γ interferon: Differential enhancement of murine γ interferon. *Cancer Research, 46*:8–13.

Fontana, A., Hengartner, H., deTribolet, N., & Weber, E. (1984). Glioblastoma cells release interleukin I and factors inhibiting interleukin II-mediated effects. *Journal of Immunology, 132*:1837–1844.

Foon, K.A., Sherwin, S.A., Abrams, P.G., Longo, D.L., et al. (1984). Treatment of advanced non-Hodgkin's lymphoma with recombinant leukocyte A interferon. *New England Journal of Medicine, 311*:1148–1152.

Foon, K.A., & Dougher, G. (1984). Increased growth of eyelashes in a patient given leukocyte A interferon. *New England Journal of Medicine, 311*:1259.

Foon, K., Bottino, G., Abrams, P.G., Fer, M., Longo, D., Schoenberger, C.S., & Oldham, R.K. (1985). Phase II trial of recombinant leukocyte A interferon in patients with advanced chronic lymphocytic leukemia. *American Journal of Medicine, 78*:216–220.

Foon, K.A., & Bunn, P.A. (1986). α interferon treatment of cutaneous T-cell lymphoma and chronic lymphocytic leukemia. *Seminars in Oncology, 13*(Suppl. 5):35–39.

Foon, K.A., Roth, M.S., & Bunn, P.A. (1986a). Alpha interferon treatment of low-grade

B-cell non-Hodgkin's lymphoma, cutaneous T-cell lymphomas, and chronic lymphocytic leukemia. *Seminars in Oncology, 13*(Suppl. 2):35–42.

Foon, K.A., Maluish, A.E., Abrams, P.G., Wrightington, S., et al. (1986b). Recombinant leukocyte A interferon therapy for advanced hairy cell leukemia. *American Journal of Medicine, 80*:351–356.

Fossati, G., Anichini, A., Taramelli, D., et al. (1986). Immune response to autologous human melanoma: Implications for class I and II MHC products. *Biochimica et Biophysica Acta: Review in Cancer, 865*:235–251.

Fuse, A., Mahmud, I., & Kuwata, T. (1982). Mechanism of stimulation by human interferon of prostaglandin synthesis in human cell lines. *Cancer Research, 42*:3209–3214.

Gams, R., Gordon, D., Guaspari, A., & Tuttle, R. (1984). Phase II trial of human polyclonal lymphoblastoid interferon in the management of malignant lymphomas. *Proceedings of the American Society of Clinical Oncology, 3*:65.

Gelmann, E.P., Preble, O.T., Steis, R., Lane, H., et al. (1985). Human lymphoblastoid interferon treatment of Kaposi's sarcoma in acquired immunodeficiency syndrome. *American Journal of Medicine, 78*:737–741.

Giacomini, P., Aguzzi, A., Pestka, S., Fisher, P., & Ferrone, S. (1984). Modulation by recombinant DNA leukocyte (α) and fibroblast (β) interferons of the expression and shedding of HLA- and tumor-associated antigens by human melanoma cells. *Journal of Immunology, 133*:1649–1655.

Goeddel, D.V., Yelverton, E., Ullrich, A., Heyneker, H.L., Miozzari, G., et al. (1980). Human leukocyte interferon produced by E. coli is biologically active. *Nature, 287*:411–416.

Goldberg, R.M., Ayoob, M., Silgals, R., Ahlgren, J.D., & Neefe, J.R. (1985). Phase II trial of lymphoblastoid interferon in metastatic malignant melanoma. *Cancer Treatment Reports, 69*:813–816.

Goldstein, D., & Laszlo, J. (1986). Interferon therapy in cancer: From imaginon to interferon. *Cancer Research, 46*:4315–4329.

Golomb, H.M., Catovsky, D., & Golde, D.W. (1978). Hairy cell leukemia—a clinical review based on 71 cases. *Annals of Internal Medicine, 89*:677–683.

Golomb, H.M. (1983). Hairy cell leukemia: Lessons learned in 25 years. *Journal of Clinical Oncology, 1*:652–656.

Golomb, H.M., Schmidt, K., & Vardiman, J.W. (1984). Chlorambucil therapy of 24 postsplenectomy patients with progressive hairy cell leukemia. *Seminars in Oncology, 11*(Suppl. 2):502–506.

Golomb, H.M., Ratain, M.J., & Vardiman, J.W. (1986a). Sequential treatment of hairy cell leukemia: A new role for interferon. In DeVita V. (Eds. Hellman S. & Rosenberg S.), *Important advances in oncology*. Philadelphia: J.B. Lippincott.

Golomb, H.M., Jacobs, A., Fefer, A., Ozer, H., Thompson, J., et al. (1986b). Alpha 2 interferon therapy of hairy cell leukemia: a multicenter study of 64 patients. *Journal of Clinical Oncology, 4*:900–905.

Golomb, H.M., & Ratain, M.J. (1987). Recent advances in the treatment of hairy cell leukemia. *New England Journal of Medicine, 316*:870–872.

Golomb, H.M., Fefer, A., Golde, D.W., Ozer, H., Portlock, C., et al. (1987). Sequential evaluation of alpha-2b-interferon treatment in 128 patients with hairy cell leukemia. *Seminars in Oncology, 14*(Suppl. 2):13–17.

Golomb, H.M. (1987). The treatment of hairy cell leukemia. *Blood, 69*:979–983.

Gray, P.W., Leung, D.W., Pennica, D., Yelverton, E., Najarian, R., et al. (1982). Expression of human immune interferon c DNA in E. coli and monkey cells. *Nature, 295*:503–508.

Green, M.D., Speyer, J., Wernz, J., Kisner, D., et al. (1985). Doxorubicin and interferon: Rationale and clinical experience. *Cancer Treatment Reviews, 12*(Suppl. B):61–67.

Gresser I. (1961). Production of interferon by suspensions of human leucocytes. *Proceedings of the Society of Experimental Biological Medicine, 108*:799–803.

Gresser, I. (1985). How does interferon inhibit tumor growth? In Gresser, I. (Ed.), *Interferon 6*, pp. 93–126. London: Academic Press.

Gresser, I., Tovey, M.G., Maury, C., & Chouroulinkov, I. (1975). Lethality of interferon preparations for newborn mice. *Nature, 258*:76–78.

Groopman, J.E., Gottlieb, M.S., Goodman, J., Mitsuyasu, R.T., et al. (1984). Recombinant alpha-2 interferon therapy for Kaposi's sarcoma associated with acquired immunodeficiency syndrome. *Annals of Internal Medicine, 100*:671–676.

Gutterman, J.U., Blumenschein, G.R., Alexanian, R., Yap, H., et al. (1980). Leukocyte interferon-induced tumor regression in human metastatic breast cancer, multiple myeloma, and malignant lymphoma. *Annals of Internal Medicine, 93*:399–406.

Gutterman, J.U., Fine, S., Quesada, J., Horning, S.J., et al. (1982). Recombinant leukocyte A interferon: Pharmacokinetics, single-dose tolerance, and biologic effects in cancer patients. *Annals of Internal Medicine, 96*:549–556.

Gutterman, J.U., & Quesada, J. (1981–82). Clinical investigation of partially pure and recombinant DNA derived leukocyte interferon in human cancer. *Texas Reports on Biology and Medicine, 41*:626–633.

Gutterman, J.U., Rosenblum, M.G., Rios, A., Fritsche, H.A., & Quesada, J.R. (1984). Pharmacokinetic study of partially pure γ-interferon in cancer patients. *Cancer Research, 44*:4164–4171.

Guyre, P.M., Morganelli, P.M., & Miller, R. (1983). Recombinant immune interferon increases immunoglobulin G Fc receptors on cultured human mononuclear phagocytes. *Journal of Clinical Investigation, 72*:393–397.

Harris, J., DasGupta, T., Vogelzang, N., Badrinath, K., et al. (1986). Treatment of soft tissue sarcoma with fibroblast interferon (β-IFN): An American Cancer Society/Illinois Cancer Council Study. *Cancer Treatment Reports 70*:293–294.

Hawkins, M.J., Krown, S.E., Borden, E.C., Krimm, M., Real, F.X., et al. (1984). American Cancer Society phase I trial of naturally produced β-interferon. *Cancer Research, 44*:5934–5938.

Hawkins, M.J., O'Connell, M.J., Schiller, J.H., Davis, T.E., Sielaff, K.M., & Aughey, J.L. (1985). Phase I evaluation of recombinant A interferon alpha (rIFN-αA) in combination with COPA chemotherapy (I-COPA). *Proceedings of the American Society of Clinical Oncology, 4*:229.

Hemmi, H., & Breitman, T.R. (1987). Combinations of recombinant human interferons and retinoic acid synergistically induce differentiation of the human promyelocytic leukemia cell line HL-60. *Blood, 69*:501–507.

Heron, I., & Berg, K. (1979). Human leucocyte interferon: Analysis of effect on MLC and effector cell generation. *Scandinavian Journal of Immunology, 9*:517–526.

Heron, I., Berg, K., & Cantell, K. (1976). Regulatory effect of interferon on T cells in vitro. *Journal of Immunology, 117*:1370–1373.

Heron, I., & Berg, K. (1978). The actions of interferon are potentiated at elevated temperatures. *Nature, 274*: 508–510.

Heron, I., Hokland, M., & Berg, K. (1978). Enhanced suppression of β-2 microglobulin and HLA antigens on human lymphoid cells by interferon. *Proceedings of the National Academy of Science USA, 75, 12*:6215–6219.

Hill, N.O., Khan, A., Pardue, A., Aleman, C., Hilario, R., & Hill, J.M. (1982). Response of a blast crisis of chronic granulocytic leukemia to interferon-alpha. *Proceedings of the American Society of Clinical Oncology, 1*:129.

Hirsch, M., Tolkoff-Rubin, N., Kelly, A.P., & Rubin, R.H. (1983). Pharmacokinetics of human and recombinant leukocyte interferons in patients with chronic renal failure who are undergoing hemodialysis. *Journal of Infectious Disease, 148*:335.

Horning, S.J., Merigan, T.C., Krown, S.E., Gutterman, J.U., Louie, A., et al. (1985). Human interferon alpha in malignant lymphoma and Hodgkin's disease—results of the American Cancer Society trial. *Cancer, 56*:1305–1310.

Horoszewicz, J.S., Leong, S.S., & Carter, W.A. (1979). Noncycling tumor cells are sensitive targets for the antiproliferative activity of human interferon. *Science, 206*:1091–1093.

Huang, K., Donahoe, R., Gordon, F., & Dressler, H. (1971). Enhancement of phagocytosis by interferon-containing preparations. *Infection and Immunity, 4*:581–588.

Idestrom, K., Cantell, K., Killander, D., Nilsson, K., Strander, H., & Willems, J. (1979). Interferon therapy in multiple myeloma. *Acta Medica Scandinavica, 205*:149–154.

Ikic, D., Brodarec, I., Padovan, I., Knezevic, M., & Soos E. (1981a). Application of human leucocyte interferon in patients with tumors of the head and neck. *Lancet, 1*:1025–1027.

Ikic, D., Maricic, Z., Oresic, V., Rode, B., et al. (1981b). Application of human leukocyte interferon in patients with urinary bladder papillomatosis, breast cancer and melanoma. *Lancet, 1*:1022–1024.

Ingimarsson, S., Bergstrom, K., Brostrom, L.A., Cantell, K., & Strander, H. (1980). Effect of long-term treatment with human leukocyte interferon on various laboratory parameters. *Acta Medica Scandinavica, 208*:155–159.

Inglot, A.D. (1983). The hormonal concept of interferon: Brief review. *Archives of Virology, 76*:1–13.

Isaacs, A., & Lindenmann, J. (1957). Virus Interference. I. The interferon. *Proceedings of the Royal Society of London: Series B, 147*:258–267.

Ito, M., & Buffett, R.F. (1981). Cytocidal effect of purified human fibroblast interferon on tumor cells in vitro. *Journal of the National Cancer Institute, 66*:819–825.

Ito, H., Murakami, K., Yanagawa, T., Ban, S., et al. (1980). Effect of human leukocyte interferon on the metastatic lung tumor of osteosarcoma. *Cancer, 46*:1562–1565.

Itoh, K., Shiiba, K., Shimizu, Y., Suzuki, R., & Kumagai, K. (1985). Generation of activated killer (AK) cells by recombinant interleukin 2 (rIL2) in collaboration with interferon-γ (IFN-γ). *Journal of Immunology, 134*:3124–3129.

Jansen, J., Hermans, J. for the Collaborative Study Group. (1981). Splenectomy in hairy cell leukemia: A retrospective multicenter analysis. *Cancer, 47*:2066–2076.

Jansen, J., Schuit, H.R., Meijer, C.J., vanNieuwkoop, J.A., & Hijmans, W. (1982). Cell markers in hairy cell leukemia studied in cells from 51 patients. *Blood, 59*:52–60.

Johnson, H.M., & Farrar, W.L. (1983). The role of a gamma interferon-like lymphokine in the activation of T cells for expression of interleukin 2 receptors. *Cellular Immunology, 75*:154–159.

Johnston, J.B., Glazer, R.I., Pugh, L., & Israels, L.G. (1986). The treatment of hairy cell leukemia with 2'-deoxycoformycin. *British Journal of Haematology, 63*:525–534.

Jones, G.J., & Itri, L.M. (1986). Safety and tolerance of recombinant interferon alfa-2a (Roferon A) in cancer patients. *Cancer, 57*:1709–1715.

Kading, V.H., Blalock, J.E., & Gifford, G.E. (1978). Effect of serum on the antiviral and anticellular activities of mouse interferon. *Archives of Virology, 56*:237–242.

Kemeny, N., Yagoda, A., Wang, Y., Field, K., et al. (1981). Randomized trial of standard therapy with or without poly 1:C in patients with superficial bladder cancer. *Cancer 48*:2154–2157.

Kirkwood, J.M., & Ernstoff, M. (1985). Melanoma: Therapeutic options with recombinant interferons. *Seminars in Oncology, 12*(Suppl. 5):7–12.

Kirkwood, J.M., & Ernstoff, M.E. (1986). Potential applications of the interferons in oncology: Lessons drawn from studies of human melanoma. *Seminars in Oncology, 13*(Suppl. 2):48–56.

Kirkwood, J.M., Ernstoff, M.S., Davis, G.A., Reiss, M., Ferraresi, R., & Rudnick, S.A. (1985a). Comparison of intramuscular and intravenous recombinant alpha-2 interferon in melanoma and other cancers. *Annals of Internal Medicine, 103*:32–36.

Kirkwood, J.M., Harris, J.E., Vena, R., Sandler, S., et al. (1985b). A randomized study of low and high doses of leukocyte α interferon in metastatic renal cell carcinoma: The American Cancer Society collaborative trial. *Cancer Research, 45*:863–871.

Koren, H., Brandt, C., Tso, C., & Laszlo, J. (1983). Modulation of natural killing activity by lymphoblastoid interferon in cancer patients. *Journal of Biological Response Modifiers, 2*:151–165.

Kraut, E.H., Bouroncle, B.A., & Grever, M.R. (1986). Low-dose deoxycoformycin in the treatment of hairy cell leukemia. *Blood, 68*:1119–1122.

Krigel, R., Poiesz, B., Comis, R., et al. (1986). A phase I study of recombinant interleukin II- (rIL-2) plus recombinant beta ser 17 interferon (IFN-β ser). *Proceedings of the American Society of Clinical Oncology, 5*:225.

Krown, S.E. (1986). Interferon and interferon inducers in cancer treatment. *Seminars in Oncology, 13*:207–217.

Krown, S.E. (1985). Therapeutics options in renal-cell carcinoma. *Seminars in Oncology, 12*(Suppl. 5):13–17.

Krown, S.E., Mintzer, D., Cunningham-Rundles, S., Niedzwiecki, D., et al. (1987). High dose lymphoblastoid interferon in metastatic colorectal cancer: Clinical results and modification of biological responses. *Cancer Treatment Reports, 71*:39–45.

Krown, S.E., Real, F.X., Lester, T., & Oettgen, H.F. (1986a). Interferon alpha-2a (IFN-α2a) ± vinblastine (VLB) in AIDS-related Kaposi's sarcoma (KS AIDS): A prospective randomized trial. *Proceedings of the American Society of Clinical Oncology, 5*:6.

Krown, S.E., Real, F.X., Vadhan-Raj, S., Cunningham-Rundles, S., et al. (1986b). Kaposi's sarcoma and the acquired immunodeficiency syndrome—treatment with recombinant interferon alpha and analysis of prognostic factors. *Cancer, 57*:1662–1665.

Krown, S.E., Burk, M.W., Kirkwood, J.M., et al. (1984). Human leukocyte (alpha) interferon in metastatic malignant melanoma: The American Cancer Society phase II trial. *Cancer Treatment Reports, 68*:723–726.

Krown, S.E., Real, F.X., Cunningham-Rundles, S., Myskowski, P.L., et al. (1983). Preliminary observations on the effect of recombinant leukocyte A interferon in homosexual men with Kaposi's sarcoma. *New England Journal of Medicine, 308*:1071–1076.

Kurzrock, R., Quesada, J.R., Rosenblum, M.G., Sherwin, S.A., & Gutterman, J.U. (1986a). Phase I study of IV administered recombinant gamma interferon in cancer patients. *Cancer Treatment Reports, 70*:1357–1364.

Kurzrock, R., Quesada, J.R., Talpaz, M., Hersh, E.M., et al. (1986b). Phase I study of multiple dose intramuscularly administered recombinant gamma interferon. *Journal of Clinical Oncology, 4*:1101–1109.

Kurzrock, R., Rosenblum, M.G., Quesada, J.R., Sherwin, S.A., et al. (1986c). Phase I study of a combination of recombinant interferon-alpha and recombinant interferon-gamma in cancer patients. *Journal of Clinical Oncology, 4*:1677–1683.

Leavitt, R.D., Ratanatharathorn, V., Ozer, H., Ultman, J.E., et al. (1987). Alpha-2b interferon in the treatment of Hodgkin's disease and non-Hodgkin's lymphoma. *Seminars in Oncology, 14*(Suppl. 2):18–23.

Lee, S., & Epstein, L. (1980). Reversible inhibition by interferon of the maturation of human peripheral blood monocytes to macrophages. *Cellular Immunology, 50*:177–190.

Legha, S.S. (1986). Interferons in the treatment of malignant melanoma: A review of recent trials. *Cancer, 57*:1675–1677.

Lembersky, B.C., Ratain, M.J., Bennett, C.L., Golomb, H.M., & Vardiman, J. (1985). Osseous complications in hairy cell leukemia. *Blood, 66*(Suppl. 1):178a.
Liberati, A.M., Puxeddu, A., Biscottini, B., Allegra, A., et al. (1985). Preliminary observation on the clinical tolerance of interferon beta in cancer patients. *Tumori,* 71:45–49.
Lindenmann, J. (1985). Personal communication. How does interferon inhibit tumor growth? In Gresser, I. (Ed.), *Interferon 6,* p.121. London: Academic Press.
Lonberg, M., Odajnyk, C., Krigel, R., Laubenstein, L., et al. (1985). Sequential and simultaneous alpha 2 interferon (IFN) and VP-16 in epidemic Kaposi's sarcoma (EKS). *Proceedings of the American Society of Clinical Oncology,* 4:2.
Lotem, J., & Sachs, L. (1978). Genetic dissociation of different cellular effects of interferon on myeloid leukemic cells. *International Journal of Cancer, 22*:214–220.
Lotzova, E., Savary, C.A., Gutterman, J.U., & Hersh, E.M. (1982). Modulation of natural killer cell-mediated cytotoxicity by partially purified and cloned interferon α. *Cancer Research, 42*:2480–2488.
Lotzova, E., Savary, C.A., Quesada, J.R., Gutterman, J.U., & Hersch, E.M. (1983). Analysis of natural killer cell cytotoxicity of cancer patients treated with recombinant interferon. *Journal of the National Cancer Institute, 71*:903–910.
Louie, A.C., Gallagher, J.G., Sikora, K., Levy, R., Rosenberg, S.A., & Merigan, T.C. (1981). Follow-up observations on the effect of human leukocyte interferon in non-Hodgkin's lymphoma. *Blood, 58*:712–718.
Ludwig, C.U., Durie, B.G., Salmon, S.E., & Moon, T.E. (1983). Tumor growth stimulation in vitro by interferons. *European Journal of Cancer and Clincal Oncology, 19*:1625–1632.
Lum, B.L., & Torti, F.M. (1985). Therapeutic approaches including interferon to carcinoma in situ of the bladder. *Cancer Treatment Reviews, 12*(Suppl. B):45–49.
Magee, M., Gee, T.S., Arlin, Z., & Clarkson, B. (1981). Androgen therapy in postsplenectomy patients with hairy cell leukemia. *Blood, 58*(Suppl. 1):145a.
Mahaley, M.S., Brooks, W.H., Roszman, T.L., Bigner, D.D., et al. (1977). Immunobiology of primary intracranial tumors. Part I: Studies of the cellular and humoral general immune competence of brain-tumor patients. *Journal of Neurosurgery, 46*:467–476.
Mahaley, M.S., Urso, M.B., Whaley, R.A., Blue, M., et al. (1985). Immunobiology of primary intracranial tumors. Part 10: Therapeutic efficacy of interferon in the treatment of recurrent gliomas. *Journal of Neurosurgery, 63*:719–725.
Maluish, A.E., Ortaldo, J.R., Conlon, J.C., Sherwin, S.A., et al. (1983). Depression of natural killer cytotoxicity after in vivo administration of recombinant leukocyte interferon. *Journal of Immunology, 131*:503–507.
Mastrangelo, M.J., Baker, A.R., & Katz, H.R. (1985). Cutaneous melanoma. In DeVita, V.T., Hellman, S., & Rosenberg, S.A. (Eds.), *Cancer: Principles and practice of oncology,* pp 1371–1423. Philadelphia: J.B. Lippincott.
Masucci, M., Szigeti, R., Klein, E., Klein, G., et al. (1980). Effect of interferon α 1 from E. coli on some cell functions. *Science, 209*:1431–1435.
Mattson, K., Niiranen, A., Iivanainen, M., Farkkila, M., et al. (1983). Neurotoxicity of interferon. *Cancer Treatment Reports, 67*:958–961.
Maxwell, B.L., Talpaz, M., & Gutterman, J.U. (1985). Down-regulation of peripheral blood cell interferon receptors in chronic myelogenous leukemia patients undergoing human interferon (Hu IFNα) therapy. *International Journal of Cancer, 36*:23–28.
McLaughlin, P., Talpaz, M., Quesada, J.R., Saleem, A., Barlogie, B., & Gutterman, J.U. (1985). Immune thrombocytopenia following alpha interferon therapy in patients with cancer. *Journal of the American Medical Association, 254*:1353–1354.
McMahon, M., & Kerr, I.M. (1983). The biochemistry of the antiviral state. In Burke,

D.C., & Morris, A.G. (Eds.), *Interferons: From molecular biology to clinical application* (pp. 89–108). London: Cambridge University Press.

Merigan, T.C., Sikora, K., Breeden, J.H., Levy, R., & Rosenberg, S. (1978). Preliminary observations on the effect of human leukocyte interferon in non-Hodgkin's lymphoma. *New England Journal of Medicine, 299*:1449–1453.

Mintz, U., & Golomb, H.M. (1979). Splenectomy as initial therapy in 26 patients with leukemic reticuloendotheliosis (hairy cell leukemia). *Cancer Research, 39*:2366–2370.

Miorner, H., Landstrom, E., Larner, E., Larsson, I., Lundgren, E., & Strannegard, O. (1978). Regulation of mitogen-induced lymphocyte DNA synthesis by human interferon of different origins. *Cellular Immunology, 35*:15–24.

Mirro, J., Kalwinsky, D., Whisnant, J., Weck, P., Chesney, C., & Murphy, S. (1985). Coagulopathy induced by continuous infusion of high doses of human lymphoblastoid interferon. *Cancer Treatment Reports* 69:315–317.

Mirro, J., Dow, L.W., Kalwinsky, D.K., Dahl, G.V., et al. (1986). Phase I–II study of continuous-infusion high-dose human lymphoblastoid interferon and the in vitro sensitivity of leukemic progenitors in nonlymphocytic leukemia. *Cancer Treatment Reports, 70*:363–367.

Mittelman, A., Krown, S., Cirrincione, C., Safai, B., Oettgen, H.F., & Koziner, B. (1983). Analysis of T cell subsets in cancer patients treated with interferon. *American Journal of Medicine, 75*: 966–972.

Murray, J.L., Rosenblum, M.G., Lamki, L., et al. (1986). Enhancement of tumor uptake of [111]Indium (^{111}In)-labeled anti-melanoma monoclonal antibody (MoAb) 96.5 in melanoma patients receiving partially purified alpha interferon (αIFN). *Proceedings of the American Society of Clinical Oncology, 5*:226.

Muss, H.B.(1987). Interferon therapy for renal cell carcinoma. *Seminars in Oncology, 14*(Suppl. 2):36–42.

Muss, H.B., Costanzi, J.J., Leavitt, R., Williams, R.D., et al. (1987). Recombinant alfa interferon in renal cell carcinoma: A randomized trial of two routes of administration. *Journal of Clinical Oncology, 5*:286–291.

Muss, H.B., Welander, C., Caponera, M., Reavis, K., et al. (1985). Interferon and doxorubicin in renal cell carcinoma. *Cancer Treatment Reports, 69*:721–722.

Naeim, F., & Jacbos, A.D. (1985). Bone marrow changes in patients with hairy cell leukemia treated by recombinant alpha 2-interferon. *Human Pathology, 16*:1200–1205.

Namba, M., Yamamoto, S., Tanaka, H., Kanamori, T., et al. (1984). In vitro and in vivo studies on potentiation of cytotoxic effects of anticancer drugs or cobalt 60 gamma rays by interferon on human neoplastic cells. *Cancer, 54*:2262–2267.

Neidhart, J.A., Gagen, M.M., Young, D., Tuttle, R., et al. (1984). Interferon-α therapy of renal cancer. *Cancer Research, 44*:4140–4143.

Ng, A.K., Giacomini, P., Kantor, R.S., Ferrone, S., et al. (1983). Recombinant human interferons alter the expression and shedding of tumor associated antigens and susceptibility to immune lysis of human melanoma cells. *Proceedings of the American Association of Cancer Research, 24*:196.

Niederle, N., Kloke, O., Osieka, R., Wandl, U., Opalka, B., & Schmidt, C. (1987). Interferon alpha-2b in the treatment of chronic myelogenous leukemia. *Seminars in Oncology, 14*(Suppl. 2):29–35.

Oberg, K., Norheim, I., Lind, E., Alm, G., et al. (1986). Treatment of malignant carcinoid tumors with human leukocyte interferon: Long term results. *Cancer Treatment Reports, 70*:1297–1304.

O'Connell, M.J., Colgan, J.P., Oken, M.M., Ritts, R.E., Kay, N.E., & Itri, L.M. (1986). Clinical trial of recombinant leukocyte A interferon as initial therapy for favorable histology non-Hodgkin's lymphoma and chronic lymphocytic leukemia—an Eastern Cooperative Oncology Group pilot study. *Journal of Clinical Oncology, 4*:128–136.

Oladipupo-Williams, C.K., Svet-Moldavskaya, I., Vikek, J., Ohnuma, T., & Holland, J.F. (1981). Inhibitory effects of human leukocyte and fibroblast interferons on normal and chronic myelogenous granulocytic progenitor cells. *Oncology, 38*:356–360.

Oldham, R.P. (1982). Toxic effects of interferon. *Science, 219*:902.

Palacios, R., Martinez-Maza, O., & DeLey, M. (1983). Production of human immune interferon (Hu IFN-γ) studied at the single cell level. Origin, evidence for spontaneous secretion and effect of cyclosporin A. *European Journal of Immunology, 13*:221–225.

Paucker, K., Cantell, K., & Henle, W. (1962). Quantitative studies on viral interference in suspended L cells. III. Effect of interfering viruses and interferon on the growth rate of cells. *Virology, 17*:324–334.

Paganelli, K.A., Evans, S.S., Han, T., & Ozer, H. (1986). B cell growth factor-induced proliferation of hairy cell lymphocytes and inhibition by type I interferon in vitro. *Blood, 67*:937–942.

Pertcheck, M., Figlin, R., & Sarna, G. (1985). Phase I study of β-ser 17 interferon by rapid intravenous push. *Proceedings of the American Society of Clinical Oncology, 4*:226.

Perussia, B., Dayton, E.T., Fanning, V., Thiagarajan, P., Hoxie, J., & Trinchieri, G. (1983). Immune interferon and leukocyte-conditioned medium induce normal and leukemic myeloid cells to differentiate along the monocytic pathway. *Journal of Experimental Medicine, 158*:2058–2080.

Pestka, S. (1983). The human interferons—from protein purification and sequence to cloning and expression in bacteria: Before, between, and beyond. *Archives of Biochemistry and Biophysics, 221*:1–37.

Pfeffer, L.M., Wang, E., & Tamm, I. (1980a). Interferon effects on microfilament organization, cellular fibronectin distribution, and cell motility in human fibroblasts. *Journal of Cell Biology, 85*:9–17.

Pfeffer, L.M., Wang, E., & Tamm, I. (1980b). Interferon inhibits the redistribution of cell surface components. *Journal of Experimental Medicine, 152*:469–474.

Quesada, J.R., Swanson, D.A., Trinidade, A., & Gutterman, J.U. (1983). Renal cell carcinoma: Antitumor effects of leukocyte interferon. *Cancer Research, 43*:940–947.

Quesada, J.R., Hawkins, M., Horning, S., Alexanian, R., et al. (1984a). Collaborative phase I–II study of recombinant DNA-produced leukocyte interferon (clone A) in metastatic breast cancer, malignant lymphoma, and multiple myeloma. *American Journal of Medicine, 77*:427–432.

Quesada, J.R., Reuben, J., Manning, J.T., Hersh, E.M., & Gutterman, J.U. (1984b). Alpha interferon for induction of remission in hairy cell leukemia. *New England Journal of Medicine, 310*:15–18.

Quesada, J.R., Rios, A., Swanson, D., Trown, P., & Gutterman, J.U. (1985). Antitumor activity of recombinant-derived interferon alpha in metastatic renal cell carcinoma. *Journal of Clinical Oncology, 3*:1522–1528.

Quesada, J.R., Talpaz, M., Rios, A., Kurzrock, R., & Gutterman, J.U. (1986a). Clinical toxicity of interferons in cancer patients: A review. *Journal of Clinical Oncology, 4*:234–243.

Quesada, J.R., Alexanian, R., Hawkins, M., Barlogie, B., et al. (1986b). Treatment of multiple myeloma with recombinant α interferon. *Blood, 67*:275–278.

Quesada, J.R., Hersh, E.M., Manning, J., Reuben, J., et al. (1986c). Treatment of hairy cell leukemia with recombinant alpha interferon. *Blood, 68*:493–497.

Ratain, M.J., Golomb, H.M., Bardawil, R.G., Vardiman, J.W., et al. (1987). Durability of response to interferon alpha-2b in advanced hairy cell leukemia. *Blood, 69*:872–877.

Ratain, M.J., Vardiman, J.W., & Golomb, H.M. (1986). The role of interferon in the treatment of hairy cell leukemia. *Seminars in Oncology, 13*(Suppl. 2):21–28.

Ratner, L., Nordlund, J.J., & Lengyel, P. (1980). Interferon as an inhibitor of cell growth: Studies with mouse melanoma cells. *Proceedings of the Society of Experimental Biology and Medicine, 163*:267–272.

Real, F.X., Oettgen, H.F., & Krown, S.E. (1986). Kaposi's sarcoma and the acquired immunodeficiency syndrome: Treatment with high and low doses of recombinant leukocyte A interferon. *Journal of Clinical Oncology, 4*:544–551.

Renton, K.W., & Mannering, G.J. (1976). Depression of hepatic cytochrome P-450-dependent monooxygenase systems with administered interferon inducing agents. *Biochemistry and Biophysical Research Communications, 73*:343–348.

Retsas, S., Priestman, T.J., Newton, K.A., & Westbury, G. (1983). Evaluation of human lymphoblastoid interferon in advanced malignant melanoma. *Cancer, 51*:273–276.

Rich, S.A. (1981). Human lupus inclusions and interferon. *Science, 213*:772–775.

Rieber, E.P., Hadam, M.R., Linke, R.P., Saal, J.G., et al. (1979). Hairy cell leukemia: Surface markers and functional capacities of the leukaemic cells analysed in eight patients. *British Journal of Haematology, 42*:175–188.

Rinehart, J., Malspeis, L., Young, D., & Neidhart, J. (1986). Phase I/II trial of human recombinant β-interferon serine in patients with renal cell carcinoma. *Cancer Research, 46*:5364–5367.

Rohatiner, A.Z., Balkwill, E.R., Malpas, J.S., & Lister, T.A. (1983a). *Cancer Chemotherapy and Pharmacology, 11*:56–58.

Rohatiner, A.Z., Prior, P.F., Burton, A.C., Smith, A.T., Balkwill, F.R., & Lister, T.A. (1983b). Central nervous system toxicity of interferon. *British Journal of Cancer, 47*:419–422.

Romagnani, S., Guidizi, G.M., Almerigogna, F., Biagiotti, R., et al. (1986). Analysis of the role of interferon-gamma, interleukin 2 and a third factor distinct from interferon-gamma and interleukin 2 on human B cell proliferation. Evidence that they act at different times after B cell activation. *European Journal of Immunology, 16*:623–629.

Rosenblum, M.G., Maxwell, B.L., Talpaz, M., Kelleher, P.J., McCredie, K., & Gutterman, J.U. (1986). In vivo sensitivity and resistance of chronic myelogenous cells to α-interferon: correlation with receptor binding and induction of 2'–5'-oligoadenylate synthetase. *Cancer Research, 46*:4848–4852.

Rossi, G.B. (1985). Interferons and cell differentiation. In Gresser, I. (Ed.), *Interferon. 6*, pp. 31–68. London: Academic Press.

Rossi, G.B., Matarese, G.P., Grappelli, C., Belardelli, F., & Benedetto, A. (1977). Interferon inhibits dimethyl sulphoxide-induced erythroid differentiation of Friend leukaemia cells. *Nature, 267*:50–52.

Rubin, B.Y., & Gupta, S.L. (1980). Differential efficacies of human type I and type II interferons as antiviral and antiproliferative agents. *Proceedings of the National Academy of Science USA, 77*:5928–5932.

Ruco, L.P., Procopio, A., Maccallini, V., Calogero, A., et al. (1983). Severe deficiency of natural killer activity in the peripheral blood of patients with hairy cell leukemia. *Blood, 61*:1132–1137.

Sagar, A.D., Pickering, L.A., Sussman-Berger, P., Stewart, W.E., & Sehgal, P.B. (1981). Heterogeneity of interferon mRNA species from Sendai virus-induced human lymphoblastoid (Namalva) cells and Newcastle disease virus-induced murine fibroblastoid (L) cells. *Nucleic Acids Research, 9*:149–159.

Saito, T., Berens, M.E., & Welander, C.E. (1986). Antitumor effects of interferon-gamma (IFN-γ) in vitro in the presence of macrophages from ovarian cancer patients. *Proceedings of the American Society of Clinical Oncology, 5*:222.

Salmon, S.E., Durie, B.G., Young, L., Liu, R.M., Trown, P.W., & Stubbing, N. (1983). Effects of cloned human leukocyte interferon in the human tumor stem cell assay. *Journal of Clinical Oncology, 1*:217–225.

Samuels, B.L., Golomb, H.M., & Brownstein, B.H. (1987). In vivo induction of proteins during therapy of hairy cell leukemia with alpha-interferon. *Blood, 69*:1570–1573.

Sarna, G., Pertcheck, M., Figlin, R., & Ardalan, B. (1986). Phase I study of recombinant β ser 17 interferon in the treatment of cancer. *Cancer Treatment Reports, 70*:1365–1372.

Sarosy, G.A., Brown, T.D., VonHoff, D.D., Spiegel, R.J., et al. (1986). Phase I study of α 2-interferon plus doxorubicin in patients with solid tumors. *Cancer Research, 46*:5368–5371.

Saxon, A., Stevens, R.H., & Golde, D.W. (1978). T-lymphocyte variant of hairy-cell leukemia. *Annals of Internal Medicine, 88*:323–326.

Schiller, J.H., Groveman, D.S., Schmid, S.M., Willson, J.K., et al. (1986). Synergistic antiproliferative effects of human recombinant α 54- or β ser-interferon with γ interferon on human cell lines of various histogenesis. *Cancer Research, 46*:483–488.

Schilsky, R.L., Davidson, H.S., Magid, D., Daiter, S., & Golomb, H.M. (1987). Gonadal and sexual function in male patients with hairy cell leukemia: Lack of adverse effects of recombinant α 2 interferon treatment. *Cancer Treatment Reports, 71*:179–181.

Schrek, R., & Donnelly, W.J. (1966). "Hairy" cells in blood in lymphoreticular neoplastic disease and "flagellated" cells of normal lymph nodes. *Blood, 27*:199–211.

Scott, G.M., Secher, D.S., Flowers, D., Bate, J., Cantell, K., & Tyrrell, D. (1981). Toxicity of interferon. *British Medical Journal, 282*:1345–1348.

Scott, G.M. (1982). Interferon: Pharmacokinetics and toxicity. *Philosophical Transactions of the Royal Society of London: Series B, 299*:91–107.

Secher, D.S., & Burke, D.C. (1980). A monoclonal antibody for large-scale purification of human leukocyte interferon. *Nature, 285*:446–450.

Seto, W., Choo, Y.C., Merigan, T.C., et al. (1984). Local interferon treatment of intraepithelial neoplasia. *Antiviral Research, 3*:35.

Shows, T.B., Sakaguchi, A.Y., Naylor, S.L., Goeddel, D.V., & Lawn, R.M. (1982). Clustering of leukocyte and fibroblast interferon genes on chromosome 9. *Science, 218*:373–374.

Sidman, C.L., Marshall, J.D., Shultz, L.D., Gray, P.W., & Johnson, H.M. (1984). γ-interferon is one of several direct B cell-maturing lymphokines. *Nature, 309*:801–804.

Siegert, W., Theml, H., Fink, V., et al. (1982). Treatment of non-Hodgkin's lymphoma of low-grade malignancy with human fibroblast interferon. *Anticancer Research, 2*:193–198.

Smalley, R.V., & Oldham, R.K. (1984). Biological response modifiers: Preclinical evaluation and clinical activity. *CRC Critical Reviews in Oncology & Hematology, 1*:259–294.

Sonnenfeld, G. (1984). Interferon and the immune system. In Vilcek, J., & DeMaeyer, E. (Eds.), *Interferon. 2*, pp. 81–99. New York: Elsevier.

Spiegel, R.J. (1985). Intron A (interferon alpha-2b): Clinical overview. *Cancer Treatment Reviews, 12*(Suppl. B):5–16.

Spiegel, R.J. (1986). Intron A (interferon alpha-2b): Clinical overview and future directions. *Seminars in Oncology, 13*(Suppl. 2):89–101.

Spiegel, R.J., Spicehandler, J.R., Jacobs, S.L., & Oden, E.M. (1986). Low incidence of neutralizing factors in patients receiving recombinant alpha-2b interferon (Intron A). *American Journal of Medicine, 80*:223–228.

Spiegel, R.J. (1987). The alpha interferons: Clinical overview. *Seminars in Oncology, 14*(Suppl. 2): 1–12.

Spiers, A.S., Parekh, S.J., & Bishop, M.B. (1984). Hairy cell leukemia; induction of complete remission with pentostatin (2'-deoxycoformycin). *Journal of Clinical Oncology, 2*:1336–1342.

Stebbing, N., & May, L. (1982). Comparisons of dose–response data for various standard and recombinant DNA-derived human interferons. *Journal of Virological Methods*, 5:309–315.

Strander, H. (1986). Interferon treatment of human neoplasia. *Advances in Cancer Research*, 46:1–265.

Szigeti, R., Masucci, M.G., Masucci, G., Klein, E., & Klein, G. (1980). Interferon suppresses antigen- and mitogen-induced leukocyte migration inhibition. *Nature*, 288:594–596.

Talpaz, M., Mavligit, G., Keating, M., Walters, R.S., & Gutterman, J.U. (1983a). Human leukocyte interferon to control thrombocytosis in chronic myelogenous leukemia. *Annals of Internal Medicine*, 99:789–792.

Talpaz, M., McCredie, K.B., Mavligit, G.M., & Gutterman, J.U. (1983b). Leukocyte interferon-induced myeloid cytoreduction in chronic myelogenous leukemia. *Blood*, 62:689–692.

Talpaz, M., Trujillo, J.M., Hittelman, W.N., Keating, M.J., & Gutterman, J.U. (1985). Suppression of clonal evolution in 2 chronic myelogenous leukemia patients treated with leukocyte interferon. *British Journal of Haematology*, 60:619–624.

Talpaz, M., Kantarjian, H.M., McCredie, K., Trujillo, J.M., et al. (1986). Hematologic remission and cytogenetic improvement induced by recombinant human interferon alpha A in chronic myelogenous leukemia. *New England Journal of Medicine*, 314:1065–1069.

Talpaz, M., Kantarjian, H.M., McCredie, K.B., Keating, M.J., Trujillo, J., & Gutterman, J. (1987). Clinical investigation of human alpha interferon in chronic myelogenous leukemia. *Blood*, 69:1280–1288.

Tamm, I., Pfeffer, L., & Murphy, J.S. (1981). Assay of the inhibitory activities of human interferons on the proliferation and locomotion of fibroblasts. *Methods in Enzymology*, 79:404–413.

Tan, Y.H., Schneider, E.L., Tischfield, J., Epstein, C.J., & Ruddle, F.H. (1974). Human chromosome 21 dosage: Effect on the expression of the interferon induced antiviral state. *Science*, 186:61–63.

Taniguchi, T., Mantei, N., Schwarzstein, M., Nagata, S., et al. (1980). Human leukocyte and fibroblast interferons are structurally related. *Nature*, 285:547–549.

Taniguchi, T., Ohno, S., & Takaoka, C. (1982). Expression of the cloned genes for human interferon β_1 in E. coli and in cultured mouse cells. *UCLA Symposium on Molecular Cellular Biology*, 25:15–25.

Targan, S., & Dorey, F. (1980). Interferon activation of "pre-spontaneous killer" (pre-SK) cells and alteration in kinetics of lysis of both "pre-SK" and active SK cells. *Journal of Immunology*, 124:2157–2161.

Taylor-Papadimitriou, J. (1984). Effects of interferons on the growth and function of normal and malignant cells. In Billiau, A. (Ed.), *Interferon 1. General and applied aspects*, pp. 109–147. Amsterdam: Elsevier.

Taylor-Papadimitriou, J., & Rozengurt, E. (1981–82). Modulation of interferons inhibitory effect on cell growth by the mitogenic stimulus. *Texas Reports on Biology and Medicine*, 41:509–516.

Taylor, J.L., Sabran, J.L., & Grossberg, S.E. (1984). The cellular effects of interferon. In Came, P.E., & Carter, W.A. (Eds.), *Interferon and their applications*, pp. 169–204. New York: Springer-Verlag.

Torrisi, J., Berg, C., Bonnem, E., & Dritschilo, A. (1986). The combined use of interferon and radiotherapy in cancer management. *Seminars in Oncology*, 13(Suppl. 2):78–83.

Torti, F.M., & Lum, B.C. (1986). Superficial carcinoma of the bladder: Natural history and the role of interferons. *Seminars in Oncology*, 13(Suppl. 2):57–60.

Tovey, M.G., Dron, M., Mogensen, K.E., Lebleu, B., Mechti, N., & Begon-Lours-Guy Marho J. (1983). Isolation of Daudi cells with reduced sensitivity to interferon. II. On the mechanisms of resistance. *Journal of General Virology, 64*:2649–2653.

Trinchieri, G., & Santoli, D. (1978). Anti-viral activity induced by culturing lymphocytes with tumor-derived or virus-transformed cells: Enhancement of natural killer cell activity by interferon and antagonistic inhibition of susceptibility of target cells to lysis. *Journal of Experimental Medicine, 147*:1314–1333.

Trown, P.W., Dennin, R.A., Kramer, M.J., Connell, E.V., et al. (1983). Antibodies to human leukocyte interferons in cancer patients. *Lancet, 1*:81–84.

Trump, D.L., Elson, P.J., Borden, E.C., Harris, J.E., et al. (1987). High-dose lymphoblastoid interferon in advanced renal cell carcinoma: An Eastern Cooperative Oncology Group study. *Cancer Treatment Reports, 71*:165–169.

Tsujimoto, M., Yip, Y.K., & Vilcek, J. (1986). Interferon γ enhances expression of cellular receptors for tumor necrosis factor. *Journal of Immunology, 136*:2441–2444.

Urba, W.J., & Longo, D.L. (1986). α interferon in the treatment of nodular lymphomas. *Seminars in Oncology, 13*(Suppl. 5):40–47.

Vadhan-Raj, S., Al-Katib, A., Bhalla, R., Pelus, L., et al. (1986). Phase I trial of recombinant interferon gamma in cancer patients. *Journal of Clinical Oncology, 4*:137–146.

Vallbracht, A., Treuner, J., Flehmig, B., Joester, K.E., & Niethammer, D. (1981). Interferon-neutralizing antibodies in a patient treated with human fibroblast interferon. *Nature, 289*:496–497.

Verma, D.S., Spitzer, G., Zander, A.R., Gutterman, J.U., McCredie, K.B., Dicke, K.A., & Johnston, D.A. (1981). Human leukocyte interferon preparation-mediated block of granulopoietic differentiation in vitro. *Experimental Hematology, 9*:63–76.

Volberding, P.A. (1986). Kaposi's sarcoma and the acquired immunodeficiency syndrome. *Medical Clinics of North America, 70*:665–675.

VonHoff, D.D., Sarosy, G., Brown, T.D. et al. (1986). Rationale for and conduct of a phase I clinical trial with interferon alfa-2b plus doxorubicin. *Seminars in Oncology, 13*(Suppl. 2):72–77.

Vugrin, D., Hood, L., Taylor, W., & Laszlo, J. (1985). Phase II study of human lymphoblastoid interferon in patients with advanced renal cell carcinoma. *Cancer Treatment Reports, 69*:817–820.

Wadell, G. (1977). Hazards of human leukocyte interferon therapy. *New England Journal of Medicine, 296*:1295–1296.

Wagstaff, J., Scarffe, J.H., & Crowther, D. (1985). Interferon in the treatment of multiple myeloma and the non-Hodgkin's lymphomas. *Cancer Treatment Reviews, 12*(Suppl. B):39–44.

Weil, J., Tucker, G., Epstein, L.B., & Epstein, C.J. (1983). Interferon induction of (2'–5') oligo-isoadenylate synthetase in diploid and trisomy 21 human fibroblasts: Relation to dosage of the interferon receptor gene (IRFC). *Human Genetics, 65*:108–111.

Welander, C., Homesley, H.M., Levin, E., & Reich, S. (1986). Phase II trial of the efficacy of human recombinant interferon gamma (rIFNγ) in recurrent ovarian adenocarcinomas. *Proceedings of the American Society of Clinical Oncology, 5*:221.

Wilkinson, M., & Morris, A. (1983). Interferon with novel characteristics produced by human mononuclear leukocytes. *Biochemical and Biophysical Research Communications, 111*:498–503.

Worman, C.P., Catovsky, D., Bevon, P.C., et al. (1985). Interferon is effective in hairy-cell leukemia. *British Journal of Haematology, 60*:759–763.

Yam, L.T., Klock, J.C., & Mielke, C.H. (1984). Therapeutic leukapheresis in hairy cell leukemia: Review of literature and personal experience. *Seminars in Oncology*, *11*(Suppl. 2):493–501.

Yam, L.T., Li, C.Y., & Lam, K.W. (1971). Tartrate-resistance acid phosphatase isoenzyme in the reticulum cells of leukemic reticuloendo-theliosis. *New England Journal of Medicine, 284*:357–360.

Yaron, M., Yaron, I., Gurari-Rotman, D., et al. (1977). Stimulation of prostaglandin E production in cultured human fibroblasts by poly (1). poly (c) and human interferon. *Nature, 267*:457–459.

Zarling, J.M. (1984). Effects of interferon and its inducers on leucocytes and their immunologic functions. In Came, P.E., & Carter, W.A. (Eds.), *Interferons and their applications*, pp. 403–431. New York: Springer-Verlag.

Zarling, J., Eskra, L., Borden, E., Horoszewicz, J., & Carter W. (1979). Activation of human natural killer cells cytotoxic for human leukemia cells by purified interferon. *Journal of Immunology, 123*:63–70.

6

Monoclonal Antibodies in Cancer Therapy

Edward H. Kaplan, Robin E. Goldman-Leikin,
James A. Radosevich, A. Michael Zimmer,
and Steven T. Rosen

The search for antigens associated with, or restricted to, human neoplasms has been motivated by the convincing demonstration of such markers in numerous experimental tumors. Both serologic and cell-mediated immunologic techniques have been utilized to detect these tumor-associated antigens. Traditional methods had limited success because they could not provide absolute specificity. Monoclonal antibodies (MoAbs) prepared by somatic cell hybridization techniques are homogenous and recognize a single antigenic determinant. Their specificity makes them ideal tools for detecting the qualitative and quantitative differences in the antigenic composition of normal and malignant cells. MoAbs are expected to have great immunodiagnostic and therapeutic value in human cancer.

PRODUCTION OF MONOCLONAL ANTIBODIES

The nobel prize-winning hybridoma technique for producing monoclonal antibodies was developed by Kohler and Milstein (1975) (Figure 6.1). Following immunization, spleen cells from a rodent are fused to a mutated mouse myeloma cell

---

The authors thank Jill Redmond and Susana Bruno for their secretarial assistance.

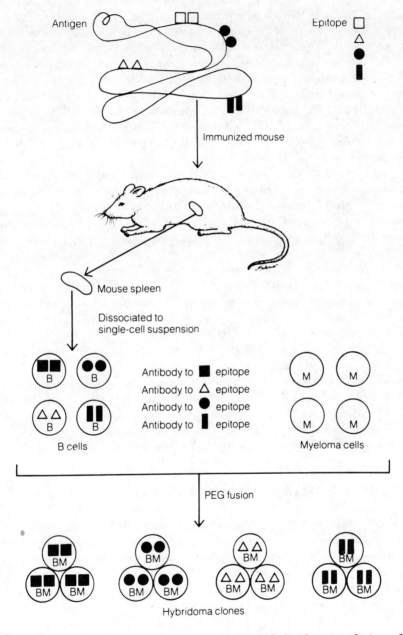

FIGURE 6.1. Diagrammatic representation of hybridoma technique for production of mouse monoclonal antibodies. PEG, polyethylene glycol. (Adapted with permission from Rosen, 1985b).

fusion process is mediated by polyethylene glycol (PEG), a wax-like substance that promotes fusion of the cell membranes. The resulting hybridomas contain genes from the B lymphocyte of the spleen that control specific antibody production and genes from the myeloma cells that allow for continuous cell proliferation. The hybridoma acts as an antibody-producing factory, which can be maintained in culture. The mouse myeloma cell line used has lost the capacity to produce its own immunoglobulin. In addition, it lacks hypoxanthine phosphoribosyltrans-ferase (HPRT), an enzyme utilized for salvage of purine nucleotides, which are needed to produce DNA. In a selective growth medium containing aminopterin, which blocks endogenous production of DNA, the unfused myeloma cell can-not survive.

The hybridoma derives its source of HPRT and the gene coding for antibody production from the sensitized splenic B lymphocyte. Spleen cells that do not fuse have a limited life span and are lost in culture within a few days. Therefore, only the spleen cell–myeloma hybridoma cells are selected for continuous propagation in media containing aminopterin. Hybridomas are dispensed into multiple culture wells. The hybridoma supernatant is tested for antibodies with desired specificity, and selected hybridomas are cloned and expanded. When large amounts of MoAbs are needed, the hybridoma clones can be injected into the peritoneal cavity of syngeneic or immunodeficient mice and ascites fluid or serum collected. Large amounts of monoclonal antibodies can also be produced utilizing fermentation, fiber systems, and growth in porous microcapsules.

MoAbs have been made against a variety of tumor-associated antigens. In most instances, these antibodies recognize differentiation or oncofetal antigens. For the immunization procedures, live or fixed whole cells or subcellular extracts have been used with or without adjuvant. Human MoAbs have been produced by fusing cells from the draining lymph nodes of cancer patients or sensitized lymphocytes in their peripheral blood to either mouse myeloma or human lymphoma cell lines (Schlom et al., 1980; Glassy et al., 1983; Haspel et al., 1985).

CLINICAL TRIALS WITH MONOCLONAL ANTIBODIES

Several reports exist of antitumor effects using xenogeneic antitumor antibody in humans (Wright et al., 1976). Dramatic responses were witnessed when polyclonal antithymocyte globulin derived from immunizing horses with T lymphocytes were administered to patients with cutaneous T cell lymphoma (Edelsen et al., 1979). In these studies toxicities included acute fever and chills, hypotension, respiratory distress, skin rashes, venous thrombophlebitis, thrombocytopenia, immune-com-plex deposition, and serum sickness. Rodent-derived monoclonal antibodies cir-cumvent many but not all of the problems associated with polyclonal antisera.

Several clinical trials using MoAbs directed against human cancers have now been completed. The earlier Phase I–II trials have utilized a variety of un-

TABLE 6.1. Toxicity in Monoclonal Antibody Clinical Trials

Anaphylactic reaction	Flushing
Arthralgias	Headache
Bronchospasm	Hypertension
Cardiac dysrhythmias	Hypotension
Chills	Myelosuppression
Coryza	Nausea/vomiting
Diaphoresis	Pain
Diarrhea	Rash
Dyspnea	Serum sickness
Fever	Urticaria

conjugated mouse MoAbs (usually of IgG type) at differing concentrations and at various infusion rates. These trials essentially established the feasibility of using xenogeneic monoclonal antibodies in humans, established a spectrum of clinical toxicity (Table 6.1), delineated mechanisms of tumor resistance to MoAb therapy (Table 6.2), and have suggested the potential for clinical response. More recently, clinical trials have focused on the use of immunoconjugates with linkage of the monoclonal antibody to radioactive isotopes, protein toxins (i.e., ricin, diphtheria, tetanus, pseudomonas), and chemotherapeutic agents. Other novel clinical approaches include the use of F(ab')$_2$ fractions of monoclonal antibody and the combination of MoAbs with other biologic response modifiers (i.e., interleukin-2 or the interferons).

The human malignancies most commonly investigated include T cell malignancies, lymphomas, acute leukemias, malignant melanoma, colorectal carcinoma, neuroblastoma, and ovarian carcinoma (Table 6.3). Preclinical experimentation has expanded this area to include potential use in cancer of the breast, prostate, bladder, as well as sarcomas and central nervous system (CNS) malignancies (Thiesen et al., 1987; Webb et al., 1987; Thor et al., 1986b; Gross et al., 1984).

TABLE 6.2. Mechanisms of Tumor Resistance to Monoclonal Antibody Therapy

Antigenic modulation
Circulating free antigen
Insufficient antigenic expression
HAMA
Heterogeneity of antigenic expression
Saturation of effector cell population
Lack of recruitment of appropriate effectors
Inadequate tumor penetration

TABLE 6.3 Combined Results of Therapeutic Trials Utilizing Monoclonal Antibodies

Disease	Antibody/class	Antigen	Responses	References
CLL	T101/IgG$_{2a}$	T65	2/33	Dillman, 1984; Foon, 1981; Bertram, 1986
	T101/RTA/IgG$_{2a}$	T65	0/4	Hertler, 1986
CTCL	T101/IgG$_{2a}$	T65	17/38	Dillman, 1984; Dillman, 1986; Bertram, 1986; Levy, 1983; Foon, 1983.
	^{131}I-T101/IgG$_{2a}$	T65	6/6	Rosen, 1987
B cell lymphomas	Anti-id	Ig	7/15	Miller, 1987; Rankin, 1985
	Chimeric Anti-id	Ig	1/1	Hamblin, 1987
	^{131}I-Anti-id	Ig	1/1	Badger, 1987
	1F5/IgG$_{2a}$	Bp35,CD20	2/4	Press, 1987
	Ab89/NS	NS	0/1	Nadler, 1980
Malignant melanoma	9.2.27/IgG$_{2a}$	MAA	0/8	Oldham, 1984
	R24/IgG$_3$	G$_{D3}$	6/21	Houghton, 1985, 1986
	MG-21/IgG$_3$	G$_{D3}$	0/8	Goodman, 1987
	96.5/IgG$_{2a}$ and 48.7/IgG$_1$	p97	0/5	Goodman, 1987
	Anti-id	Anti-MAA MoAb	1/4	Mittleman, 1987
	96.5-RTA/IgG$_{2a}$	P97	5/22	Spitler, 1987
	3F8/IgG$_3$	G$_{D2}$	4/9	Cheung, 1987
		C	NS/9	Baiorin, 1987

Cancer	MoAb	Antigen	Response	Reference
Neuroblastoma	3F8/IgG$_3$	G$_{D2}$	2/8	Cheung, 198?
Colorectal carcinoma	17-1A/IgG$_{2a}$	Surface glycolipid	7/44	Sears, 1982, 1984, 1985
	28A32/human IgM	Cell membrane and cytoplasmic antigen	0/5	Smith, 1987
	17-1A/IgG$_{2a}$ and rIF-gamma	Surface glycolipid	(NS/27)	Weiner, 1986
	^{131}I-AUA1/IgG	Cell–surface antigen	1/1	Epenetos, 1986a
Ovarian carcinoma	^{131}I-HFMG$_2$/IgG	Carbohydrate on milk-fat globule membrane		
	^{131}I-tumor Associated MoAb	NS	9/12	Epenetos, 1986

Anti-id: anti-idiotype monoclonal antibody; Ig: immunoglobulin; MAA: melanoma-associated antigen; MoAb: monoclonal antibody; NS: not specified; rIF-gamma: recombinant gamma interferon; RTA: ricin A chain.

Chronic Lymphocytic Leukemia and Cutaneous T Cell Lymphoma

T101, a murine IgG_{2a} monoclonal antibody, has been the most extensively studied MoAb in clinical trials. T101 recognizes T65, a 65,000-dalton antigen present on T lymphocytes, thymocytes, and chronic lymphocytic leukemia (CLL) cells (Bertram et al., 1986; Foon et al., 1985; Dillman et al., 1985). Dillman and coworkers (1984) reported results from a preliminary trial of T101 in four patients with CLL and four patients with cutaneous T cell lymphoma (CTCL). Immunofluorescence studies verified that circulating cells did bind to the antibody *in vivo* and were subsequently removed from the circulation. Seven patients received multiple infusions of the antibody. All patients showed a substantial drop in circulating target cells during treatment, and two patients with CTCL had clinical improvement in their skin lesions. However, clinical responses were short-lived, lasting from days to a few weeks. Tumor lysis appeared to be mediated by removal of opsonized target cells in the reticuloendothelial system, especially the spleen. Similar observations have been made by other groups using murine IgG monoclonal antibodies directed against leukemia and lymphoma-associated antigens (Levy & Miller, 1983; Nadler et al., 1980; Foon et al., 1984). In these studies, monoclonal antibody dosages ranged from 1 to 1500 mg.

Because of the suggestion of a possible clinical advantage to high dose and prolonged infusion, Dillman and associates (1986) subsequently conducted a trial using 24-hour infusions of T101 at doses from 10 to 500 mg. Six patients with CLL and ten with CTCL were treated at doses of 10, 50, 100, or 500 mg. A brief objective response was seen in four of ten CTCL patients and two of six CLL patients.

Toxicity was similar at all dose levels and consisted of fever, sweats, and chills. Allergic reactions as manifested by pruritus and urticaria occurred in one-third of the patients. These side effects were generally not associated with demonstrable IgE allergic reactions and could usually be well controlled with diphenhydramine hydrochloride. Patients who developed urticaria did not appear to be at increased risk for more serious allergic-type reactions upon subsequent exposure to the monoclonal antibody. The most significant toxicities seen were bronchospasm in a patient with CLL and an acute immune complex-mediated reaction in a CTCL patient. Antigenic modulation was rapid and persisted throughout the 24-hour infusions (Shawler et al., 1985). Human anti-mouse antibody (HAMA) was seen in no patients with CLL and in five of the patients with CTCL within 2 weeks of the treatment. This was associated with a decreased effect on peripheral lymphocytes. A dose of 500 mg was not tolerated because both patients who received that dose developed high titers of anti-mouse antibodies. This study clearly demonstrated the following: (1) a 24-hr infusion of monoclonal antibody is safe; (2) relatively specific *in vivo* toxicity can be expected; (3) high sustained levels of free T101 can be obtained with continuous infusion; and (4) HAMA can develop regardless of dose.

Bertram and associates (1986) treated eight patients with CTCL and five with various other T cell malignancies using T101 at weekly 2-hr infusions of 1 to 500 mg. One complete remission of convoluted T cell lymphoma (lasting 6 weeks) and one partial remission of CTCL (lasting 3 months) were observed. Generally, complete targeting of peripheral blood T cells was seen with a dose of 1 mg of antibody. Free antibody was present in the circulation at a dose of 10 mg or greater and persisted for as long as 6 weeks at the higher dose levels. This excess antibody induced antigenic modulation, which was of concern when it persisted until the next treatment. Three of the 13 patients developed HAMA. Toxicities were generally similar to those of other trials. One patient developed an anaphylactic reaction. This reaction occurred during a third dose of 500 mg T101. The patient had demonstrable HAMA, which may have been responsible for this reaction. Other toxicities not previously noted included blood pressure instability, premature atrial contractions, atrial fibrillation, and atrioventricular conduction disturbances. These toxicities occurred only at 10 mg or greater dose levels and seemed to be related to the rapid (2-hr) rate of infusion. Moderate to severe dyspnea was observed in all patients in this trial. Two of the patients demonstrated transient defects on perfusion lung scan or chest x-ray supporting the hypothesis of lymphocyte aggregation causing microemboli. Transient lymphocyte depletion was observed at all dose levels with the best mean peripheral blood T cell reduction occurring at the 10-mg dose level. It was concluded that rapid infusion of nonmodulating doses of T101 demonstrated excellent targeting and transient removal of peripheral blood T cells. However, because of the minimal response demonstrated it was assumed that this approach would be more beneficial if treatment employed the use of immunoconjugated T101. A similar conclusion was reached by others who investigated unconjugated T101.

Our laboratory embarked on a Phase I–II trial using ^{131}I-labeled T101 for radioimmunodetection and therapy of patients with CTCL (Rosen et al., 1987). T101 was radiolabeled with Na[131]I, using chloramine-T at an iodine/antibody ratio of 1.0, with only a partial loss in immunoreactivity. All patients received a diagnostic dose of ^{131}I-T101, ranging from 5.0 to 13.1 mCi on 10 mg of antibody. Radiation dosimetry estimates were obtained from biodistribution data as well as diagnostic imaging data. Radioimmunotherapeutic doses of ^{131}I-T101, ranging from 98.3 to 150.1 mCi on 10 mg of antibody, were then administered to all patients 1 week later. All of the five patients who received a therapeutic dose had an objective response to their initial therapy, and two patients responded when they were retreated. Regression of skin lesions and decrease in peripheral adenopathy was seen. All patients reported resolution of their chronic pruritus. The duration of response ranged from 3 weeks to 3 months with relapses generally occurring in areas not previously involved. Acute toxicity included fever, pruritus, and mild dyspnea. Myelosuppression was seen in patients receiving over 140 mCi of ^{131}I-T101; blood counts returned to normal within 10 weeks after therapy. All patients developed a HAMA response, which was detected by 14 days after the radioimmunodetection injection and persisted for more than 22 months. Using a competition radioimmunoassay, we found that in the case of four of the five patients, 50% to 75% of HAMA was directed against antigenic determinants common to all mouse IgG_{2a} antibodies. The remaining 25% to 50% of HAMA was idiotypic, being specific for T101 epitopes. In the case of one patient the HAMA showed little specificity for T101, reacting equally well with all IgG_{2a} antibodies tested. In all patients, 0% to 24% of HAMA reacted with IgG_1 antibodies, demonstrating that HAMA specifically recognized epitopes common to IgG_{2a} molecules (Goldman-Leikin et al., 1987).

HAMA responses were of both IgG and IgM isotypes. Because HAMA titers persisted at the time of disease progression, patients underwent plasmapheresis prior to retreatment. Plasmapheresis was effective in reducing the IgM component of HAMA but was less efficient in removing the IgG portion of HAMA. High pressure liquid chromatography (HPLC) quantitative analysis determined that plasmapheresis reduced total HAMA levels by 28% to 61% (Zimmer et al., 1988). Residual HAMA probably accounted for the enhanced T101 antibody clearance rates observed and for the little clinical improvement derived from retreatment.

The preliminary data from this trial demonstrated a definite therapeutic benefit to radiolabeled monoclonal antibody with myelosuppression as the limiting toxicity. Optimization of dose scheduling, dosimetry quantitation, and improved radiolabeling methodologies may lead to improved therapeutic outcome.

Recently, Hertler and associates (1986) treated four CLL patients refractory to alkylating agents with T101 linked to ricin A chain (T101-RTA). Each patient received eight infusions of 3 mg/M^2 T101-RTA over 1 hr. All four patients had rapid fall in WBC count of less than 24 hours duration after each infusion. No sustained benefit was demonstrated in any patient. *In vivo* binding of T101-RTA to tumor cells was demonstrated by flow cytometric analysis and saturation of target sites was seen. No significant toxicity was noted and no HAMA was detectable.

In the combined analysis of all trials reported to date, 33 patients with CLL (Hertler et al., 1986; Dillman et al., 1986; Bertram et al., 1986; Dillman et al., 1984; Foon et al., 1984; Foon et al., 1983) and 46 patients with CTCL or other T cell malignancies (Rosen et al., 1987; Bertram et al., 1986; Dillman et al., 1986; Dillman et al., 1984; Levy et al., 1983; Foon et al., 1983) have been treated with T101 monoclonal antibody therapy. Two of 33 CLL patients have demonstrated some response and 23 of 44 CTCL patients have responded. No CLL patients had detectable HAMA, whereas 20 of 36 with CTCL had HAMA.

B Cell Lymphomas

Human B cell lymphomas usually express an immunoglobulin molecule that is unique to that tumor. Highly specific monoclonal antibodies can be generated by immunizing mice with either purified idiotype or with whole cells that express the idiotype on their surface. Miller and colleagues (1982) used a novel approach to produce these antibodies by fusing a patient's malignant B lymphoma cells with a mouse myeloma cell line. The resulting heterohybridomas secrete large quantities of human immunoglobulin, which is identical to that found on the patient's tumor cells. This immunoglobulin can then be used as the immunogen to generate a mouse monoclonal "anti-idiotype" antibody. These antibodies are essentially tumor-specific and may avoid the limitation inherent in most monoclonals by not cross-reacting with normal tissues.

Miller and colleagues (1987) have treated 13 patients with B cell lymphomas using anti-idiotypes. Six of the patients had clinically significant, but short-lived, objective responses beginning 8–16 days after initiation of therapy. One patient, however, had a complete remission, which has been sustained for more than 50 months without further therapy. Toxicities were seen in patients with either circulating tumor cells, serum idiotype levels of greater than 1 mg/ml, or demonstrable HAMA. Toxicity, which was similar to that discussed previously, was generally mild and easily controlled.

HAMA was detected in five patients after which further infusions of antibody failed to reach the tumor or induce tumor regression. The patients who did not develop HAMA had received large initial doses of anti-idiotype ranging from 200 to 500 mg, which implied that large doses may induce immunologic tolerance. This is similar to the observations from the Netherlands Cancer Institute in which no HAMA was detected in two patients receiving 3.8 g or 5.8 g of anti-idiotype antibody (Rankin et al., 1985). Biopsies of residual disease in four patients with partial remissions showed nonreactivity with the anti-idiotype antibody. This implied selective destruction of idiotype-positive cells with emergence of idiotype-negative tumor cell variants.

Further evaluation of the responding patients showed that the therapeutic outcome correlated with the number of nontumor cells (mostly mature T cells) infiltrating the tumor (Lowder et al., 1987). This suggested that the preexisting host–tumor interaction is important in the effect of anti-idiotype antibodies. One patient with prolymphocytic leukemia showed a direct antiproliferative effect of the anti-idiotype antibodies *in vitro*. The isotype of the monoclonal antibodies, their avidity, the number of antigen sites per cell, and surface immunoglobulin modulation ability were not predictive of clinical response.

Rankin and co-workers (1985) reported on the treatment of two refractory B cell lymphoma patients with very large doses of anti-idiotype monoclonal antibodies. Both patients showed transient decreases in the levels of circulating malignant cells and free antigen. The appearance of unbound monoclonal antibody was detected in the serum. However, only minimal clinical response was seen in these patients. Antigenic modulation, heterogeneity of tumor cells, and HAMA were not detected.

Recently, Hamblin et al. (1987) reported on the treatment of a single patient with a chimeric univalent derivative of an anti-idiotype monoclonal antibody (FabIgG). The chimeric derivative consists of Fab fragments from a mouse monoclonal anti-idiotype linked by thioether bonds to human normal IgG (Oi and Morrison, 1986; Stevenson et al., 1985). The preparation is univalent and therefore avoids rapid antigenic modulation. By possessing a human Fc region it optimizes recruitment of effector cells, prolongs the metabolic half-life of the molecule, and minimizes the immunogenicity of the mouse-derived component. A previously untreated patient with a nodular B cell lymphoma received four intravenous infusions of 380 to 580 mg over 11 weeks. Four days after each injection, swollen and tender lymph nodes were reported, which gradually subsided over 5–8 days. The patient experienced a partial response with demonstration of greater than 50% decrease in tumor burden. There was no significant toxicity, and there was a fall in the number of tumor cells with each infusion.

There is only one preliminary report of treatment with radiolabeled anti-idiotype antibodies (Badger et al., 1987). After dosimetry studies of trace labeled anti-idiotype antibodies using increasing doses of antibody (50–1000 mg), a patient received an infusion of 232 mCi ^{131}I-labeled antibody (1000 mg). The estimated radiation dose was 615 cGy to the tumor and 120 cGy whole body exposure. The patient was reported as being in complete remission for more than 3 months after therapy. The major toxicity was bone marrow suppression, which required autologous bone marrow rescue.

MoAbs that recognize other B cell markers have been investigated in clinical trials (Press et al., 1987; Ritz and Schlossman, 1982; Nadler et al., 1980). Recently, Press et al. (1987) treated four refractory B cell lymphoma patients with the monoclonal antibody 1F5; a murine IgG$_{2a}$ that recognizes a 35,000-dalton antigen (Bp35,CD20) present on the surface of normal and malignant B cells. This antigen is unique in that it reportedly is not shed from the cell surface and does not modulate after binding to 1F5. The MoAb also appears not to bind to any other normal tissues. Patients were treated by continuous infusions over 5–10 days with 50–2380 mg of 1F5. Low doses of 1F5 (5–10 mg/M^2/day) were adequate for depleting circulating tumor cells, but high antibody doses (100–800 mg/M^2/day) and high serum 1F5 levels were required to coat tumor cells in bone marrow and lymph nodes. Clinical response correlated directly with dose; a total dose of 52.4 mg was associated with progressive disease, 104.8 mg resulted in stable disease, 1032 mg produced a minor response, and 2380 mg caused a partial response with 90% reduction in evaluable lymph node disease lasting 6 weeks. There was minimal toxicity reported. IgG HAMA was seen in only one patient which became detectable 5 months after therapy.

Recently two unique monoclonal antibodies (Lym-1 and Lym-2) have been described (Epstein et al., 1987). These were produced using tumor nuclei as immunogens. Because of their specificity for B cells, their avidity for lymphoma cells, and their chemical stability after radiolabeling procedures, they hold promise for therapeutic potential. Clinical trials with these antibodies are soon to be initiated.

Acute Leukemia

Therapeutic use of MoAbs directed against the CALLA antigen for patients with acute lymphoblastic leukemia (Ritz et al., 1981) and myeloid differentiation antigens in acute myelogenous leukemia (Ball et al., 1986) have shown similar toxicity and short-lived incomplete responses as those seen with the other hematologic malignancies discussed above. The greatest potential for the use of MoAbs in the leukemias is in bone marrow purging prior to autologous bone marrow transplantation. A complete review of this area was published by Reading and Takaue (1986).

Malignant Melanoma

Malignant melanoma provides a unique model for study of monoclonal antibody therapy in a solid tumor. Cutaneous tumor nodules are easily accessible for biopsy, and relatively specific MoAbs have been raised against a variety of melanoma cell antigens. Preclinical studies with human melanoma xenografts in nude mice have shown selective localization (Hwang et al., 1985; Fritzberg et al., 1987). MoAb-toxin conjugates (vinca alkaloids, diphtheria A toxin, abrin, ricin, gelonin) have shown impressive suppression of tumor growth *in vivo* with tolerable toxicity (Bumol et al., 1983, 1987; Sivam et al., 1987; Fritzberg et al., 1987).

Six MoAbs (9.2.27, 96.5, 48.7, R24, MG-21, and 3F8) with specificity to human melanoma cells have been studied in Phase I and pilot clinical trials; 9.2.27 is a murine IgG_{2a} MoAb that recognizes a 250,000-dalton melanoma-associated antigen (chondroitin sulfate proteoglycan core glycoprotein) present on 90% of melanomas. Because of this MoAb's prevalence, selectivity for tumor cells (Morgan et al., 1981) and selective localization in preclinical trials (Hwang et al., 1985), Oldham et al. (1984) chose 9.2.27 for a pilot clinical trial. In this study, eight patients with metastatic malignant melanomas were treated intravenously. Biopsies were performed 24 hours to 4 days after the infusion. No antibody was detected in the tumors after 1 or 10 mg of 9.2.27, but 50 mg or greater demonstrated localization. When a 200-mg dose was given, almost 100% of the viable tumor cells were stained with antibody as determined by flow cytometry. No major toxicity was seen; however, there were no clinical responses. Forty percent of the patients demonstrated a transient HAMA response. No increase in HAMA was detected after the 200 mg infusion, implying a potential tolerogenic effect of higher doses of MoAb. Higher doses of the antibody were associated with prolonged circulating levels of 9.2.27.

Twenty-one patients have been entered into a Phase I trial utilizing R24, an IgG_3 MoAb that recognizes the G_{D3} ganglioside found on the surface of melanoma cells as well as other cells of neuroectodermal origin (Houghton et al., 1985, 1986). R24 was given intravenously as eight doses over 2 weeks with doses ranging from 1 mg/M^2 to 50 mg/M^2. Partial or minor responses were seen in six patients lasting 6–44 weeks. Most of the responding patients had doses of 1 mg/M^2 or 10 mg/M^2. Toxicity was related to dose and rate of infusion. All patients receiving 10 mg/M^2 or greater of this MoAb developed urticaria and pruritus, which was often localized to tumor sites. Marked nausea, vomiting and diarrhea were seen at 50

mg/M^2. Most patients developed HAMA after 8–50 days (mean of 16 days). Because R24 is able to activate human complement, the authors concluded that the MoAb was responsible for complement-mediated cytotoxicity and cell-mediated cytotoxicity with tumor cell injury occurring secondary to an inflammatory reaction in the tumor bed. It was also noted that in nude mice studies, the antitumor effect of R24 is potentiated by adriamycin and other drugs, providing another potential model for further studies in humans.

Goodman et al. (1985) treated five patients with disseminated melanoma using two MoAbs, 96.5 and 48.7. The MoAb 96.5 is an IgG_{2a} that is specific for p97, a surface glycoprotein present on many normal cells but found in much greater density on most human melanoma cells. The MoAb 48.7 is an IgG_1 that is directed against a cell surface proteoglycan expressed on 90% of melanomas. The antigen is also seen on benign nevi and is detectable in small amounts on some endothelial cells. Four patients received 212 mg of each antibody and one patient received only the MoAb 96.5 in escalating doses over 6–10 days. Biopsies performed 2–240 hours after treatment demonstrated immunohistologic evidence of extensive binding to melanoma cells but not to normal cells; however, no clinical responses were seen. There was no treatment-related toxicity. Four of the patients developed HAMA. In one patient, the HAMA apparently rose from a tumor-imaging dose of Fab fragments of MoAb 48.7 given 3 months prior to the current trial. This appeared to be associated with a decrease in the elimination half-life of the antibody. A subsequent trial has investigated the clinical use of MG-21, an IgG_3 MoAb directed against the G_{D3} ganglioside. This MoAb can mediate the lysis of antigen-positive melanoma cells when in the presence of human complement or mononuclear cells (Goodman et al., 1987). Eight patients were treated with daily infusions of $5\ mg/M^2$ to $100\ mg/M^2$ MG-21 as a 4- to 12-hour intravenous infusion. There was no detectable antitumor response in this study. Urticaria, pruritus, nausea, and coryza were dose-limiting at $50\ mg/M^2$ over 6 hr. HAMA was detected in most patients by 3–4 weeks after treatment.

Recently, Cheung and colleagues (1987) reported the results of a Phase I study in which nine patients with malignant melanoma and eight with neuroblastoma were treated with a murine IgG_3 MoAb. This MoAb, 3F8, is specific for the G_{D2} ganglioside, activates human complement, and is involved in antibody-dependent cell-mediated cytotoxicity. Six of the 17 patients treated had significant responses to therapy. Two patients with advanced neuroblastoma that had failed conventional chemotherapy and allogeneic bone marrow transplantation experienced complete responses to intravenous 3F8. One of the patients, originally treated with $5\ mg/M^2$ of 3F8, died after 63 weeks of interstitial pneumonitis but without clinical evidence of recurrent neuroblastoma. The second patient, treated with $20\ mg/M^2$ of 3F8, developed an isolated asymptomatic area of uptake in the skull on bone scan 28 weeks after therapy but continued to be free of widespread disease at 45 weeks. Although a biopsy of the lesion showed neuroblastoma cells to be G_{D2}-positive and ^{131}I-3F8 imaging visualized involved lesions, she failed to respond to a subsequent treatment.

Two patients with malignant melanoma sustained partial responses lasting 22 to 56+ weeks after treatment with 20 mg/M^2 and 50 mg/M^2 of 3F8, respectively. Two other melanoma patients obtained mixed responses lasting 16 weeks and 6 weeks after treatment with 20 mg/M^2 and 100 mg/M^2, respectively. Response did not appear to correlate with amount and type of pretreatment or with MoAb dose used.

Aside from urticaria, fever, and nausea observed in most MoAb trials, toxicity in this study also included severe pain, transient hypertension, and arthralgias. The pain was seen in all patients and required analgesic therapy. It typically involved the abdomen, lower back, and occasionally the chest with peripheral spreading to the ankles and feet. There were no long-term neurologic deficits and the pain resolved after cessation of antibody infusion. Two patients described slight decrease in temperature sensitivity lasting 4 weeks after the treatment. The authors postulated that reactivity of pain fibers with 3F8 may have been responsible for the pain reactions seen.

Peak serum 3F8 correlated with amount of MoAb infused. HAMA was seen in all patients but did not increase with higher doses of 3F8. Patients with lower levels of HAMA reportedly were more likely to respond to retreatment.

Although MoAbs are mostly used for passive immunization or as site-directed carriers of toxins, there is some experimental evidence suggesting that anti-idiotype MoAbs may actually promote active immunization leading to immune responses against tumors (Kennedy et al., 1985; Gorczynki et al., 1984). It is postulated that the anti-idiotypes mirror the binding sites of MoAbs specific for tumor antigens and, acting as antigens themselves, stimulate the host's immune system to react with the tumor's epitopes. This theory has been applied in a Phase I clinical trial of patients with malignant melanoma, the preliminary results of which were recently reported (Mittelman et al., 1987). Murine anti-idiotype MoAbs raised against three anti-high molecular weight–melanoma-associated antigen (HMW–MAA) MoAbs were tested in four patients. One patient demonstrated reduction in the size and extent of cutaneous melanoma lesions. There was no detectable toxicity. Further studies of this approach are clearly warranted.

Conjugates of antimelanoma MoAbs and radioactive isotypes have mostly been investigated as an imaging tool. [111]Indium-labeled MoAb ZME-018, a mouse IgG$_{2a}$, which recognizes a 240,000-dalton antigen (gp240) found on the surface of most melanomas, was recently investigated for radioimmunoscintigraphy in 30 patients with biopsy-proven metastatic melanoma (Murray et al., 1987). Patients were given a single IV infusion of 0.6–40 mg ZME–018 labeled with 5 mCi [111]In. Uptake was seen in 110 of 171 previously diagnosed metastases for a sensitivity of 64%. Nonspecific uptake was consistently seen in the liver and spleen and less frequently in other organs. This appears to be the major drawback to ^{111}In-labeled antibodies. The sensitivity increased significantly with higher doses of MoAB; 73% of lesions imaged at 20 mg as compared to 29% imaging at 2–5 mg ($P < 0.005$). Soft tissue lesions imaged better than visceral lesions, and no tumor smaller than 1 cm was visualized. No toxicity was reported. There were 22 instances in which uptake occurred in areas that were not confirmed by biopsy. One patient did have a positive radioimaging scan seen before the appearance of lymphadenopathy on physical examination.

Other studies using whole antibodies conjugated to ^{111}In revealed very poor sensitivity and specificity as diagnostic aids (Engelstad et al., 1986; Frontiera et al., 1987). However, studies investigating the use of radiolabeled F(ab')$_2$ or Fab fragments of MoAbs have been encouraging (Abrams et al., 1987; Siccardi et al., 1986; Buraggi, 1986; Larson et al., 1983). Siccardi et al. (1986) from the National Cancer Institute in Milan, Italy recently reported the results of a multicenter study analyzing [99m]Tc- and ^{111}In-labeled F(ab')$_2$ fragments of the MoAb 225.28S. The MoAb 225.28S is a mouse IgG$_{2a}$ reactive with an HMW–MAA. In a study of 206 patients, 377 lesions were visualized. Of these, 250 lesions were in known sites of disease, 95 were occult, and 32 areas were visualized but not biopsy confirmed. The major limitation appeared to be nonspecific accumulation in bone marrow, spleen, liver, and kidneys; subcutaneous injection of the conjugated antibody fragments appeared to decrease nonspecific background. The stage of disease appeared to have significance with an increased frequency of false-negative scans seen in patients with Stage IV disease. The percentage of visualized lesions was significantly higher (74% versus 59%) when F(ab')$_2$ fragments were labeled with ^{99m}Tc rather than [111]In. There was good agreement in the results among the ten nuclear medicine departments involved in the study, suggesting that the procedure was reliable. The National Cancer Institute in Milan has subsequently initiated a prospective trial and has reported their preliminary findings (Buraggi, 1986). In 29 patients with 38 suspected axillary involvement sites, the sensitivity of the radioimmunodetection is 71%. The predictive value of a positive test is 100%, while that of a negative test is 81%. Of all the studies performed by the Milan group, F(ab')$_2$ labeled with ^{99m}Tc provides the best results with sensitivity at 70% to 85% and specificity of approximately 100%. The results of these studies suggest imminent widespread clinical applicability.

The results of one preliminary clinical trial using a MoAb (96.5)-ricin A chain immunoconjugate (xomazyme-mel) has recently been reported (Spitler et al., 1987). In this trial, 22 patients with Stage III metastatic melanoma received a total dose of 3.2–300 mg of immunotoxin. One patient had a complete response with disappearance of pulmonary metastases, which lasted longer than 13 months. Four patients had mixed responses and five had stabilization of disease. The observed responses were noteworthy in that they continued to regress for prolonged periods following a single course of immunotoxin without any additional therapy.

The severity of the side effects was generally related to the dose of immunotoxin. All patients receiving at least 0.2 mg/kg/day of immunotoxin experienced a reversible fall in serum albumin and total protein. Weight gain and fluid shifts were noted which resulted in clinical signs of edema in some patients. There was no pulmonary edema. Patients receiving greater than or equal to 0.5 mg/kg/day of immunotoxin demonstrated signs of mild hypovolemia with tachycardia and a drop in orthostatic blood pressure. The patients' weights and serum albumin levels returned to baseline within 48 hr of the last immunotoxin treatment.

The decrease in albumin was thought to be related to the ricin A chain. The mechanism was postulated to include either decreased albumin synthesis, loss from the intravascular compartment, increased catabolism, or increase in the circulating fluid volume. Proteinuria and diarrhea were not noted excluding a urinary or gastrointestinal loss as an etiology.

In most of the patients toxicity included fever, malaise, fatigue, and decreased appetite. Also noted was decreased voltage on electrocardiogram and sinus tachycardia. Possible allergic reactions as manifested by rash, pruritus, or eosinophilia were seen in three patients. Two of these had received a prior radioimmunoimaging dose of murine MoAb.

Immunologic analysis demonstrated that almost all of the patients developed an immune response to both the MoAb and the ricin A chain components of the immunotoxin.

Colorectal Carcinoma

Sears and co-workers (1984, 1985) have used an IgG_{2a} mouse MoAb (17-1A) for therapy in patients with metastatic gastrointestinal malignancies. The antibody had been shown to mediate lysis of colorectal carcinoma cells in tissue culture by human or mouse effector cells and specifically inhibited the growth of human colon carcinoma xenografts in athymic nude mice. Collectively, the investigators reported results of 40 patients in Phase I–II trials. Overall seven patients were reported to have responded to this therapy. In the earlier study, 20 patients were treated with a single injection of 15–1000 mg. The patients studied had large tumor burdens, a short life expectancy, and many had received MoAb incubated with an autologous leukocyte preparation. In addition, many received surgery, chemotherapy, or radiation after receiving the MoAb. Three of the patients (one with rectal cancer and lung metastases, one with colon cancer and peritoneal metastases, and one with metastatic pancreatic cancer) had between 10 to greater than 24 months (or more) disease-free survival.

The more recent study (Sears et al., 1985) evaluated a more homogenous population of 20 patients with metastatic colorectal carcinoma treated with a single 200–850 mg IV infusion. Of these patients, there were three partial responses and one mixed response. Of the 40 patients in the two studies, toxicity was mild or nonexistent and similar to that previously described in other MoAb studies. HAMA was detected in approximately one-half of the patients.

Smith and associates (1987) have reported preliminary results of a clinical trial using a human monoclonal antibody in five patients with metastatic colorectal cancer. The MoAb 28A32 is an IgM that recognizes a cell membrane and cytoplasmic antigen present in colon cancer cells. This MoAb was produced from a human–mouse heterohybridoma resulting from the fusion of NS-1 mouse myeloma cells with B lymphocytes from a patient previously immunized with a mixture of irradiated autologous colon cancer cells and Bacille Calmette-Guérin. The initial phase of the protocol utilized 8 mg of 28A32 labeled with 5 mCi of ^{131}I. This was given IV twice (1 week apart) for radioimmunoscintigraphy. Four of the five patients had positive images of metastatic lesions. Sites of metastases included liver, lung, and bone and could still be imaged on day 17. After imaging doses with radiolabeled MoAb the patients received weekly injections of either 10 mg or 50 mg of unlabeled MoAb. No toxicity was noted, yet there have been no responses reported.

Other groups have investigated various radiolabeled MoAbs for purposes of immunodetection (Farrands et al., 1982; Epenetos et al., 1982; Leyden et al., 1986; Colcher et al., 1987b). These studies have generally shown a good correlation between biopsy-proven metastases and MoAb localization. A significant amount of unlabeled antibody in appropriate proportions to the labeled MoAb may be necessary to assure visualization of otherwise "cold" liver metastases (Patt et al., 1987). Some researchers contend that the partial blocking of nonspecific uptake by normal liver may account for the observed improved MoAb nuclear scans. The optimal MoAb and immunoscintigraphic technique for a clinically useful nuclear scan has yet to be determined.

There is preclinical evidence that recombinant human leukocyte interferons (especially alpha interferon) can increase the amount of tumor antigen expressed (Greiner et al., 1987). This causes the tumor cell population to become more homogenous and thus augments MoAb binding. A Phase I trial was recently described in which patients with metastatic colon cancer were treated with 400 mg of the MoAb 17-1A after four daily infusions of varying doses of recombinant gamma interferon (Weiner & Comis, 1986). Toxicity appeared to be directly related to the interferon dose; clinical results have yet to be published.

A Phase I clinical trial investigating the use of MoAb XMMCO-791 conjugated to ricin A chain (RTA) has recently been initiated (Byers et al., 1987). XMMCO-791 reacts with a gp72 antigen expressed on colorectal carcinoma cells. The immunotoxin XMMCO-791-RTA is cytotoxic to antigen-positive tumor cells *in vitro* and has been shown to suppress growth of colon cancer xenografts in nude mice.

Ovarian Cancer

Although intravenous injections of radiolabeled MoAbs have successfully imaged ovarian cancer masses (Granowska et al., 1986; Epenetos et al., 1987), the amount of MoAb actually reaching the tumor is very small (Epenetos, 1986). Because adenocarcinoma of the ovary is confined to the peritoneal cavity throughout most of its course, the intracavitary administration of MoAbs, as with other therapeutic agents, is a reasonable approach to therapy. Studies have shown a distinct advantage in tumor uptake when MoAbs or MoAb fragments are administered intraperitoneally (IP) as opposed to intravenously both in animal studies with human xenografts (Wahl et al., 1987) and in human subjects (Haisma et al., 1987). The preliminary data from one study suggest that simultaneous administration of IP and IV MoAb may be complementary (Colcher et al., 1987a).

To date, there are no published reports of clinical trials for ovarian cancer using unconjugated MoAbs. Epenetos et al. (1987) has reported the preliminary results of a Phase I clinical trial utilizing IP administration of ^{131}I-labeled MoAbs in patients with chemotherapy and/or radiation therapy resistant advanced ovarian cancer. Nine of 12 patients obtained some benefit from the therapy. The patients with minimal disease (< 2 cm^2 tumor volume) appeared to benefit the most. Four of six patients achieved a complete remission lasting 3 to more than 24 months. Toxicity was related to the dose of radioactivity administered and was seen at 100 mCi in patients with ascites and 150 mCi in patients without ascites. Because of tumor heterogeneity, it has been suggested that a cocktail of MoAbs may be efficacious (Epenetos et al., 1986a). A patient with ovarian cancer had ascites with tumor cells reactive to two tumor-associated MoAbs, AUAI and HMFG$_2$. The patient underwent IP therapy with ^{131}I-AUAI resulting in a partial response. Subsequent ascites reaccumulation contained tumor cells reactive only to HMFG$_2$. After further IP treatment with the other MoAb, ^{131}I-HMFG$_2$, the patient sustained a complete response.

Pilot clinical trials using intraperitoneal injections of ^{111}In and ^{90}Y conjugates of (Fab')$_2$ fragments of the OC125 MoAb have been initiated (Griffin et al., 1987). The IP administration was well tolerated, and external imaging has demonstrated 70% of the activity remaining in the peritoneal cavity for up to 6 days.

At Northwestern University, we have recently initiated a trial using IP administration of labeled B72.3 for radioimmunodetection and radioimmunotherapy in patients with refractory ovarian cancer. B72.3 is a murine IgG$_1$ MoAb reactive with TAG-72, a high molecular weight glycoprotein. TAG-72 has been shown immunohistologically to be commonly expressed in most cases of epithelial ovarian cancer (Thor et al., 1986a).

Various MoAbs have been developed into immunotoxins active against ovarian cancer cell lines (Pirker et al., 1985) and efficacious in inhibiting human ovarian cancer xenograft growth in a mouse model (Willingham et al., 1987); however, these have yet to reach clinical trials.

SUMMARY

Initial enthusiasm for the use of monoclonal antibodies as "magic bullets" for the selective destruction of cancer cells has been tempered. Key problems and potential benefits with this approach have been identified. Preliminary trials have illustrated that these antibodies can be administered safely, that tumor binding can be achieved, and that therapeutic responses can occur. The potential limitations of rodent monoclonal therapy are now being addressed and will, it is hoped, be overcome. Monoclonal antibodies offer great promise in the therapy of malignant disease. Further investigation using innovative approaches and in combination with other therapies may help attain this goal.

REFERENCES

Abrams, P., Eary, J., Schroff, R., et al. (1987). Successful imaging of metastatic melanoma with ^{99m}Tc labeled monoclonal antibodies and its implications for therapy. *Second International Conference on Monoclonal Antibody Immunoconjugates for Cancer*, San Diego.

Badger, C.C., Eary, J., Brown, S., et al. (1987). Therapy of lymphoma with ^{131}I-labeled anti-idiotype antibodies (Anti-Id). *Proceedings of the Amercian Association of Cancer Research, 28*:338.

Bajorin, D., Chapman, P., Kunicka, J., et al. (1987). Phase I trial of a combination of R24 mouse monoclonal antibody and recombinant interleukin-2 in patients with melanoma. *Proceedings of the American Society of Clinical Oncology, 6*:210.

Ball, E.D., Mills, L.E., Coughlin, C.T., et al. (1986). Autologous bone marrow transplantation in acute myelogenous leukemia: In vitro treatment with myeloid cell-specific monoclonal antibodies. *Blood, 68*:1311–1315.

Bertram, J.H., Gill, P.S., Levine, A.M., et al. (1986). Monoclonal antibody T101 in T cell malignancies. A clinical, pharmacokinetic, and immunologic correlation. *Blood, 68*:752–761.

Bumol, T.F., Laguzza, B.C., DeHerdt, S.V., et al. (1987). Preclinical studies with 9.2.27-4-desacetyl vinblastine-3-carboxhydrazine (9.2.27-DAVLB-HYDRAZIDE) for site-directed therapy of human melanoma. *Second International Conference on Monoclonal Antibody Immunoconjugates for Cancer*, San Diego.

Bumol, T.F., Wang, O.C., Reisfeld, R.A., et al. (1983). Monoclonal antibody and an antibody-toxin conjugate to a cell surface proteoglycan of melanoma cells suppress in vivo tumor growth. *Proceedings of the National Academy of Sciences USA, 80*:529–533.

Buraggi, G.L. (1986). Radioimmunodetection of malignant melanoma with the 225.285 monoclonal antibody to HMW-MAA. *Nuklearmedizin, 25*:220–224.

Byers, V.S., Rodvien, R., Grant, K., et al. (1987). Monoclonal antibody XMMCO 791-ricin: A chain immunotoxin in the treatment of colorectal cancer. *Second International Conference on Monoclonal Antibody Immunoconjugates for Cancer*, San Diego.

Cheung, N.-K. V., Lazarus, H., Miraldi, F.D., et al. (1987). Ganglioside G_{D2} specific monoclonal antibody 3F8: A Phase I study in patients with neuroblastoma and malignant melanoma. *Journal of Clinical Oncology, 5*:1430–1440.

Colcher, D., Esteban, J.M., Carrasquillo, J.A., et al. (1987a). Complementation of intracavitary and intravenous administration of a monoclonal antibody (B72.3) in patients with carcinoma. *Cancer Research, 47*: 4218–4224.

Colcher, D., Esteban, J.M., Carrasquillo, J.A., et al. (1987b). Quantitative analysis of selective radiolabeled monoclonal antibody localization in metastatic lesions of colorectal cancer patients. *Cancer Research, 47*:1185–1189.

Dillman, R.O., Shawler, D.L., Dillman, J.B., et al. (1986). Monoclonal antibody in patients with chronic lymphocytic leukemia and cutaneous T-cell lymphoma. *Journal of Cellular Biochemistry, 9*:108A.

Dillman, R.O., Shawler, D.L., Dillman, J.B., et al. (1984). Therapy of chronic lymphocytic leukemia and cutaneous T-cell lymphoma with T101 monoclonal antibody. *Journal of Clinical Oncology, 2:*881–891.

Edelsen, R.L., Raafat, J., Berger, C.L., et al. (1979). Antithymocyte globulin in the management of cutaneous T-cell lymphoma. *Cancer Treatment Reports, 63:*675–680.

Engelstad, B.L., Spitler, L.E., Del Rio, M.J., et al. (1986). Phase I immunolymphoscintigraphy with an [111]I_n labeled antimelanoma monoclonal antibody. *Radiology, 161:*419–422.

Epenetos, A.A. (1986). Intraperitoneal therapy of ovarian cancer: *International Conference on Monoclonal Antibody Immunoconjugates for Cancer,* San Diego, CA.

Epenetos, A.A., Hooker, G., Krausz T, et al. (1986a). Antibody-guided irradiation of malignant ascites in ovarian cancer: A new therapeutic method possessing specificity against cancer cells. *Obstetrics and Gynecology, 88:*71S–74S. 1986.

Epenetos, A.A., Britton, K.E., Mather, S., et al. (1982). Targeting of iodine-123 labelled tumour-associated monoclonal antibodies to ovarian, breast, and gastrointestinal tumours. *Lancet, 2:*999–1004.

Epenetos, A.A., Lavender, J.P., Kenemans, P., et al. (1987). Early results of the monoclonal antibody OVTL3 in specific detection of ovarian cancer. *Journal of Clinical Oncology, 4:*160.

Epstein, A.L., Marder, R.J., Winter, J.N., et al. (1987). Two new monoclonal antibodies, Lym-1 and Lym-2, reactive with human B-lymphocytes and derived tumors, with immunodiagnostic and immunotherapeutic potential. *Cancer Research, 47:*830–840.

Farrands, P.A., Perkins, A.C., Pimm, M.V., et al. (1982). Radioimmunodetection of human colorectal cancers by an anti-tumor monoclonal antibody. *Lancet, 2:*397–400.

Foon, K.A., Schroff, R.W., Bunn, P.A., et al. (1984). Effects of monoclonal antibody therapy in patients with chronic lymphocytic leukemia. *Blood, 64:*1085–1093.

Foon, K.A., Schroff, R.W., & Bunn, P.A. (1985). Monoclonal antibody therapy for patients wth leukemia and lymphoma. In Morgan, A.C. Jr., & Foon, K.A. (Eds.), *Monoclonal antibody therapy of human cancer* (pp. 85–101). Bingham, MA: Martinas Nijhoff.

Foon, K.A., Shcroff, R.W., Mayer, D., et al. (1983). Monoclonal antibody therapy in chronic lymphocytic leukemia and cutaneous T cell lymphoma: Preliminary observations. In Boss, B.D., Langman, R., Trowbridge, I., et al. (Eds.), *Monoclonal antibodies and cancer* (pp. 39–52). San Diego: Academic Press.

Fritzberg, A.R., Vanderheyden, J.-L., Rao, T.N., et al. (1987). Rhenium labelling of antimelanoma 9.2.27 for radioimmunotherapy. *Second International Conference on Monoclonal Antibody Immunoconjugates for Cancer.* San Diego.

Frontiera, M., Schmelter, R., Chu, H., et al. (1987). Immunolymphoscintigraphy with radiolabeled monoclonal antibodies in patients with malignant melanoma. *Proceedings of the American Society of Clinical Oncology, 6:*231.

Glassy, M.C., Handley, H.H., Hagiwara, H., et al. (1983). UC 729-6, human lymphoblastoid B-cell line useful for generating antibody-secreting human–human hybridomas. *Proceedings of the National Academy of Sciences USA, 80:*6327–6331.

Goldenberg, D.M., & DeLand, F.H. (1984). Clinical studies of prostatic cancer imaging with radiolabeled antibodies against prostatic acid phosphatase. *Urological Clinics of North America 11:*277–281.

Goldman-Leikin, R.E., Marder, R., Kaplan, E.H., et al. (1987). Immunologic studies in a trial evaluating ^{131}I-T101 for radioimmunoimaging and radioimmunodetection of cutaneonous T-cell lymphoma. *Recent Advances in Leukemia and Lymphoma,* a UCLA Symposium.

Goodman, G.E., Hellstrom, I., Hummel, D., et al. (1987). Phase-I trial of monoclonal antibody MG-21 directed against a melanoma associated GD3 ganglioside antigen. *Proceedings of the American Society of Clinical Oncology, 6:*209.

Goodman, G.E., Hellstrom, I., Hummel, D., et al. (1985). Pilot trial of murine monoclonal antibodies in patients with advanced melanoma. *Journal of Clinical Oncology, 3*:340–352.

Gorczynski, R.N., Kennedy, M., Polidoulis, I., et al. (1984). Altered tumor growth in vivo after immunization of mice with anti-tumor antibodies. *Cancer Research, 44*:3291–3298.

Granowska, M., Britton, K.E., Shepard, J.H., et al. (1986). A prospective study of ^{123}I-labeled monoclonal antibody imaging in ovarian cancer. *Journal of Clinical Oncology, 4*:730–736.

Greiner, J.W., Guadagni, F., Noguchi, P., et al. (1987). Recombinant interferon enhances monoclonal antibody-targeting of carcinoma lesions in vivo. *Science, 235*:895–898.

Griffin, T., Raso, V., Hnatowich, D., et al. (1987). Intraperitoneal therapy with ricin A chain and yttrium conjugates: Preclinical and clinical studies. *Second International Conference on Monoclonal Antibody Immunoconjugates for Cancer*, San Diego, CA.

Gross, M.D., Skinner, R.W.S., & Grossman, H.B. (1984). Radioimmunodetection of a transplantable human bladder carcinoma in a nude mouse. *Investigations in Radiology, 19*:530–534.

Haisma, H.J., Battaile, A., Moseley, K., et al. (1987). Favorable tumor uptake of ^{131}I-labeled monoclonal antibody OC125 after I.P. administration as opposed to IV administration in ovarian cancer patients. *Second International Conference on Monoclonal Antibody Immunoconjugates for Cancer*, San Diego, CA.

Hamblin, T.J., Cattan, A.R., Glennie, M.J., et al. (1987). Initial experience in treating human lymphoma with a chimeric univalent derivative of monoclonal anti-idiotype antibody. *Blood, 69*:790–797.

Haspel, M.V., McCabe, R.P., Pomato, N., et al. (1985). Generation of tumor cell-reactive human monoclonal antibodies using peripheral blood lymphocytes from actively immunized colorectal carcinoma patients. *Cancer Research, 45*:3951–3961.

Hertler, A.A., Schlossman, D.M., Bosowitz, M.J., et al. (1986). A Phase I study of T101 RTA immunotoxin in refractory chronic lymphocytic leukemia. *Blood, 68*:223A.

Houghton, A.N., Mintzer, D., Cordon-Cardo, C., et al. (1985). Mouse monoclonal IgG3 antibody detecting G_{D3} ganglioside: A Phase I trial in patients with malignant melanoma. *Proceedings of the National Academy of Sciences USA, 82*:1242–1246.

Houghton, A.N., Vadhan, S., Wong, G., et al. (1986). Clinical study of a mouse monoclonal antibody directed against G_{D3} ganglioside in patients with melanoma. *Proceedings of the American Society of Clinical Oncology, 5*:231.

Hwang, K.M., Fodstad, O., Oldham, R.K., et al. (1985). Radiolocalization of xenografted human malignant melanoma by a monoclonal antibody (9.2.27) to a melanoma-associated antigen in nude mice. *Cancer Research, 45*:4150–4155.

Kennedy, R.C., Dreesman, G.R., Butel, J.S., et al. (1985). Suppression of in vivo tumor formation induced by simian virus 40-transformed cells in mice receiving antidiotype antibodies. *Journal of Experimental Medicine, 161*:1432–1449.

Kohler, G., & Milstein, C. (1975). Continuous culture of fused cells secreting antibody of predefined specificity. *Nature, 256*:495–497.

Larson, S.M., Brown, J.P., Wright, P.W., et al. (1983). Imaging of melanoma with ^{131}I-labeled monoclonal antibodies. *Journal of Nuclear Medicine, 24*:123–129.

Levy, R., & Miller, R.A. (1983). Tumor therapy with monoclonal antibodies. *Federation Proceedings, 42*:2650–2656. 1983.

Levy, R., Miller, R.A., Stratte, P.T., et al. (1983). Therapeutic trials of monoclonal antibody in leukemia and lymphoma: Biologic considerations. In Boss, B.D., Langman, R., Trowbridge, I., et al. (Eds.), *Monoclonal antibodies and cancer* (pp. 5–16). San Diego: Academic Press.

Leyden, M.J., Thompson, C.H., Lichtenstein, M., et al. (1986). Visualization of metastases from colon carcinoma using an ^{131}I-radiolabeled monoclonal antibody. *Cancer, 57*:1135–1139.

Lowder, J.N., Meeker, T.C., Campbell, M., et al. (1987). Studies on B lymphoid tumors treated with monoclonal anti-idiotype antibodies: Correlation with clinical responses. *Blood, 69*:199–210.

Miller, R.A., Lowder, J., Meeker, T.C., et al. (1987). Anti-idiotypes in B-cell tumor therapy. *National Cancer Institute Monographs, 3*:131–134.

Miller, R.A., Maloney, D.G., Warnke, R., et al. (1982). Treatment of B-cell lymphoma with monoclonal anti-idiotype antibody. *New England Journal of Medicine, 306*:517–522.

Mittleman, A., Ferrone, S., Kageshita, T., et al. (1987). A Phase I clinical trial of murine anti-idiotypic monoclonal antibodies to anti-human high molecular weight-melanoma associated antigen monoclonal antibodies in patients with malignant melanoma. *Proceedings of the American Association of Cancer Research, 28*:390.

Morgan, A.C., Galloway, D.R., & Reisfeld, R.A. (1981). Production and characterization of monoclonal antibody to a melanoma-specific glycoprotein. *Hybridoma, 1*:27–36.

Murray, J.L., Rosenblum, M.G., Lamki, L., et al. (1987). Radioimmunoimaging in malignant melanoma patients with the use of ^{111}In-labeled antimelanoma monoclonal antibody (ZME-018) to high-molecular-weight antigen. *National Cancer Institute Monographs, 3*:3–9.

Nadler, L.M., Stashenko, P., Hardy, R., et al. (1980). Serotherapy of a patient with a monoclonal antibody directed against a human lymphoma-associated antigen. *Cancer Research, 40*:3147–3154.

Oi, V.T., & Morrison, S.C. (1986). Chimeric antibodies. *Biotechnology, 4*:214–221.

Oldham, R.K., Foon, K.A., Morgan, A.C., et al. (1984). Monoclonal antibody therapy of malignant melanoma: In vivo localization in cutaneous metastasis after intravenous administration. *Journal of Clinical Oncology, 2*:1235–1244.

Patt, Y.Z., Lamki, L., & Haynie, T.P. (1987). Improved ^{111}In monoclonal anti-CEA 2CE-025 localization in colorectal cancer: Liver metastases by the addition of unlabeled 2CE-025. *Proceedings of the American Association of Cancer Research, 28*:390.

Pirker, R., Fitzgerald, D.J.P., Hamilton, T.C., et al. (1985). Characterization of immunotoxins active against ovarian cancer cell lines. *Journal of Clinical Investigation, 76*:1261–1267.

Press, O.W., Appelbaum, F., Ledbetter, J.A., et al. (1987). Monoclonal antibody 1F5 (Anti-CD20) serotherapy of human B cell lymphomas. *Blood, 69*:584–591.

Rankin, E.M., Hekman, A., Somers, R., et al. (1985). Treatment of two patients with B cell lymphoma with monoclonal anti-idiotype antibodies. *Blood, 65*:1373–1381.

Reading, C.L., & Takaue, Y. (1986). Monoclonal antibody applications in bone marrow transplantation. *Biochimica et Biophysica Acta, 865*:141–170.

Ritz, J., Pesando, J.M., Sallan, S.E., et al. (1981). Serotherapy of acute lymphoblastic leukemia with monoclonal antibody. *Blood, 58*:141–152.

Ritz, J., & Schlossman, S.F. (1982). Utilization of monoclonal antibodies in the treatment of leukemia and lymphoma. *Blood, 59*:1.

Rosen, S.T., Zimmer, A.M., Goldman-Leikin, R., et al. (1987). Radioimmunodetection and radioimmunotherapy of cutaneous T-cell lymphomas using an ^{131}I-labeled monoclonal antibody: An Illinois Cancer Council Study. *Journal of Clinical Oncology, 5*:562–573.

Rosen, S.T., Goldman-Leikin, R.E., Zimmer, A.M., et al. (1985). Monoclonal antibodies in cancer therapy. *Laboratory Medicine, 16*:310–314.

Rosen, S. T., Lambiase, E. A., Ma, Y., Radosevich, J. A., & Epstein, A. L. (1985b). Monoclonal antibodies: Their promise for tumor diagnosis, staging, and therapy. *Postgraduate Medicine, 77*: 129–134.

Schlom, J., Wunderlich, D., & Teramoto, Y.A. (1980). Generation of human monoclonal antibodies reactive with human mammary carcinoma cells. *Proceedings of the National Academy of Sciences USA*, 77:6841–6845.

Schroff, R.W., Farrell, M.M., Klein, R.A., et al. (1984). T65 antigen modulation in a phase I monoclonal antibody trial with chronic lymphocytic leukemia patients. *Journal of Immunology*, 133:1641–1648.

Sears, H.F., Herlyn, D., Steplewski, Z., et al. (1984). Effects of monoclonal antibody immunotherapy on patients with gastrointestinal adenocarcinoma. *Journal of Biological Response Modifiers* 3:138–150.

Sears, H.F., Herlyn, D., Steplewski, Z., et al. (1985). Phase II clinical trial of a murine monoclonal antibody cytotoxic for gastrointestinal adenocarcinoma. *Cancer Research*, 45:5910–5913.

Shawler, D.L., Miceli, M.C., Wormsley, S.B., et al. (1984). Induction of in vitro and in vivo antigenic modulation by the anti-human T-cell monoclonal antibody T101. *Cancer Research*, 44:5921–5927.

Siccardi, A.G., Buraggi, G.L., Callegaro, L., et al. (1986). Multicenter study of immunoscintigraphy with radiolabeled monoclonal antibodies in patients with melanoma. *Cancer Research*, 46:4817–4822.

Sivam, G., Pearson, J.W., Bohn, W., et al. (1987). Immunotoxins to a human melanoma-associated antigen: Comparison of gelonin with ricin and other A chain conjugates. *Cancer Research*, 47:3169–3173.

Smith, J., Bookman, M., Carrasquillo, J., et al. (1987). Evaluation of a human anti-colorectal carcinoma monoclonal antibody in patients with metastatic colorectal cancer. *Proceedings of the American Society of Clinical Oncology*, 6:250.

Spitler, L.E., del Rio, M., Khentigam, A., et al. (1987). Therapy of patients with malignant melanoma using a monoclonal antimelanoma antibody-ricin A chain immunotoxin. *Cancer Research*, 47:1717–1723.

Stevenson, G.T., Glennie, M.J., Paul, F.C., et al. (1985). Preparation and properties of FabIgG, a chimeric univalent antibody designed to attack tumor cells. *Bioscience Reports*, 5:991.

Thiesen, H.-J., Juhl, H., & Arndt, R. (1987). Selective killing of human bladder cancer cells by combined treatment with A and B chain ricin antibody conjugates. *Cancer Research*, 47:419–423.

Thor, A., Gorstein, F., Ohuchi, N., et al. (1986a). Tumor-associated glycoprotein (TAG-72) in ovarian carcinomas defined by monoclonal antibody B72.3. *Journal of the National Cancer Institute*, 76:995–1006.

Thor, A., Weeks, M.O., & Schlom, J. (1986b). Monoclonal antibodies and breast cancer. *Seminars in Oncology*, 13:393–401.

Wahl, R.L., Liebert, M., Caino, L., et al. (1987). Intraperitoneal ovarian carcinoma: IP delivery of specific monoclonal antibodies is superior to IV delivery. *Journal of Nuclear Medicine*, 28:651–652.

Webb, K.S., Sussman, E.M., & Walther, P.J. (1987). Production and partial characterization of a prostate carcinoma-directed MAB. *Proceedings of the American Association of Cancer Research*, 28:15–47.

Weiner, L.W., & Comis, R.L. (1986). Phase I trial of murine monoclonal antibody administration preceded by recombinant gamma interferon therapy in patients with advanced gastrointestinal carcinoma. *Proceedings of the American Society of Clinical Oncology*, 5:225.

Willingham, M.C., Fitzgerald, D.J., & Pastan, I. (1987). Pseudomonas exotoxin coupled to a monoclonal antibody against ovarian cancer inhibits the growth of human ovarian cancer cells in a mouse model. *Proceedings of the National Academy of Sciences USA*, 84:2474–2478.

Wright, P.W., Hellstrom, K.E., Hellstrom, I., et al. (1976). Serotherapy of malignant disease in "immunotherapy of malignant disease." *Medical Clinics of North America,* *60*:607–622.

Zimmer, A.M., Rosen, S.T., Spies, S.M., et al. (1988). Radioimmunotherapy retreatment of patients with cutaneous T-cell lymphoma using an ^{131}I-labeled monoclonal antibody: Antibody analysis of retreatment following plasmapheresis. *Journal of Nuclear Medicine, 29*:174–180.

7

Treatment of Solid Tumors with High-Dose Chemotherapy and Autologous Marrow Rescue

William A. Knight, III

More than a quarter of a century has passed since infusion of autologous marrow was first used in an attempt to ameliorate myelosuppression in the treatment of neoplastic disease (Kornick et al., 1958). In the early 1960s, many patients with refractory malignancies were treated with such therapy in hopes of increasing tumor response and avoiding fatal marrow toxicity (Kornick et al., 1958; McFarland et al., 1959; McGovern et al., 1959; Newton et al., 1959; Clifford et al., 1961; Pegg et al., 1962). The results of these initial studies were disappointing. Lack of tumor response or protection from myelosuppression led to little interest in further exploration as a viable treatment modality for cancer. That these studies were destined to fail is now obvious in retrospect because the doses of radiation and chemotherapy utilized were only moderate by today's standards and would not have been expected to induce a degree of myelosuppression to demonstrate an effect on autologous marrow. Moreover, the amount and handling of the marrow was quite variable such that in some instances only trivial numbers of viable stem cells were infused.

During the next 10 years clinical trials focused on more intensive chemotherapy using combinations of agents to treat hematopoietic neoplasms (Henderson & Samayo, 1969; DeVita et al., 1970). Aggressive combination chemotherapy for solid tumors met with varying degrees of success in the induction of remission

(Cohen et al., 1977; Young et al., 1975; DeVita et al., 1975). Associated with the advent of increasingly intensive chemotherapy was the appearance of increasing morbidity and mortality rates from toxicity. The toxicity from these regimens is enhanced, with myelosuppression and thrombocytopenia being dose-limiting toxicities.

The renewed interest in autologous marrow transplantation has arisen for several reasons. First, and perhaps most important, is the demonstration that 15% of patients with refractory acute leukemia are cured with intensive chemotherapy and total body irradiation followed by allogeneic bone marrow transplantation (Thomas et al., 1977). Autologous marrow has the additional advantage of avoiding the problems that plague allogeneic grafts including acute and chronic graft versus host disease and graft rejection (Thomas et al., 1977; Thomas et al., 1975). In addition, the technology now exists to manage patients with protracted cytopenias. An understanding of the use of blood product support, sterile environments, and antibiotic management in aplastic patients has developed over the last decade and is necessary for the success of intensive therapy. Finally, there is an overriding fascination with the attempt to enhance tumor cytoreduction with more intensive therapy.

In this setting, it is important to realize that autologous bone marrow infusion is a rescue technique and is not by itself a therapy of malignancy. The central issue that will determine its usefulness is whether it is possible to overcome tumor resistance with higher doses of chemotherapy. The use of autologous marrow will then be dictated by the degree and duration of myelosuppression induced by the potentially effective chemotherapeutic regimen.

AUTOLOGOUS BONE MARROW INFUSION AS SUPPORT: TECHNICAL ASPECTS

The procedure for procurement of bone marrow for infusion has been well described (Thomas & Sturb, 1970). Marrow is removed by repeated aspirations from the posterior and, if necessary, anterior iliac crests. The aspirated marrow, a mixture of fat, blood, bone, and nucleated cells, is immediately passed through a sterile wire mesh screen and suspended in anticoagulated culture media. Under ideal circumstances, enough aspirations are performed to yield between 2 and 5 × 10^8 nucleated cells/kg. Previous studies indicated that 0.4–0.8 × 10^8 nucleated cells/kg are necessary to repopulate the marrow following lethal therapy (Van Patten, 1965). The minimum dose of marrow in humans has not been firmly established. Using animal models as a guide, most transplant centers infuse a minimum dose of at least 1 × 10^8 nucleated cells/kg to allow a margin of safety.

The capability to cryopreserve and store marrow is required if one intends to utilize intensive therapy as a means of consolidation or as an approach to relapse. From a practical standpoint such preservation is necessary even in the adjuvant setting because treatment regimens may take 2–10 days to administer and bone marrow loses viability at 4°C after approximately 4 days. The first evidence that animals could be protected from marrow lethal therapy by the use of cryopreserved bone marrow was demonstrated in 1954 (Barnes & Lootit), but the physiology of cryopreservation is still not fully understood. After harvest, marrow is centrifuged to separate nucleated cells from erythrocytes, the buffy coat is suspended in plasma and the cryoprotectant DMSO is added. Although differentiated cells may lyse during the freezing process, a rate of cooling of 1°C/min appears to protect stem cells (Schlater, 1972; Major, 1970). As the cells change from liquid to solid phase, heat is released. Programmable freezing chambers are used to maintain a linear freeze, thus protecting cells from the damaging effects of crystallization. Marrow cells frozen in this fashion may be stored at −196°C for prolonged periods with little loss of viability.

HIGH-DOSE CHEMOTHERAPY: THE DOSE–RESPONSE RELATIONSHIP AND THEORETICAL LIMITATIONS

Clinical experience with neoplasms sensitive to chemotherapy has confirmed the critical dependence of the curability of these tumors upon the ability to deliver full doses and the ability to adhere to schedule (Frei & Canellos, 1980; Brindley et al., 1964; Frei et al., 1965; Cullen et al. 1977; Pinkel et al., 1971; Gehan & Coltman, 1980; Bonadonna & Valagossa, 1980; DeVita et al., 1970; Young et al., 1973; Lewis & DeVita, 1978). The assumption that increased doses of chemotherapy yields increased tumor response has not been confirmed clinically for human solid tumors. Toxicity is clearly related to dose; thus, it might be argued that lower doses with less attendant toxicity can be used effectively and more safely (Bross et al., 1966; Tattersall & Tobias, 1976).

Current principles of chemotherapy have, in part been guided by animal models, such as those developed by Skipper and his co-workers (Skipper et al., 1964; Skipper, 1978). Their experiments established the foundation of the fractional cell kill hypothesis, which simply states that a given concentration of drug applied for a specified period of time will kill a constant fraction of cells, regardless of tumor size. Each treatment cycle is expected to kill a specific fraction of the remaining cells. Given a sensitive tumor, the results of treatment are a function of drug dose and the frequency with which cycles are repeated (Skipper et al., 1964).

Tumor cell kill can be modulated in this system by varying the dose of the chemotherapeutic agent. For high growth fraction tumors such as the mouse L1210 leukemia and AKR lymphoma, a linear log relationship does exist between dose of chemotherapy and tumor cytoreduction (Skipper et al., 1964; Skipper, 1978; Skipper et al., 1950; Bruce et al., 1966; Bruce et al., 1967; Steel, 1977). In such sensitive tumors, the number of tumor cells surviving exposure to a chemotherapeutic agent declines as a logarithmic function of drug concentration (Bruce et al.,

1966; Bruce et al., 1967; Steel, 1977). Hence, simply doubling the dose of an agent may lead to an increase in cell kill by a full log or greater (Bruce et al., 1966; Bruce et al., 1967). These steep linear dose–response curves exist for such drugs as the anthracycline antibiotics, the alkylating agents, and other drugs such as procarbazine and DTIC (Frei & Canellos, 1980). The dose–response curve for cell cycle-specific agents (e.g., antimetabolites and vinca alkaloids) is complicated by cytokinetic heterogeneity; therefore, these curves exhibit a plateau in dose–response (Frei & Canellos, 1980; Herzig, 1981). Extending the duration of exposure in this setting will increase cytoreduction following the destruction of the mitotically active component and the recruitment of arrested cells into cycle, again yielding a steep dose–response curve (Steel, 1977).

Using this hypothesis one can define resistance as a shallow dose–response curve. Herzig has pointed out the significance of this observation as it applies to high dose chemotherapy. In the instance in which the tumor is sensitive to drugs at conventional therapeutic doses, a modest dose increase may markedly increase cell kill and possibly effect remission induction and cure. Should the tumor have a more shallow dose–response curve, a considerably greater dose may be required such that nonhematologic toxicities become dose-limiting. Finally, it appears for some tumors there is initially a shallow dose–response curve, but when a certain threshold is reached the curve becomes steep (Herzig, 1981).

Unfortunately, there is conclusive evidence in both experimental systems and in humans that toxicity is dose-related (Frei & Canellos, 1980; Deisseroth & Abrams, 1979). Because of the morbidity and mortality rates associated with protracted myelosuppression (Bodey et al., 1966), the potential benefit of dose escalation has not been extensively studied in clinical trials. The use of the technology available for marrow harvest, storage, and infusion should allow circumvention of prolonged myelosuppression as the dose-limiting toxicity and should allow examination of the role of chemotherapy at levels five to ten times the conventional dose.

Chabner has recently explored the considerations in the selection of agents for high-dose chemotherapy (Chabner, 1980). Antimetabolites such as the antifolates and purine and pyrimidine antagonists are not attractive agents for dose escalation because of limiting gastrointestinal toxicity. Avoiding the gastrointestinal mucosal denudement associated with these agents is critical because of the likelihood of infection with enteric intestinal flora. Moreover, pharmacokinetic considerations for drugs, such as methotrexate, which depend on an active membrane transport, make extension of exposure duration more attractive than dose escalation (Pinedo et al., 1977). The saturation kinetics of enzymes that activate nucleoside analogues are such that prolonging exposure rather than increasing dose beyond the threshold of these enzymes may also be preferable (Chabner, 1980).

Drugs suitable for consideration in high-dose regimens include the alkylating agents, the antitumor antibiotics, and the nitrosoureas. Almost all of these agents exhibit the exponential relationship between dose and cytoreduction upon which the success of intensive therapy is predicated (Bruce et al., 1966; Bruce et al., 1967; Salmon et al., 1978; Chabner, 1980). These agents also display relatively low gastrointestinal toxicity. For some drugs, such as the antibiotics and plant alkaloids, the toxicities have been predictable: cardiac (anthracyclines), neurologic (vinblastine), and lung (bleomycin). For other drugs, such as the alkylating agents, the toxicities have not been predicted in animal models, presumably owing to variation among species: lung (Cytoxan, BCNU), heart (Cytoxan), and liver (BCNU). In the selection of any chemotherapeutic agent for the intensive treatment of malignancy, the focus must be on the potential for success in treating the tumor, not necessarily on the agent that is most marrow–ablative.

From the preceding discussion two observations about high-dose chemotherapy can be made:

1. The neoplasm under treatment should be sensitive to chemotherapy at a higher dose; i.e., the tumor should have a steep dose–response curve.
2. The agents used must have some activity at a dose below which nonhematologic toxicity occurs.

SELECTED RESULTS IN SOLID TUMORS

Many studies in high-dose chemotherapy and autologous marrow support in solid tumors have explored the toxicities of single agents in Phase I type studies. Another avenue of investigation has been to examine escalation of combination chemotherapy in tumors that have failed standard therapy. Philip et al. (1982) have recently catalogued the published studies by tumor type.

For tumors that have demonstrated sensitivity to several myelosuppressive drugs, effective combinations have been compromised by the need to lower drug dosage and to avoid some active agents because of overlapping toxicities. The tumors for which intensification of combination chemotherapy coupled with autologous marrow support has yielded the best results are refractory non-Hodgkin's lymphomas. Appelbaum et al. (1978a,b) initially reported the results of intensive therapy with BACT (BCNU, Ară-C, Cytoxan, 6-thioguanine) in 22 patients with lymphoma refractory to combination chemotherapy. Of these patients, 18 were evaluable for response and ten patients achieved complete remission. Four patients with Burkitt's lymphoma were long-term responders (Appelbaum et al., 1978). Since this report more than 70 patients with refractory lymphoma have received intensive therapy with combination chemotherapy or a single agent with or without total body irradiation. The complete responses have been between 60% and 80% with these regimens. More importantly, up to one-third of these patients, most with Burkitt's lymphoma, are free of disease at 1 year (Philip et al., 1982).

Long-term responses have also been generated in other resistant solid tumors. Neuroblastoma has been treated with high-dose melphalan and intensive combination chemotherapy. Although the inability totally to irradicate residual disease with intensive therapy is disappointing, the low morbidity in this group allowed McElwain et al. (1979) to propose early additional treatment in this group. Theoretically, the ability to treat patients while their tumor burden is small can make a difference in response to therapy and cure. This is underscored by the increased survival seen in patients who attain remission with intensive therapy (Pritchard et al., 1982).

Nonseminomatous carcinoma of the testes is another solid tumor now considered curable with combination chemotherapy. A number of patients with refractory tumors have now been treated with a variety of intensive protocols. A common feature of these protocols is the utilization of alkylating agents in high doses. Although interpretation of these studies is hindered by the heterogeneity of intensive regimens and previous treatment, the early results are comparable with other salvage regimens (Philip et al., 1982). In these heavily pretreated patients, there is also a high rate of early death owing to treatment-related toxicities (Buckner et al., 1972; Tobias et al., 1977; Dover et al., 1981; Gorin et al., 1981; Bligham et al., 1981; Sarna et al., 1982; Gale, 1980; Spitzer et al., 1980).

Small cell carcinoma of the lung is presumed to be a suitable model for testing the effects of high-dose chemotherapy. This tumor has demonstrated a higher frequency of response to more intensive therapy (Cullen et al., 1977). Despite improvements in response, however, few patients survive beyond 2 years. A number of studies have examined intensive single agent or combination therapy in heavily treated patients who have failed to enter remission or have relapsed. Although nearly 90% of these patients will respond to these increasing doses, the responses are of short duration, with few patients alive 1 year after treatment (Philip et al., 1982; Buckner et al., 1972; Gale, 1980; Spitzer et al., 1980; Klatersky et al., 1982; Glade et al., 1982; Souhami et al., 1982; Dicke et al., 1980; Zander et al., 1981). Moreover, there are about 20% to 30% early deaths in this group, primarily related to progressive disease and treatment-related complications. Because of these failures in advanced disease, some investigators are examining the utility of including intensive therapy in induction regimens as a means of late intensification or even as initial therapy. The European Organization for Research and Therapy in Cancer (EOTRC) Lung Cancer Working Party reported their experience in 13 patients who had undergone induction with CAV and received intensification with the same regimen at higher doses with and without bone marrow support (Klatersky et al., 1982). There were two treatment-related deaths. Two patients had an upgrading of their response status from no response (NR) to partial response (PR) and PR to complete response (CR), respectively. Results from this study are comparable, but no better than reported standard therapy. Bone marrow support probably was not needed at most of the dosages used, and it is possible that further dose escalations would yield better tumor response. This has been the experience at the University of Colorado as well for small cell carcinoma of the lung (Glade et al., 1982). Souhami et al. (1982) have reported their experience with high-dose Cytoxan as initial therapy. No maintenance therapy was given in this study. When compared with combination chemotherapy, the results are encouraging as 81% of patients responded with 44% CR. Seven of the 16 patients remained relapse-free at the time of report. The patients who relapsed were sensitive to standard combination chemotherapy (Souhami et al., 1982). These results warrant further exploration.

As has been highlighted several times, more intensive therapy must overcome tumor resistance in order to be successful. Although the results previously reviewed are promising, one must realize that these tumors share the common feature of being sensitive to chemotherapy at standard dose. For the majority of solid tumors, curative chemotherapy is not available. Before high-dose therapy can have a role in the treatment of such tumors, activity of chemotherapeutic agents alone or in combination must be demonstrated.

Results from Phase I studies examining single agents in increasing dose are variable. In melanoma, for example, it is clear that agents such as AMSA have little activity at high dose and should not be pursued for this tumor (Philip et al., 1982). Melphalan, and most recently BCNU, have been used in the treatment of melanoma with some success. Over 30 patients have been treated with melphalan in high dose, with 60% of patients responding and 20% enjoying CR (Philip et al., 1982; McElwain et al., 1979). Phillips et al. (1983) have recently reported 32 patients treated with BCNU; although there were three toxic deaths, 14 patients responded and five entered complete remission.

Melphalan in high dose has also been used with some success in another tumor for which curative chemotherapy is not available, adenocarcinoma of the colon. Nine patients with metastatic colon carcinoma have been treated with melphalan at a dose of 180 mg/M^2 with autologous marrow given 24 hr later. Of six evaluable patients, five have had greater than 50% reduction in tumor size (Knight et al., 1983). These data, while exciting, are still preliminary and require confirmation. What may be taken from these early results obtained in refractory neoplasms is an indication that occasional tumors that are considered refractory may respond to chemotherapy at a higher dose.

CONCLUSIONS AND FUTURE DIRECTIONS

There are several requirements for the use of high-dose chemotherapy and autologous marrow infusion.

1. The neoplasm should be sensitive to more intensive therapy than to conventional therapy.
2. The choice of agents should be made on the basis of their extent of activity against the tumor.
3. The use of autologous marrow should be restricted to agents/regimens that produce myelosuppression lasting longer than 2–3 weeks because the

hematopoietic recovery for stem cells infused in autologous marrow requires 14–21 days.

4. The collection of marrow should occur at a time when contamination with cancer cells will be minimal.

The oncologist must be cognizant of these requirements when developing protocols to evaluate intensive chemotherapy for selected tumors because the group at risk and natural history for a given tumor may preclude them from such therapy. These criteria become even more important in the selection of individual patients. Although the age restrictions that apply for allogeneic bone marrow transplantation are not as rigid for autologous protocols, performance status is a critical consideration in determining eligibility. Because intensive chemotherapy frequently demonstrates dose-limiting toxicity in the form of cardiac or pulmonary complications, patients must be selected carefully (Buckner et al., 1972; Hronin et al., 1980; Spitzer et al., 1979). Moreover, they must be capable of enduring the consequences of prolonged aplasia.

The limited studies with single agents performed to date suggest that only moderate increments in dose can be made prior to limiting toxicity to other organ systems. For most agents, increases rarely exceed three times the maximum dose. Escalation of this magnitude is unlikely to impact the response of solid tumors. These single-agent studies are imperative, however, because the experience with conventional therapy can predict neither the spectrum of activity nor the extramedullary toxicity seen at high dose. Even with the modest response and short duration of the CR that are achieved, it may be that once activities and toxicities are defined, intensive protocols utilizing combinations of agents in high dose will provide durable responses.

What is now clear is that patients can be successfully rescued from what is presumed to be marrow-ablative therapy, allowing the investigation of more intensive therapy in overcoming the resistance seen in many solid tumors. It is also clear that selected tumors, such as the non-Hodgkin's lymphomas will respond to high dose chemotherapy.

As has been noted, the morbidity and mortality rates of intensive regimens are directly related to the duration of aplasia. Even if intensive therapy is not marrow lethal, autologous marrow infusion may be useful in hastening hematologic recovery, thereby decreasing morbidity. Presumably, there may be a long-term advantage in repopulating marrow with stem cells that have been protected from intensive chemotherapy. As a rule, physicians have a tendency to underestimate the capacity of bone marrow to regenerate, and the exact role of this expensive support technique remains to be defined. The definition can be achieved only through Phase I studies of single agents given in increasing doses.

When innovative therapies become available, it is common to utilize them first in the care of patients with high tumor burdens and refractory disease. As the boundaries of such therapies become defined, then they are utilized earlier in the course of disease. Whether high-dose chemotherapy will ultimately prove beneficial in the treatment of solid tumors remains to be seen. It is likely that once the activity of single agents given at high dose is defined for a given tumor, intensive chemotherapy may be useful either as initial treatment or as a mechanism for early intensification in some tumors.

REFERENCES

Appelbaum, F.R., Deisseroth, A.B., Graw, R.G., Herzig, G.P., Levine, A.S., Magrath, I.T., Pizzo, P.A., Poplack, D.G., Ziegler, J.L. (1978a). Prolonged complete remission following high dose chemotherapy of Burkitt's lymphoma in relapse. *Cancer, 41*:1059–1063.

Appelbaum, F.R., Herzig, G.P., Ziegler, J.L., Graw, R.G., Levine, A.S., & Deisseroth, A.B. (1978b). Successful engraftment of cryopreserved autologous bone marrow in patients with malignant lymphoma. *Blood, 52*:85–95.

Barnes, D.W.H., & Lootit, J.F. (1954). The radiation recovery factor: Preservation by the Polge-Smith-Parks technique. *Journal of the National Cancer Institute, 15*:901–905.

Bligham, G., Spitzer, G., Litan, J., Zanter, A.R., Verma, D.S., Vellekoop, L., Samuels, M.L., McCredle, K.B., & Dicke, K.A. (1981). The treatment of advanced testicular carcinoma with high dose chemotherapy and autologous marrow support. *Environmental Journal of Cancer, 17*:441–443.

Bodey, G.P., Buckley, M., Sathe, Y.S., & Freireich, E.J. (1966). Quantitative relationships between circulating leukocytes and infection in patients with leukemia. *Annals of Internal Medicine, 64*:328–340.

Bonadonna, G., & Valagossa, P. (1980). Dose response effect of CMF in breast cancer. *Proceedings of the American Society of Clinical Oncology, 21*:413.

Brindley, C.O., Salvin, L.G., Potee, K.G., Lipowska, B., Shinder, B.I., Regelson, W., & Colsky, J. (1964). Further comparative trial of thio-phosphoramide and mechlorethamine in patients with melanoma and Hodgkin's disease. *Journal of Chronic Diseases, 17*:19.

Bross, I., Rimm, A.A., Slack, W.H., Ausman, R.K., & Jones, R. (1966). Is toxicity really necessary? *Cancer, 19*:1780–1804.

Bruce, W.B., Valeriote, F.A., & Merker, B.E. (1967). Survival of mice bearing a transplanted syngeneic lymphoma following treatment with cyclophosphamide, 5-fluorouracil, or 1,3-bis (2 chloroethyl)-1-nitrosourea. *Journal of the National Cancer Institute, 39*:257–266.

Bruce, W.R., Meeker, B.E., & Valeriote, F.A. (1966). Comparison of the sensitivity of normal hematopoietic and transplanted lymphoma colony-forming cells to chemotherapeutic agents in vivo. *Journal of the National Cancer Institute, 37*:233–245.

Buckner, C.D., Rudolph, R.H., Fefer, A., Cliff, R.A., Epstein, R.B., Funk, D.D., Neiman, P.E., Skichler, J.J., Storb, R., & Thomas, E.D. (1972). High dose cyclophosphamide therapy for malignant disease. *Cancer, 29*:357–365.

Chabner, B.A. (1980). Pharmacological considerations in autologous bone marrow transplant regimens. In Gale, R.P., & Fox, C.F. (Eds.), *Biology of bone marrow transplantation* (pp. 37–143). San Diego: Academic Press.

Clifford, P., Clift, R.A., & Duff, J.K. (1961). Nitrogen mustard therapy combined with autologous marrow infusion. *Lancet, 1*:687–690.

Cohen, M.H., Creavan, P.J., Fossieck, B.E., Jr., Broder, L.E., Selawry, O.S., Johnston, A.V., Williams, C.L., & Minna, J.D. (1977). Intensive chemotherapy of small cell bronchogenic carcinoma. *Cancer Treatment Reports, 61*:349–354.

Cullen, M.H., Creaven, P.S., Fossieck, J.R., Brodes, L.E., Dewary, O.S., Johnston, A.R., Williams, C.L., & Minna, J.D. (1977). Intensive chemotherapy of small cell bronchogenic carcinoma. *Cancer Treatment Reports 61*:349–353.

Deisseroth, A., & Abrams, R. A. (1979). The role of autologous stem cell reconstitution in intensive therapy for resistant neoplasms. *Cancer Treatment Reports 63*:461–471.

DeVita, V.T., Serpick, A., & Carbone, P.P. (1970). Combination chemotherapy in the treatment of advanced Hodgkin's disease. *Annals of Internal Medicine, 73*:881–895.

DeVita, V.T., Jr., Young, R.C., & Canellos, G.P. (1975). Combination versus single agent chemotherapy: A review of the basis for selection of drug treatment of cancer. *Cancer, 35*:98–110.

Dicke, K.A., Vellekoop, L., Spitzer, G., Zander, A.R., Schell, F., & Verma, D.S. (1980). Autologous bone marrow transplantation in neoplasia. Gale, R.P., and Fox, C.F., (eds.). In *Biology of bone marrow transplantation*, (pp. 159–165). San Diego, Academic Press.

Dover, D., Champlin, R.E., Ho, W.N., Sarna, G.P., Wells, J.H., Graze, P.R., Cline, M.J., & Gale, R.P. (1981). High dose combined modality therapy and autologous bone marrow transplantation in resistant cancer. *American Journal of Medicine, 71*:973–976.

Frei, E. III, & Canellos, G.P. (1980). Dose: A critical factor in cancer chemotherapy. *American Journal of Medicine, 69*:585–593.

Frei, E. III, Spurr, C.L., Brindley, C.O., Selawry, D., Holland, J.F., Rall, D.P., Wasserman, L.R., Houystralen, B., Shnider, B.I., McIntyre, O.R., Matthews, L.B., & Miller, S.P. (1965). Clinical studies of dichloromethotrexate (NSC 29630). *Clinical Pharmacology and Therapeutics, 6*:160–171.

Gale, R.P. (1980). Autologous bone marrow transplantation in patients with cancer. *Journal of the American Medical Association, 243*:540–542.

Gehan, E., & Coltman, C. (1980). Southwest Oncology Group unpublished observations.

Glade, L.M., Robinson, W.A., Hartmann, D.W., Klein, J.J., Thomas, M.R., & Morton, W. (1982). Autologous bone marrow transplantation in the therapy of small cell carcinoma of the lung. *Cancer Research, 42*:4270–4275.

Gorin, W.C., David, R., Stachowiak, J., Salmon, C., Petit, J.C., Parlier, Y., Najman, A., & Duhamel, G. (1981) High dose chemotherapy and autologous bone marrow transplantation in acute leukemias, malignant lymphomas and solid tumors. *Environmental Journal of Cancer, 17*:557–568.

Henderson, E.S., & Samayo, R.J. (1969). Evidence that drugs in multiple combinations have materially advanced the treatment of human malignancies. *Cancer Research, 29*:2272–2280.

Herzig, G.P. (1981). Autologous marrow transplantation in cancer chemotherapy. *Progress in Hematology, 12*:1–23.

Hronin, P.A., Mahaley, M.S., & Rudnick, S.A. (1980). Prediction of BCNU toxicity in patients with malignant glioma: An assessment of risk factors. *New England Journal of Medicine, 303*:183–188.

Klatersky, J., Wicaise, C., Longerail, E., Stryckman, P., & the EOTRC Lung Cancer Working Party. (1982). Cisplatinum, adriamycin, and etoposide (CAV) for remission induction in small cell carcinoma of the lung. *Cancer, 50*:652–658.

Knight, W.A., III, Page, C.P., Kuhn, J.G., Clark, G.M., Bell, B.S., & Newcomb, T.F. (1983). High dose melphalan with autologous bone marrow infusion in Dukes D colorectal carcinoma. *Proceedings of the American Society of Clinical Oncology, 2*:118A.

Kornick, W.B., Montano, A., Gerdes, J.C., & Feder, B.H. (1958). Preliminary observations on the treatment of postirradiation hematopoietic depression in man by the infusion of stored autogenous bone marrow. *Annals of Internal Medicine, 49*:973–986.

Lewis, B.J., & DeVita, V.T. (1978). Combination chemotherapy of the lymphomas. *Seminars in Hematology, 15*:431–462.

Major, P. (1970). Cryobiology: The freezing of biological systems. *Science, 168*:939–949.

McElwain, T.J., Hedley, D.W., Burton, G., Clink, H.M., Gordon, M.Y., Jarman, M., Juttner, C.A., Millar, J.L., Milstead, R.A.V., Prentice, G., Smith, I.E., Spence, D., & Woods, M. (1979). Marrow autotransplantation accelerates haematological recovery in patients with malignant melanoma treated with high dose melphalan. *British Journal of Cancer, 40*:72–80.

McFarland, W.F., Granville, W.B., & Dameshek, W. (1959). Autologous bone marrow infusion as an adjunct in therapy of malignant disease. *Blood, 260*:675–683.

McGovern, J.J., Jr., Russell, P.S., Atkins, L., & Webster, E. (1959). Treatment of terminal leukemia relapse by total body irradiation and intravenous infusion of stored autologous bone marrow obtained during remission. *New England Journal of Medicine, 260*:675–683.

Newton, L.A., Humble, J.B., Wilson, C.W., Pegg, D.E., & Skinner, M.E.G. (1959). Total thoracic supervoltage irradiation followed by the intravenous infusion of stored autogenous marrow. *British Medical Journal, 1*:531–535.

Pegg, D.E., Humble, J.G., & Newton, K.A. (1962). The clinical application of bone marrow grafting. *British Journal of Cancer, 16*:417–435.

Philip, T., Herve, P., Racadot, E., Cahn, J.Y., Biron, P., Brunat-Mentigny, M., Peters, A., & Mayer, M. (1982). Intensive cytoreductive regimen and autologous bone marrow transplantation in leukemia and solid tumors (a review): Immunology of transplantation, *Excerpta Medica, 14*: 89–109.

Phillips, G.L., Fay, J.W., Herzig, G.P., Herzig, R.H., Weiner, R.S., Wolff, S.N., Lazarus, H.M., Karanes, C., Ross, W.E., & Kramer, B.S. (1983). A Phase I–II study: Intensive BCNU and cryopreserved autologous marrow transplantation for refractory cancer. *Cancer, 52*:1792–1802.

Pinedo, H.R., Bull, J.M., Zaharko, D.S., & Chabner, B.A. (1977). The relative contribution of drug concentration and duration of exposure to mouse bone marrow toxicity during continuous methotrexate infusion. *Cancer Research, 37*:445–447.

Pinkel, D., Harnandez, K., Bovella, L., Holton, C., Aur, R., Samoy, G., & Pratt, C. (1971). Drug dose and remission duration in childhood lymphocytic leukemia. *Cancer, 27*:247–256.

Pritchard, J., McElwain, T.J., & Graham, B.L.J. (1982). High dose melphalan with autologous marrow for treatment of advanced neuroblastoma. *British Journal of Cancer, 45*:86–94

Salmon, S.E., Hamburger, A.W., Soehnlen, B., Durie, B.G.M., Alberts, D.S., & Moon, T.E. (1978). Quantitation of differential sensitivity of human tumor stem cells to anticancer drugs. *New England Journal of Medicine, 298*:1321–1327.

Sarna, G.P., Champlin, R., Wells, J., & Gale, R.P. (1982). Phase I study of high dose mitomycin with autologous bone marrow support. *Cancer Treatment Reports, 66*:277–282.

Schlater, M. (1972). Drugs that modify cellular responses to low temperature. *Federation Proceedings, 36*:2950–2959.

Skipper, H.E. (1978). Reasons for success and failure in treatment of murine leukemias with the drugs now employed in treating human leukemias. In *Cancer chemotherapy*, Vol. 1 (pp. 1–166). Ann Arbor, MI: University Microfilms International.

Skipper, H.E., Schlabel, F.M. Jr., Mellet, L.B., Montgomery, J.A., Willkoff, L.J., Lloyd,

A.H., & Brockman, R.W. (1950). Implications of biochemical, cytokinetic, pharmacologic and toxicologic relationships in the design of optional therapeutic schedules. *Cancer Chemotherapy Reports, 54*:431–450.

Skipper, H.E., Schlabel, F.M., Jr., & Wilcox, W.S. (1964). Experimental evaluation of potential anticancer agents. XII. On the criteria and kinetics associated with "curability" of experimental leukemia. *Cancer Chemotherapy Reports 35*:1–111.

Souhami, R.L., Harper, P.G., Linch, D., Trask, C., Golstone, A.H., Tobias, J.L., Spiro, S.G., Gedeles, D.M., Richards, J.D.M. (1982). High dose cyclophosphamide with autologous marrow transplantation as initial treatment of small cell carcinoma of the bronchus. *Cancer Chemotherapy and Pharmacology, 8*:31–34.

Spitzer, G., Dicke, K.A., Litam, J., Verna, S., Zander, A., Lanzotti, V., Valdirieso, M., McCredle, K.B., & Samuels, M.L. (1980). High dose combination chemotherapy with autologous bone marrow transplantation in adult solid tumors. *Cancer, 43*:3075–3085.

Spitzer, G., Dicke, K.A., Verma, D.S., Zander, A., & McCredle, K.B. (1979). High dose BCNU therapy with autologous bone marrow infusion. *Cancer Treatment Reports, 63*:1257–1264.

Steel, G.G. (1977). Growth and survival of tumor stem cells. In *Growth kinetics of tumors*. Oxford: Clarendon Press.

Tattersall, M.H.N., & Tobias, J.S. (1976). How strong is the case for intensive cancer chemotherapy? *Lancet, 2*:1071–1072.

Thomas, E.D., Buckner, C.D., Banaji, M., Cliff, R.A., Fefer, A., Flournay, W., Goodell, B., Hickman, R.D., Lerner, K.G., Weiman, P.E., Sale, G.E., Sanders, J.E., Singer, J., Stevens, M., Sturb, R., Weiden, P.L. (1977). One hundred patients with acute leukemia treated by chemotherapy, total body irradiation, and allogeneic marrow transplantation. *Blood, 49*:511–533.

Thomas, E.D., Sturb, R., Cliff, R.A., Fefer, A., Johnson, L., Neiman, P.E., Lerner, K.G., & Glucksburg, H. (1975). Bone marrow transplantation. *New England Journal of Medicine 292*:832–902.

Thomas, E.D., & Sturb, R. (1970). Technique for human marrow grating. *Blood, 36*:507–515.

Tobias, J.S., Weiner, R.S., Griffiths, C.T., Richman, C.M., Parker, L.M., & Yankee, R.A. (1977). Cryopreserved autologous marrow infusion following high dose cancer chemotherapy. *European Journal of Cancer, 13*:269–277.

Van Patten, L.M. (1965). Quantitative aspects of the storage of bone marrow cells for transplanation. *European Journal of Cancer, 1*: 15–22.

Young, R.C., Canellos, G.P., Chabner, B.A., Schein, P.S., & DeVita, V.T. (1973). Maintenance chemotherapy for advanced Hodgkin's disease in remission. *Lancet, 1*:1339.

Young, R.C., Chabner, B.A., Hubbard, S.P., Canellos, G.P., & DeVita, V.T. (1975). Preliminary results of trials of chemotherapy in advanced ovarian carcinoma. *National Cancer Institute Monographs, 42*:145–148.

Zander, A.R., Spitzer, G., Vellekoop, L., Verma, D., Minhaar, G., & Dicke, K.A. (1981). New developments in bone marrow transplantation. *Cancer Bulletin, 33*:286–295.

PART III
Pharmacological Aspects of Cancer in the Elderly

8

Age-Related Changes in Drug Disposition

Linda S. Birnbaum

The elderly represent not only the fastest growing segment of our population, but the largest users of drugs (Reidenberg, 1980). Altered therapeutic responses are often observed in older people (Ouslander, 1981). Evidence has accumulated suggesting that adverse reactions and altered responsiveness increase with age (Sellers et al., 1983). Such changes can result from either pharmacokinetic or pharmacodynamic factors, i.e., what the body does to the drug or what the drug does to the body, respectively. Recent experimental work has suggested that the effect of drugs at the target site may show age-related changes in receptor number or affinity (Rogh & Hess, 1982). However, changes in tissue sensitivity are not the subject of this review. Rather, the focus is on the hypothesis that changes in drug disposition that occur during the aging process result in altered concentrations of drugs at the site of action leading to variations in drug response. There have been a number of reviews on this topic (Blumberg, 1985; Schmucker, 1979, 1985; Sellers et al., 1983). Therefore, the emphasis will be on recent results in experimental animals with the potential for extrapolation to the human situation.

Drug disposition can be divided into four stages: absorption, distribution, metabolism, and excretion. At times the last two stages may be grouped under the heading of elimination because both result in the removal of the parent chemical from the body. However, although early studies of drug metabolism viewed this process as one of detoxification, current knowledge reveals that biotransformation may often result in activation of a compound to a toxic metabolite. Therefore, it is more helpful to consider metabolism as a process distinct from excretion. These pharmacokinetic parameters will be discussed in relation to the aging process.

ABSORPTION

Absorption can be defined as the processes in which an exogenous chemical enters the bloodstream. Thus, absorption is 100% when compounds are given intravenously, (IV). However, for most environmental chemicals as well as most drugs exposure is *via* the oral, dermal, or respiratory route. Very little is known about age-related changes in pulmonary absorption. There appears to be a slight reduction of respiratory efficiency in old hamsters or rats but no dramatic loss of lung function with age (Mauderly, 1979a, 1982). This is in contrast to the linear decline observed in both humans and dogs (Mauderly, 1979b). The actual rate of gas exchange across the air sacs into the pulmonary capillaries has been shown to be reduced with age in humans and dogs (Mauderly, 1979b). It appears difficult to extrapolate from small laboratory animals to humans to understand age-related changes in pulmonary absorption.

The data on age-related changes in dermal absorption are also limited. It is known that the structure of skin changes throughout the life span. In humans, skin thickness increases during maturation and then decreases with advancing age (Vogel, 1983). A similar decrease was observed in skin thickness of aged rats. However, this thinning does not appear to compromise the barrier ability of senescent human skin (Lauker et al., 1987).

Behl et al. (1987) have recently reviewed the influence of age on the percutaneous absorption of drugs. The most dramatic age effects observed *in vivo* occur between the neonatal and young adulthood period and involve the structure of the skin itself. Skin of infants is much more permeable than that of any other age group. After maturity absorption appears to decline. Christophers and Kligman (1965) observed a 67% decrease in the dermal absorption of testosterone in young (24 years) as compared to old (75 years) humans. Similar results were observed *in vitro* for tri-*n*-propylphosphate (Marzulli, 1962). There are few studies on the effects of senescence on dermal absorption in experimental animals. Kohn (1969) observed a decrease in the absorption of Evans blue dye in old rats as compared to middle-aged rats. Using the hairless mouse as a model, Behl and co-workers (1987) have shown that permeability reaches a maximum value around weaning, declines sharply during maturation, and remains relatively constant from young adulthood through senescence. This pattern was shown to be the same for simple straight-chain alcohols, as well as hydrocortisone (Behl et al., 1984). No sex-related differences were observed. Recent studies from our laboratory (Banks, Brewster, & Birnbaum, unpublished) have shown an age-related decrease in the dermal absorption of 2,3,4,7,8-pentachlorodibenzofuran, a potent promotor of hepatocarcinogenesis (Nishizumi and Masuda, 1986), closely related in structure and toxicity to 2,3,7,8-tetrachlorodibenzo-*p*-dioxin (TCDD; dioxin). Whether these changes are due to structural differences in the skin or to changes in clearance owing to an alteration in blood flow with age, as suggested earlier by Christophers and Kligman (1965), remains to be determined.

Most emphasis in both experimental animals and humans has been on age-related changes in oral absorption. There are several physiologic changes that occur in the gastrointestinal (GI) tract that could impact on absorption. These changes include increased gastric pH, decreased splanchnic blood flow, decreased absorptive surface area, and reduced motility of the GI tract.

The gastric pH affects not only the ionizability but also the solubility of certain drugs. Therefore, the age-related decrease in acid secretion in the stomach, resulting in a rise in pH, can result in altered drug absorption after oral exposure (Israeli and Wenger, 1981; Kekki et al., 1982). This could contribute to a reduction in gastric motility, resulting in an increase in transit time through the gut. Varga (1976) observed age-related delay in transit through the large intestines in old as compared to young rats. Lin and Hayton (1983) observed a similar increase in transit time through the small intestine when comparing middle-aged to senescent rats. However, no evidence was found for a decrease in the rate of gastric emptying. A slower rate of transport might compensate for the age-related decline in splanchnic blood flow owing to reduced cardiac output (Varga & Csakey, 1977). However, although subepithelial blood flow through the intestines appears to decrease during maturation (Csakey & Varga, 1975), there is no evidence of a further decline with senescence (Lin & Hayton, 1983).

Structural changes have also been reported in the absorptive surface of the intestines. A recent report has indicated that the intestinal mucosa represent a significantly larger proportion of the intestinal weight in old than in young rats (Hebert and Birnbaum, 1987). This is compatible with the study of Holt et al. (1984) who observed that total small intestinal length, weight, and gut mucosal mass were greater in old than in young rats. However, these workers observed that the epithelial cells might be functioning less effectively. Such a phenomenon would clearly impact on the absorptive capacity of the intestines.

Oral absorption can occur either *via* active or passive processes unlike the situation in the skin or lungs in which diffusion provides the only mechanism for absorption. Many small molecules are actively transported from the intestinal lumen into the blood. In elderly people the active transport of galactose, calcium, thiamine, and iron is reduced (Reidenberg, 1980). Similar decreases have been observed for rats in the active absorption of glucose (Birnbaum, 1987; Eastin & Lindi et al., 1985; Vinardell & Bolufer, 1984) as well as calcium and phosphorus (Ambrecht, 1986). However, passive transport, i.e., simple diffusion, of glucose shows no age-related decline (Eastin & Birnbaum, 1987). Most foreign chemicals are absorbed passively, and a recent study using the highly toxic environmental contaminant TCDD revealed no effect of age on its intestinal absorption (Hebert & Birnbaum, 1987). In contrast, the intestinal absorption of endogenous lipophilic compounds such as cholesterol (Hollander & Morgan, 1979a), vitamin A (Hollander & Morgan, 1979b), and oleic acid (Hollander & Dadufalza, 1983) appears to increase with age in rats, possibly owing to changes in the unstirred water layer. However, more recent studies from the same laboratory revealed that age did not affect vitamin A absorption in mice (Hollander et al., 1986), which is in agreement with the results of Fleming and Barrows (1982a) in rats. Absorption of vitamins D, B_{12}, and niacin have also been shown to remain unchanged during aging (Fleming & Barrows, 1982a,b). Conflicting results have also been reported concerning amino acid absorption and aging. Penzes (1974a,b) observed no change in the absorption of neutral or basic amino acids between young, middle-aged, and senescent rats. More recent studies, however, have shown that older animals have a decreased absorption of tyrosin (Huang et al., 1985; Navab et al., 1984). In humans absorption of xylose only declines in senescence (Mayersohn, 1982). However, the functional significance of this observation is open to question (Weiner et al., 1984) because aged humans do not usually suffer from carbohydrate malabsorption. Age-related changes in the oral absorption of a variety of drugs have not been observed (Castleden et al., 1977).

DISTRIBUTION

Various factors can affect the manner in which drugs and other chemicals are distributed throughout the body. These include changes in body size and composition, plasma protein binding of drugs, and blood flow. Changes in body composition include a decrease in the lean body mass in the elderly (Edelman et al., 1952). This is coupled with an increase in the amount of body fat (Novack, 1972) and a loss in body water (Edelman and Leibman, 1959). Such changes in body composition may influence the volume of distribution (Vd) of compounds, affecting the concentration reaching the target site. For drugs that are relatively water-soluble, their tissue distribution may be less extensive in the elderly. For lipophilic compounds, however, the increase in adipose tissue may result in a larger Vd.

Similar changes in body composition occur in aging animals (Lesser et al., 1973). Whereas young adult rats generally have between 6% and 12% of the body weight as fat (depending on strain and sex differences), senescent Sprague-Dawley rats have been reported to have as much as 34% of their body weight as dissectable adipose tissue (Birnbaum, 1983), which resulted in increased retention of the highly lipophilic environmental pollutants polychlorinated biphenyls in old as compared to young rats. York (1982) observed a negative relationship between the percent of body water and increasing age, 59% in young adults versus 49% in senescent rats. This change in body composition resulting in a decrease in Vd appeared to explain the greater ethanol sensitivity observed in old rats. Similar observations were made by Yang et al. (1984) concerning the pharmacokinetic behavior of ethylenediamine. The Vd decreased with age for this chemical resulting in higher blood levels and potentially greater toxicity in the older rats during chronic exposure. The opposite result was reported following long-term exposure to methylchloroform, an extremely lipophilic volatile solvent (Schumann et al., 1982). An increase in the body burden was mainly attributable to an increase in the Vd of this compound.

Changes in plasma protein binding can also influence the distribution of many compounds, especially those that are extensively bound. Most drugs are transported in the blood in bound form, but it is only the free drug that can exert its effect at the target site. Albumin is the major binding protein in the blood, and its concentration has been reported to decrease in both aging humans (Bender et al., 1975; Wallace et al., 1976) and mice (Rogers & Gass, 1983). However, albumin synthesis actually increases during senescence (Van Benzooijen, 1984) in aging rats, whereas total plasma albumin levels remain unchanged (Horback et al., 1983).

As mentioned earlier in regard to gastrointestinal absorption, cardiac output declines with age. The pattern of blood flow also changes with the proportions of cardiac output received by the kidneys, skin, GI tract, and liver decreasing in older rats (Yates & Hiley, 1979). Such reductions in blood flow will clearly alter the distribution of compounds to and from these tissues.

METABOLISM

Age-dependent changes in the metabolism of drugs in both humans and experimental animals have been recently reviewed (Birnbaum, 1987; Schmucker, 1985; Van Bezooijen, 1984). There were few general patterns that emerged from these analyses other than that age, species, strain, and sex all contributed to the metabolic picture. For a given compound metabolism might decrease, increase, or remain unchanged with age. Most of the available information concerned hepatic metabolism, but some data are available from other organs, including kidney, lungs, and intestines. The focus here is on the most recent findings not previously reviewed.

Contradictory age-related changes have been reported to occur in the components of the mixed-function oxidase (MFO) system. Recently, it has become clear that the major changes observed in rats in cytochrome P450 are due to an age-related loss in the male-specific forms (Kamataki et al., 1985; Sun et al., 1986). This may be a result of the decrease in circulating testosterone in old male rats. Specific changes in inducibility were also observed, with hepatic cytochrome P450c being less inducible by β-naphthoflavone in old rats while induction of cytochrome P450b by phenobarbital did not change with age (Sun et al., 1986). In contrast to liver, cytochrome P450c was more inducible in colon, kidney, and lung tissue from old rats as compared to young rats (Sun & Stobel, 1986). NADPH cytochrome c (P450) reductase activity has been reported to decrease from young to middle-aged to old rats (Devasagayam, 1986). In contrast, no decline was observed in this enzyme in the Rhesus monkey (Schmucker & Wang, 1987). The third component, lipid, was recently examined by Baird and Hough (1987) who observed no changes in the sensitivity of cytochrome P450 to phospholipase digestion, suggesting no major changes in membrane structure in aged rats.

Several recent studies have also examined the effect of aging on coordinated

MFO activities. Hepatic microsomes from senescent rats (Prasanna et al., 1986) were less able to demethylate the potent hepatocarcinogen dimethylnitrosamine. This could be attributed to an age-related decrease in cytochrome P450. However-rats. Metabolism of the local anesthetic bupivacaine decreased in senescent rats (Thompson et al., 1987), as did that of p-nitro-anisol (Galinsky et al., 1986; Sweeney & Weiner, 1986). Metabolism of haloperidol and phenobarbital also appears to decline in old rats (Kapetanovic et al., 1982a,b). In contrast, the metabolism of the carcinogen benzo(a)pyrene (BP) increased in lung, kidney, and colon of old rats (Sun & Strobel, 1986). Although colonic metabolism of BP increased throughout the age span evaluated of rats, no change was detected in this activity in small intestines (McMahon et al., 1987). Phenobarbital induction of BP hydroxylation was greater in the colon of old than young rats (Sun & Strobel, 1986). Recent studies from humans also indicate that the ability of oxidative metabolism to be induced is maintained in old age (Vestal et al., 1987).

Alcohol dehydrogenase activity was examined in livers from aging male and female rats using allyl alcohol as the substrate. Whereas the activity increased 35% in middle-aged and 53% in old male rats as compared to young adult males, no change with age was observed in the females (Rikans & Moore, 1987). No change with age was seen in ADH activity in the colon of male rats (McMahon et al., 1987).

The activity of Phase II enzymes, those involved in conjugation or deconjugating the primary metabolites, may also change with age. Recent studies have indicated that conjugation of glutathione with the model substrate 1-chloro-2,4-dinitro-benzene remains unchanged in the liver (Galinsky ct al., 1986), and declines in the colon (McMahon et al., 1987). This occurred without a decrease in colonic glutathione concentrations. Hepatic glutathione conjugation with the oxidative product of aflatoxin B_1 also decreased in old rats (Prasanna et al., 1986). A smiliar decline in the conjugation of glutathione with sulfobromophthalein was observed in old male, but not female, rats in liver cytosol (Kanai et al., 1985).

Age-related changes in sulfate conjugation are also substrate-specific. Sulpho-transferase activity declines with age in rat hepatocytes when p-nitrophenol (PNP) is the substrate (Sweeney and Weiner, 1986), and in hepatic cytosol preparations with acetaminophen-phenol as the sulfate acceptor (Galinsky et al., 1986). Similar results were observed *in vivo* in which the fraction of the administered dose recovered as the acetaminophen-sulfate decreased with age (Galinsky & Corcoran, 1986). In contrast, sulfation of the bile salt glycolithocholate doubled in senescent male rats as compared to young or middle-aged animals (Galinsky et al., 1986). Support for the presence of at least two distinct sulphotransferases in respect to changes with age come from the studies of Iwasaki et al. (1986). Using β-naphthol as a phenol substrate, these workers observed a decrease in its conjugation with sulfate in old males but an increase in female rats with age. In contrast, sulpho-conjugation with an alcohol, tiaramide, and several amines, including desmethylimipramine, increased in the senescent males while remaining unchanged in aging females. Thus, sulphoconjugation of phenolic groups in rat liver differs temporarily from that of amines and alcoholic groups.

The opposite effects caused by aging on the metabolism of substrates metabolized by different conjugation enzymes is also observed in the glucuronyl transferases. At least three patterns of age-related changes have been observed. Conjugation of estrone by rat liver microsomes and of acetaminophen *in vivo* with glucuronic acid was shown to increase with age (Galinsky et al., 1986; Galinsky & Corcoran, 1986). No change with age was observed, however, when naphthol, morphine, or testosterone were the substrate for UDPGA conjugation by rat liver microsomes (Galinsky et al., 1986) or with PNP when rat hepatocytes were used (Sweeny and Weiner, 1986). In contrast, Borghoff et al. (1987) observed a decrease in the formation of the glucuronide of 4,4'thiobis-(6-*t*-butyl-m-cresol), a major antioxidant in the rubber industry. This decline occurred both *in vivo* and *in vitro*. The conjugation of PNP with glucuronic acid also showed a decrease in microsomes from the colon of aging rats (McMahon et al., 1987). The levels of the cofactor, UDPGA, were shown to drop in senescent rats (Borghoff et al., 1987), suggesting that this factor, along with a decrease in glucuronyl transferase activity, would limit *in vivo* glucuronidation.

Another possible route of metabolism that could be affected with age is deconjugation, which releases the oxidized (less polar) metabolites. One enzyme involved in this reaction is beta-glucuronidase (BG), which is primarily a lysosomal enzyme. Its activity has been shown to increase with age in rat hepatocytes (Van Manen et al., 1983). However, McMahon et al. (1987) failed to observe any change in BG activity in cytosol from the large intestines of rats.

Thus, as concluded in other reviews published recently (Birnbaum, 1987; Schmucker, 1985; Van Benzooijen, 1984), there are few generalities that can be made *a priori* about age-related changes in drug metabolism. The recent observation of major age differences really being sex-linked in the rat does raise the need for caution in extrapolating any changes observed in rodents to the human situation.

EXCRETION

There are three major routes of excretion: renal; hepatic; and pulmonary. In addition, there are minor routes involving hair, sweat, and saliva as well as sex-linked routes such as milk. For certain classes of compounds, these routes may play a major role in reducing the body burden of a chemical. However, sex-linked routes are not appreciable in senescence. There is little, it anything, known about age-related changes in the function of the minor routes, although parameters such as hair growth do change with age.

The pulmonary route plays a role in the elimination of volatiles and gases, either parent compound or metabolites such as carbon monoxide or carbon dioxide. Therefore, changes in age-related pulmonary physiology (Mauderly, 1982) will affect excretion in an opposite way in which such changes impact on absorption. For example, although a decreased rate of respiration may impede absorption of an inhaled chemical, it will also slow exhalation. A recent study with methylchloroform, a poorly metabolized solvent, indicated that age-related changes in its disposition in rats and mice were in part related to a decreased rate of pulmonary elimination (Schumann et al., 1982). There is also data suggesting that blood flow to the lungs, as a percentage of total cardiac output, may actually increase with age (Yates & Hiley, 1979).

The major function of the kidney is elimination of wastes from the body. An impairment of renal function with age has long been known (Davies & Shock, 1950; McLachlan, 1978). Much of the age-related decline in renal function is due to a reduction in blood flow to the kidney resulting in a lower glomerular filtration rate (Schmucker, 1979, 1985). There is also an age-related decrease in the number of functional nephrons. Therefore, for drugs subject to renal clearance, physicians must anticipate a need to reduce dosage to prevent accumulation and hence toxicity (Sellers et al., 1983).

The kidneys of aging experimental animals, especially rats, are compromised with advancing age. Chronic glomerulonephropathy is a common age-related change occurring in laboratory rodents (Coleman et al., 1977). Yacobi et al. (1982) observed a decrease in the renal elimination of N-acetylprocainamide, a major metabolite of the anti-arrhythmia drug procainamide, during a 2-year chronic toxicity study in rats. Similarly, Young and Norvell (1984) observed decreased renal elimination of 2-acetylaminofluorene in old mice following 18 months of treatment.

Elimination of many compounds in the kidney occurs, in addition to ultrafiltration in the nephron, by active secretion in the renal tubules. Galinsky and Corcoran (1986) recently showed an age-related decline in the active transport of acetaminophen-sulfate out of the kidney without any effect on the secretion of the glucuronide conjugate. This suggests that age-related changes in renal elimination may be substrate-specific, just as are metabolic changes. In contrast, urinary elimination of albumin appears to increase in old rats (Horbach et al., 1983). This may reflect alteration in the structure of the nephron, resulting in poorer exclusion of larger molecules. The kidney, in part because of functional alterations, may thus exhibit enhanced sensitivity in the older organism. Gentamicin, an aminoglycoside antibiotic that may be nephrotoxic in the aged, is actively reabsorbed in the tubules and results in greater toxicity in old versus young rats (McMartin & Engel, 1982).

The liver is the other major excretory organ. A number of hepatobiliary functions have been reported to decline with age. Like the kidneys, reduction in blood flow plays a major role in reduced elimination in the liver (Yates & Hiley, 1979). Recent studies have demonstrated a reduction in bile flow with age (Borghoff et al., 1987; Kanai et al., 1985; Schmucker et al., 1985). These studies were in male rats, and a lack of reduction with age in bile flow and bile acid secretion has also been reported in female rats (Kitani et al., 1981). Transport into the bile from the liver may be either by simple diffusion or carrier-mediated. The biliary transport for ouabain progressively decreased with age (Kitani et al., 1978, 1982). However, the biliary elimination of digoxin and digitoxin, other neutral cardiac glycosides, contrasts with that seen for ouabain, suggesting that a different mechanism may be involved (Kitani et al., 1985). The biliary excretion of ouabain, which while neutral is also polar, is most affected by aging, whereas that of the very nonpolar digitoxin is least altered. Major sex differences were also seen in the effects of age on biliary transport.

A decrease with age in the transport into the bile of an organic anion, sulfobro-mophthalein (SBP) has been reported (Kitani et al., 1981). The hepatic handling of SBP in older rats resulted in a decreased biliary elimination owing both to the age-related effects on the biliary transport mechanism as well as the decrease in bile flow rate (Kanai et al., 1985). Decrements were observed in both sexes, although the decline in male biliary transport was much greater than that observed in females. These data suggest that biliary excretion does change with age and calls for further study of the basis of such change. The result on rats is especially important in light of the recent observations that decreases in biliary excretion as well as bile acid synthesis also occur in aging humans (Einarsson et al., 1985).

CONCLUSIONS

Although it is clear that the disposition of drugs and other chemicals changes during the aging process, the basis for these changes remains unclear. Absorption seems to be the process least sensitive to age, although active transport in the GI tract does appear to decline. Distribution is affected by changes in body composition, blood flow, and protein binding. Changes in the Vd can have major impact on tissue levels of drugs. Metabolism is extremely complex, and age-related changes cannot be generalized between substrates, species, and sex, and biotransformation reactions. Only excretion seems to show some consistent changes with age, owing in large part to the altered blood flow and physiology of the kidney. Hepatic and pulmonary elimination may decline only in some instances.

Thus, no broad generalizations can be made about pharmacokinetic changes with age, other than the observation that alterations may occur. The situation with pharmacodynamic effects resulting in altered tissue sensitivity is even less clear.

REFERENCES

Armbrecht, H.J. (1986). Age-related changes in calcium and phsophorus uptake by rat small intestines. *Biochimica et Biophysica Acta, 882*:281–286.

Baird, M.B., & Hough, J.L. (1987). Phospholipase A_2-catalyzed conversion of hepatic cytochrome P_{450} to P_{420} in microsomal membranes prepared from young and old rats. *Age, 10*:90–95.

Behl, C.R., Bellantone, N.H., & Flynn, G.L. (1987). Influences of age on percutaneous absorption of drug substances. In Kydonieuks, A.F., & Berner, B. (Eds.) *Transdermal delivery of drugs*, Vol. 2, pp. 109–132. Boca Raton, Florida: CRC Press.

Behl, C.R., Flynn, G.L., Linn, E.E., & Smith, W.M. (1984). Percutaneous absorption of corticosteroids: Age, site and skin sectioning of hydrocortisone through hairless mouse skins. *Journal of Pharmaceutical Sciences, 73*:1287–1290.

Bender, A., Post, A., Meier, J., Higson, J., & Reichard, G. (1975). Plasma protein binding of drugs as a function of age in adult human subjects. *Journal of Pharmaceutical Sciences, 64*:1711–1713.

Birnbaum, L.S. (1987). Age-related changes in carcinogen metabolism. *Journal of the American Geriatric Society, 35*:51–60.

Birnbaum, L.S. (1983). Distribution and excretion of 2,3,6,2',3', 6'- and 2,4,5,2', 4', 5'-hexachlorobiphenyl in senescent rats. *Toxicology and Applied Pharmacology, 70*:262–272.

Blumberg, J.B. (1985). A discussion of drug metabolism and actions in the aged. *Drug–Nutrient Interactions, 4*:99–106.

Borghoff, S.J., Stefanski, S.A., & Birnbaum, L.S. (1988). The effect of age on the glucuronidation and toxicity of 4,4'-thiobis(6-*t*-butyl-*m*-cresol). *Toxicology and Applied Pharmacology, 92*:453–466.

Castelden, C.M., Volans, C.N., & Raymond, K. (1977). The effect of aging on drug absorption from the gut. *Age and Ageing, 6*:138–143.

Christophers, E., & Kligman, A.M. (1965). Percutaneous absorption in aged skin. In Montagna, W. (Ed.), Advances in the biology of skin, Vol. 6, Aging (pp. 163–175). Oxford: Pergamon Press.

Coleman, G.L., Barthold, S.W., Osbaldiston, G.W., Foster, S.J., & Jonas, A.M. (1977). Pathological changes during aging in barrier-reared Fischer 344 male rats. *Journal of Gerontology, 32*:258–278.

Csakey, T., & Varga, F. (1975). Subepithelial blood flow estimated from blood-to-lumen flux of barbital in ileum of rats. *American Journal of Physiology, 229*:549–552.

Davies, D.F., & Shock, N.W. (1950). Age changes in glomerular filtration rate, effective renal plasma flow, and tubular excretory function in adult males. *Journal of Clinical Investigation, 29*:496–507.

Devasagayam, T.P.A. (1986). Senescence-associated decrease of NADPH-induced lipid peroxidation in rat liver microsomes. *FEBS Letters, 205*:246–250.

Eastin, W.C., Jr., & Birnbaum, L.S. (1987). Intestinal absorption of two glucose analogues in rats of different ages. *Experimental Gerontology, 22*:351–357.

Edelman, I., Haley, H., Schloerb, P., Sheldon, D., Fris-Hansen, B., Stol, G., & Moore, F. (1952). Further observations on total body water. I. Normal values throughout the life span. *Surgery, Gynecology and Obstetrics, 95*:1–12.

Edelman, I.S., & Leibman, J. (1959). Anatomy of body water and electrolytes. *American Journal of Medicine, 27*:256–277.

Einarsson, K., Nilsell, K., Leijd, B., & Angelin, B. (1985). Influence of age on secretion of cholesterol and synthesis of bile acids by the liver. *New England Journal of Medicine, 313*:277–282.

Fleming, B.B., & Barrows, C.H., Jr. (1982a). The influence of aging on intestinal absorption of vitamins A and D by the rat. *Experimental Gerontology, 17*:115–120.

Fleming, B.B., & Barrows, C.H., Jr. (1982b). The influence of aging on intestinal absorption of vitamin B_{12} and niacin in rats. *Experimental Gerontology, 17*:121–126.

Galinsky, R.E., & Corcoran, G.B. (1986). Influence of advanced age on the formation and elimination of acetaminophen metabolites by male rats. *Pharmacology, 32*:313–320.

Galinsky, R.E., Kane, R.E., & Franklin, M.R. (1986). Effect of aging on drug-metabolizing enzymes important in acetaminophen elimination. *Journal of Pharmacology and Experimental Therapeutics, 237*:107–113.

Hebert, C.D., & Birnbaum, L.S. (1987). The influence of aging on intestinal absorption of TCDD in rats. *Toxicology Letters, 37*:47–55.

Hollander, D., & Dadufalza, V. D. (1983). Increased intestinal absorption of oleic acid with aging in the rat. *Experimental Gerontology, 18*:287–292.

Hollander, D., Dadufalza, V., Weindruch, R., & Walford, R.L. (1986). Influence of life-prolonging dietary restriction on intestinal vitamin A absorption in mice. *Age, 9*:57–60.

Hollander, D., & Morgan, D. (1979a). Increase in cholesterol intestinal absorption with aging in the rat. *Experimental Gerontology, 14*:201–204.

Hollander, D., & Morgan, D. (1979b). Aging: Its influence on vitamin A intestinal absorption *in vivo* by the rat. *Experimental Gerontology, 14*:301–305.

Holt, A.R., Pascal, R.R., & Kotler, D.P. (1984). Effect of aging upon small intestinal structure in the Fischer rat. *Journal of Gerontology, 39*:642–647.

Horbach, G.J.M.J., Yap, S.H., & Van Bezooijen, C.F.A. (1983). Age-related changes in albumin elimination in female WAG/RIJ rats. *Biochemistry Journal, 216*:309–315.

Huang, J.T., Nakajima, T., & Maito, S. (1985). Age-related changes of intestinal absorption of α-aminoisobutyric acid, tyrosine and tyr-D-ala-gly in rats. *Age, 8*:64–68.

Israeli, Z., & Wenger, J. (1981). Aging, gastrointestinal disease and response to drugs. In L. Jarvik (Ed.), *Clinical pharmacology and the aged patient*, pp. 131–155. New York: Raven Press.

Iwasaki, K., Chiraga, T., Tada, K., Noda, K., & Noguchi, H. (1986). Age- and sex-related changes in amine sulphoconjugations in Sprague Dawley strain rats. Comparison with phenol and alcohol sulphconjugations. *Xenobiotica, 16*:717–723.

Kamataki, T., Maeda, K., Shimada, M., Kitani, K., Nagai, T., & Kato, R. (1985). Age-related alteration in the activities of drug-metabolizing enzymes and contents of sex-specific forms of cytochrome P-450 in liver microsomes from male and female rats. *Journal of Pharmacology and Experimental Therapeutics, 233*:222–228.

Kanai, S., Kitani, K., Fujita, S., & Kitagawa, H. (1985). The hepatic handling of sulfobromophthalein in aging Fischer-344 rats: *in vivo* studies. *Archives of Gerontology and Geriatrics, 4*:73–85.

Kapetanovic, I.M., Sweeney, D.J., & Rapoport, S.I. (1982a). Age effects on haloperidol pharmacokinetics in male, Fischer 344 rats. *Journal of Pharmacology and Experimental Therapeutics, 221*:434–438.

Kapetanovic, I.M., Sweeney, D.J., & Rapoport, S.I. (1982b). Phenobarbital pharmacokinetics as a function of age. *Drug Metabolism and Disposition, 10*:586–589.

Kekki, M., Samloff, I., Ihamaki, T., Varis, K., & Siurala, M. (1982). Age and sex-related behavior of gastric acid secretion at the population level. *Scandinavian Journal of Gastroenterology, 17*:737–743.

Kitani, D., Kanai, S., Mirua, R., Morita, Y., & Kasahara, M. (1978). The effect of aging on the biliary excretion of ouabain in the rat. *Experimental Gerontology, 13*:9–17.

Kitani, D., Soto, Y., Kanai, S., & Nokubo, M. (1982). Biliary elimination of cardiac glycosides in aging rats—sex and strain differences. In Kitani, K. (Ed.), *Liver and Aging*, pp. 179–190. Amsterdam: Elsevier Press.

Kitani, K., Ohta, M., Kanai, S., & Sato, Y. (1985). Sex difference in the biliary excretion of digoxin and its metabolites in aging Wistar rats. *Archives of Gerontology and Geriatrics, 4*:1–12.

Kitani, K., Zurcher, C., & Van Bezooijen, C.F.A. (1981). The effect of aging on the hepatic metabolism of sulfobromophthalein in BN/Bi Female and WAG/Rij male and female rats. *Mechanisms of Ageing and Development, 17*:381–393.

Kohn, R. (1969). Age variation in rat skin permeability. *Proceedings of the Society for Experimental Medicine and Biology, 131*:521–522.

Lauker, R.M., Zheng, P., & Dong, G. (1987). Aged skin: A study by light, transmission electron and scanning electron microscopy. *Journal of Investigative Dermatology, 88*:44S–51S.

Lesser, G.T., Deutsch, S., & Markofsky, J. (1973). Aging in the rat: Longitudinal and cross-sectional studies of body composition. *American Journal of Physiology, 225*:1472–1478.

Lin, C.F., & Hayton, W.L. (1983). GI motility and subepithelial blood flow in mature and senescent rats. *Age, 6*:48–51.

Lindi, C., Marciani, P., Faelli, A., & Esposito, G. (1985). Intestinal sugar transport during aging. *Biochimica et Biophysica Acta, 816*:411–414.

Marzulli, F.N. (1962). Barriers to skin penetration. *Journal of Investigative Dermatology, 39*:387–393.

Mauderly, J.L. (1979a). Ventilation, lung volumes, and lung mechanics of young adult and old Syrian hamsters. *Experimental Aging Research, 5*:497–508.

Mauderly, J.L. (1979b). Effect of age on pulmonary structure and function of immature and adult animals and man. *Federation Proceedings, 38*:173–177.

Mauderly, J.L. (1982). The effect of age on respiratory function of Fischer 344 rats. *Experimental Aging Research, 8*:31–36.

Mayersohn, M. (1982). The "Xylose Test" to assess gastrointestinal absorption in the elderly: A pharmacokinetic evaluation of the literature. *Journal of Gerontology, 37*:300–305.

McLachlan, M.S.F. (1978). The aging kidney. *Lancet, 2*:143–145.

McMahon, T.F., Beierschmitt, W.P., & Weiner, M. (1987). Changes in Phase I and Phase II biotransformation with age in male Fischer 344 rat colon: Relationship to colon carcinogenesis. *Cancer Letters, 36*:273–282.

McMartin, D.N., & Engel, S.G. (1982). Effect of aging on gentimicin nephrotoxicity and pharmacokinetics in rats. *Research Communications in Chemical Pathology and Pharmacology, 38*:193–207.

Navab, F., Reis, R.J.S., Konduri, K., & Texter, E.C., Jr. (1984). Effect of aging on intestinal absorption of aromatic amino acids in the rat. *Gastroenterology, 86*:1193.

Nishizumi, M., & Masuda, Y. (1986). Enhancing effect of 2,3,4,7,8-pentachlorodibenzofuran and 1,2,3,4,7,8-hexachlorodibenzofuran on diethylnitrosamine hepatocarcinogenesis in rats. *Cancer Letters, 33*:333–339.

Novak, L.P. (1972). Aging, total potassium, fat free mass and cell mass in males and females between the ages of 18 and 85 years. *Journal of Gerontology, 27*:438–443.

Ouslander, J.G. (1981). Drug therapy in the elderly. *Annals of Internal Medicine, 95*:711–722.

Penzes, L. (1974a). Intestinal absorption of glycine, L-alanine and L-leucine in the old rat. *Experimental Gerontology, 8*:245–252.

Penzes, L. (1974b). Further data on the age-dependent intestinal absorption of dibasic amino acids. *Experimental Gerontology, 9*:259–262.

Prasanna, H.R., Lotlilkar, P. D., Hacobian, N., & Magee, P.N. (1986). Differential effects on the metabolism of dimethylnitrosamine and aflatoxin B_1 by hepatic microsomes from senescent rats. *Cancer Letters, 33*:259–267.

Reindenberg, M.M. (1980). Drugs in the elderly. *Bulletin of the New York Academy of Medicine, 56*:703–714.

Rikans, L.E., & Moore, D.R. (1987). Age- and sex-determined differences in allyl alcohol hepatotoxicity: Relation to liver alcohol dehydrogenase activity (ADH). *Pharmacologist, 29*:177.

Rodgers, J., & Gass, G. (1983). The effect of age on serum proteins in mice. *Experimental Gerontology, 14*:169–173.

Roth, G.S., & Hess, G.D. (1982). Changes in the mechanisms of harinone and neurotransmitter action during aging: Current status of the role of receptor and post-receptor alteration. A review. *Mechanics of Ageing and Development, 20*:175–194.

Schmucker, D.L. (1979). Age-related changes in drug disposition. *Pharmacological Reviews, 30*:445–456.

Schmucker, D.L. (1985). Aging and drug disposition: An update. *Pharmacological Reviews, 37*:133–148.

Schmucker, D.L., Gilbert, R., Jones, A.L., Hradek, G.T., & Bazin, H. (1985). Effect of aging on the hepatobiliary transport of dimeric immunoglobulin A in the male Fischer rat. *Gastroenterology, 88*:436–443.

Schmucker, D.L., & Wang, R.K. (1987). Effects of aging on the properties of Rhesus monkey liver microsomal NADPH-cytochrome c (P-450) reductase. *Drug Metabolism and Disposition, 15*:225–232.

Shumann, A.M., Fox, T.R., & Watanabe, P.G. (1982). A comparison of the fate of inhaled methyl chloroform (1,1,1-trichloroethane) following single or repeated exposure in rats and mice. *Fundamentals of Applied Toxicology, 2*:27–32.

Sellers, E.M., Frecker, R.C., & Romach, M.K. (1983). Drug metabolism in the elderly: Confounding of age, smoking, and ethanol effects. *Drug Metabolism Reviews, 14*:225–250.

Sun, J., & Strobel, H.W. (1986). Aging affects the drug metabolism systems of rat liver, kidney, colon, and lung in a differential fashion. *Experimental Gerontology, 21*:523–534.

Sun, J., Lau, P.O., & Strobel, H.W. (1986). Aging modifies the expression of hepatic microsomal cytochrome P-450 after pretreatment of rats with β-naphthoflavone or phenobarbital. *Experimental Gerontology, 21*:65–73.

Sweeney, D.J., & Weiner, M. (1986). Effect of aging on the metabolism of p-nitroanisole and p-nitrophenyl in isolated rat hepatocytes. *Age, 9*:95–98.

Thompson, G.A., Myers, J.A., Turner, P.A., Coyle, D.E., Ritschel, W.A., & Denson, D.D. (1987). Influence of age on intrinsic clearance of bupivacaine and its reduction by cimetidine in elderly male rats. *Drug Metabolism and Disposition, 15*:130–137.

Van Bezooijen, C.F.A. (1984). Influence of age-related changes in rodent liver morphology and physiology on drug metabolism—a review. *Mechanics of Ageing and Development, 25*:1–22.

Van Manen, R., De Priester, W., & Knook, D.L. (1983). Lysosomal activity in aging rat liver: I. Variation in enzyme activity within the liver lobule. *Mechanics of Ageing and Development. 22*:159–165.

Varga, F. (1976). Transit time changes in age in the gastrointestinal tract of the rat. *Digestion, 14*:319–324.

Varga, F., & Csakey, T. (1977). Changes in the blood supply of the gastrointestinal tract in rats with age. *Pfluegers Archiv. European Journal of Physiology, 364*:129–133.

Vestal, R.E., Cusack, B.J., Mercer, G.D., Dawson, G.W., & Park, B.K. (1987). Aging and drug Interactions. I. Effect of cimetidine and smoking on the oxidation of theophylline and cortisol in healthy men. *Journal of Pharmacology and Experimental Therapeutics, 241*:488–500.

Vinardell, P., & Bolufer, J. (1984). Age-dependent changes on jejunal sugar absorption by rat *in vivo*. *Experimental Gerontology, 19*:73–78.

Vogel, H.B. (1983). Effects of age on the biomechanical and biochemical properties of rat and human skin. *Journal of the Society of Cosmetic Chemistry, 34*:453–463.

Wallace, S., Whiting, B., & Runcie, J. (1976). Factors affecting drug-binding in plasma of elderly patients. *British Journal of Clinical Pharmcology, 3*:327–330.

Weiner, R., Dietze, F., & Laue, R. (1984). Age-dependent alterations of intestinal absorption. II. A clinical study using a modified D-xylose absorption test. *Archives of Gerontology and Geriatrics, 3*:97–108.

Yacobi, A., Kamath, B.L., & Lau, C.M. (1982). Pharmacokinetics in chronic animal toxicity studies. *Drug Metabolism Reviews, 13*:1021–1051.

Yang, R.S.H., Tallant, M.J., & McKelvey, J.A. (1984). Age-dependent pharmacokinetic changes of ethylenediamine in Fischer 344 rats parallel to a two-year chronic toxicity study. *Fundamentals of Applied Toxicology, 4*:663–670.

Yates, M.S., & Hiley, C.R. (1979). The effect of age on cardiac output and its distribution in the rat. *Experientia, 35*:78–79.

York, J.L. (1982). Body water content, ethanol pharmacokinetics, and the responsiveness to ethanol in young and old rats. *Developmental Pharmacology and Therapeutics, 4*:106–116.

Young, J.F., & Norvell, M.J. (1984). Dietary and age influences on the pharmacokinetic parameters of 2-acetylaminofluorene in BALB/c mice. *Fundamentals of Applied Toxicology, 4*:164–169.

9

Cancer Chemotherapy in the Elderly: Clinical Pharmacologic Considerations

Ian G. Kerr and Carlo DeAngelis

Cancer is a common disease in the elderly; approximately 50% of all cancers occur in the age segment over 65 years of age (Yancik, 1983). In addition, age has become an important prognostic factor with respect to treatment outcome as well as the selection of treatment. Many older patients have been excluded from clinical trials because of the widespread belief that they tolerate chemotherapy relatively poorly. It is indeed difficult to separate the role of various factors that may contribute to altered response of the elderly to chemotherapy. These factors include the natural history of tumors in older individuals, physiologic changes that take place in the host with aging, co-morbid conditions, as well as purely treatment-related factors (Table 9.1). Many chemotherapeutic agents and protocols have a low therapeutic/toxic index and therefore must be administered with appropriate care. However, administered dose, dose rate, and dose intensity may also be important factors for treatment outcome. For example, some data are available for tumors conventionally thought of as responsive, such as the leukemias and lymphomas, as well as for some of the solid tumors such as breast cancer and ovarian cancer, that dose and dose intensity may be important (Dembo, 1987; DeVita, 1986; Frei & Canellos, 1980; Gehan, 1984; Hryniuk & Bush, 1984; Hryniuk & Levine, 1986; Levin & Hyrniuk, 1987).

If elderly patients do indeed tolerate chemotherapy less well than younger patients, then it may be justified to attenuate doses to avoid excessive toxicity. Is the increased toxicity from "usual" doses seen in the elderly owing to altered host

**TABLE 9.1 Issues That Relate to Cancer Chemotherapy
Trials in the Elderly**

Tumor
   Natural history
   Extent of disease
Host
   Patient selection
   Physiologic changes with aging
   Co-morbid states
   Performance status
   Psychologic and social impact
Drugs
   Choice of treatment
   Dose changes
   Pharmacokinetic changes
   Pharmacodynamic changes
   Compliance (patient and physician)
   Retrospective data

---

responsiveness or drug elimination capabilities? If their tolerance to chemotherapy is not significantly different from somewhat younger patients, assuming reasonable elimination organ function, then many patients may be underdosed with the very real possibility of suboptimal treatment. If impaired drug elimination is responsible for excessive drug exposure and therefore toxicity, drug doses could be adjusted appropriately to give equal drug exposure, assuming equal responsiveness of the host (e.g. as would be provided in a younger population). Good data regarding these issues are presently limited. However, empirical decisions are often made not only for the entry of patients into clinical trials but also for arbitrary dose reductions and choice of treatment owing to age and/or organ dysfunction (Mor, et al., 1985; Sulkes & Collins, 1987). Problems with compliance, therefore, not only rest with the older patient but also with the physician.

The use of chemotherapy unfortunately has various trade-offs that have to be considered. Tumors that are common in the elderly (e.g. lung cancer, colon cancer, breast cancer, prostate cancer) generally are less responsive than tumors seen in younger adults (e.g. germ cell tumors, childhood tumors) and may in fact not have a steep clinically achievable dose–response curve (Frei & Canellos, 1980). The second part of this equation is that of the possibility of decreased tolerance to the administered drugs as well as the perceived quality of life of the elderly patient. These factors include not only the side effects of the drug but also various psychologic factors and inconvenience of intensive treatments (Winograd, 1986). In addition, there may be important differences between the "old" (e.g. 65–75 years) and the "very old" (e.g. 75 years and older) with respect to treatment decisions. Many of these factors have to be considered before embarking on a course of intensive chemotherapy in the elderly population. This review will discuss the issues that deal with clinical trials involving the elderly, host–drug interactions that could affect the tolerance and toxicity to the administered drugs, and information on selected drugs.

CLINICAL TRIALS AND THE ELDERLY CANCER PATIENT

Patient age has become a major prognostic factor for selecting treatments, the outcomes of treatments, and the survival of patients with cancer. Why are the elderly less likely to accrue benefit from chemotherapy than a younger subset of patients? Several possibilities exist. The first is that of a change in the natural history of the cancer itself. It is clear, for example, that breast cancer in the elderly may respond somewhat differently to various hormonal therapies, possibly owing to changes in the relative content of estrogen and progesterone receptor positive tumors (Stoll, 1973; Kennedy, 1986). Patients may also delay in seeking medical attention until the time a tumor has become very advanced. Associated with treatment outcome, the patient may have a poor physiologic reserve particularly if other co-morbid conditions are present (e.g. congestive heart failure, renal disease, liver disease) (Leventhal, 1986; Winograd, 1986). Finally, one must wonder whether some of these age related changes in prognosis are related to inadequate treatments based on the assumption that the elderly tolerate chemotherapy less well than younger patients. For example, it is not uncommon for an *a priori* dosage reduction to take place for myelosuppressive agents in the elderly patient. Many studies still contain downward dose modifications even for starting doses before it is clear what the tolerance of the patient is for that particular form of chemotherapy. It has only been in recent years that the National Cancer Institute (NCI) has abolished age restrictions on many of its studies. This is obviously an important step because it will allow us to examine the effects of drugs on patients as they age in a prospective clinical trial setting. However, this will not necessarily remove the bias of patient selection whereby "healthier" elderly patients may be entered on trials.

Tolerance of Anticancer Drugs by the Elderly

Although it has been well documented in the noncancer literature that the elderly patient often has major changes in drug disposition and degrees of drug toxicity when compared to younger individuals (Mayersohn, 1986; Ouslander, 1981; Schmucker, 1985), there are relatively few published data in the cancer literature that specifically address the problem of differences in disposition, efficacy, and toxicity of anticancer drugs in the elderly host and how these factors interact (Kelly, 1986; Kennedy, 1986; Kerr & Chabner, 1983). In addition, most reported clinical trials have selected their patients for favorable features often with an upper age limitation. As a result, most chemotherapy is administered to elderly patients in an empirical fashion with the belief that they tolerate treatment poorly. Is this conclusion justified? If this conclusion is justified, what are the factors that contribute to this phenomenon?

An analysis of six terminated studies of the Eastern Cooperative Oncology Group (ECOG) was undertaken in an attempt to describe specific problems encountered by elderly patients receiving chemotherapy (Begg et al., 1980). The conclusion of this retrospective review was that elderly patients with cancer did not experience any increase in the frequency or severity of toxicity or have any significant differences in compliance or response rates as compared to middle-aged patients when treated for breast, colorectal, or lung cancer. However, in this retrospective review relatively few patients were actually elderly: only 22% of breast cancer patients were over age 60 and only 9.7% and 14.5% of patients with lung and colorectal cancer, respectively, were over 70 years of age. As a large percentage of patients with these common diseases are over age 65 it must also be questioned whether a selection process took place for patient entry into these trials that were reviewed.

A subsequent retrospective study also using data from the ECOG looked at toxicity rates of elderly patients (> 70 years) and compared them with nonelderly controls for each of eight disease sites of advanced cancer (Begg et al., 1983). The results again indicated that in general the elderly patient had identical rates of severe toxicity as their younger counterparts. The only exception was that for hematologic reactions in a few of the sites studied. The agents that appeared to be responsible for these specific adverse effects were methotrexate and methyl-CCNU. Whether the changes in methotrexate toxicity are due to changes in renal function with aging is unclear. Changes in drug distribution, and hence possibly clearance, may be responsible for the change in the toxicity pattern of methyl-CCNU. Although it is known that there are changes in body fat content with aging, it is unclear whether this is the major contributing factor in altered drug pharmacokinetics for lipid-soluble drugs (Mayersohn, 1986; Ouslander, 1981).

Other commonly used drugs that were also in this analysis did not show an age trend in toxicity and included cyclophosphamide, mitomycin-C, bleomycin, cis-platin, vincristine, and VP-16. None of these drugs, however, is highly dependent on renal function for their elimination or toxicity profiles (Balis et al., 1983; Grygiel et al., 1983). The data from this report also indicated that elderly patients had a similar response rate and survival expectancy compared to the nonelderly control patients. Their conclusion was that the apparent discrimination of not treating elderly patients as aggressively as younger patients, and in excluding elderly patients from protocols, did not appear to be justified. These investigators suggested that exclusions should be based on physiologic functional parameters such as renal and liver function (Begg et al. 1983). However, physiologic parameters of organ function may not necessarily correlate with the ability to eliminate the drug (especially drugs metabolized by the liver) or toxicity.

Dosage Levels and Therapeutic Outcomes

If dose, dose rate, and dose intensity are important variables for therapeutic success, there is a clear disadvantage in delaying or limiting drug administration because of empiric notions regarding the tolerance of chemotherapy in the elderly. In addition, presently available dosage adjustment guidelines for organ dysfunction are themselves tenuous at best because of the relative lack of prospective confirmatory trials that also take pharmacokinetic factors into account (Sulkes & Collins, 1987). Relative drug underdosing may therefore have significant effects not only with the middle-aged host if inappropriate dose reductions are made, but also for the elderly in whom even fewer guidelines are available.

Are dose and dose intensity really important in the treatment of many of the tumors seen in the elderly? Unfortunately, good data are sparse and mainly retrospective in nature. Bonadonna and Valagussa (1981), for example, have reported that postmenopausal women receiving aggressive adjuvant chemotherapy with cyclophosphamide, methotrexate, and 5-FU (CMF) may benefit in a similar fashion to premenopausal women. These investigators proposed that CMF was useful only when given in full or nearly full doses (greater than 85% of the planned dose). However, this conclusion was based on a retrospective analysis and left unanswered questions such as why many of the older patients were unable to tolerate full drug doses. The authors suggested that some of these patients may not have received full doses for the fear that "aggressive" adjuvant chemotherapy might produce excessive toxicity in an older patient who might be cured through surgery.

Another study utilizing CMF in elderly women (over 65) with metastatic breast cancer found that if the initial doses of cyclophosphamide and methotrexate were calculated using a linear function of creatinine clearance, as both drugs or their metabolites do undergo renal excretion, and if the initial 5-FU dose was two-thirds that of younger patients, then there were no significant age trends in response or in toxicity (Gelman et al., 1984). Patients older than 65 years in this study subsequently had their doses decreased less quickly than did patients younger than 65 years and that by the sixth chemotherapy cycle the young and the elderly patients were receiving almost the same amount of methotrexate and 5-FU.

Similar trends have appeared for the treatment of hematologic malignancies as in the foregoing examples for solid tumors. In the treatment of acute myelogenous leukemia (AML) it was initially believed that response rate and survival were adversely affected by advanced age. However, some recent studies have suggested that the elderly can tolerate aggressive chemotherapy with a high survival benefit (Gale et al., 1981; Reiffers et al., 1980). However, in these reports patients who did not achieve a complete remission experienced a high incidence of treatment-related deaths during the chemotherapy induction phase. A study carried out by Kahn and colleagues (1984) compared the administration of daunorubicin, ara-C, and 6-thioguanine in full dosage versus an attenuated schedule of the same drugs for patients 70 years of age or older. They concluded that attenuated chemotherapy was the preferred induction regimen for elderly patients because it caused few early deaths and allowed a better quality of life with survival times as durable as those obtained with intensive therapy. However, in more recent studies carried out by Bern and colleagues (1987) utilizing etoposide, ara-C, doxorubicin, and 6-thioguanine for the treatment of AML using an age adjusted protocol for patients older than 50 years of age (oldest patient being 78-years-old), remissions were fewer and less durable and toxicity less for the attenuated program. It is therefore unclear from these studies what is the optimal policy for treating older patients with AML. Although they should not be denied therapy, it is unclear how much dose attenuation (if any) should be carried out. This needs to be addressed in further prospective trials with investigators willing to utilize intensive support services that will be required to handle the toxicities associated with aggressive chemotherapy.

Hodgkin's Disease: A Case Example

The analysis of the interaction of drug doses, toxicity, and therapeutic effect is instructive for the treatment of Hodgkin's disease in the elderly. Lokich et al. (1974) reported on a retrospective review of 47 patients with Hodgkin's disease presenting after age 60. They noted significant differences in both clinical and pathologic features of this elderly group of patients when compared to the younger group of patients treated in the same institution. For example, "B" symptomatology occurred in 55% of the elderly group versus only 18% in the unmatched control group. These investigators noted a significantly shorter median duration of survival in the older group of patients. However, the majority of patients in the older age group were treated with palliative intent. Of the 47 elderly patients only nine were treated with curative intent versus 42 of the 47 younger patients. Within the small group of optimally treated elderly patients there was a complete remission rate of 66%. Although Hodgkin's disease may in fact be a different clinicopathologic entity in an older group of patients (Lokich et al., 1974; MacMahon, 1957; Newell et al., 1970), it is also important, as suggested in this retrospective review, that older patients be optimally staged and treated before firm conclusions can be made regarding differences in toxicity and therapeutic outcome.

To further this end the CALGB (Peterson et al. 1982) analyzed their data from two Phase III trials involving 385 previously untreated patients with advanced stage Hodgkin's disease receiving multidrug chemotherapy. Seventy-three patients in this analysis were 60 years of age or older. They noted that even when the analysis was restricted to the older patients who received more than 90% of projected drug doses, the complete remission rate; median time for recurrence, and duration of survival were still shorter than in the younger patients. They also suggested that age was associated with an increased frequency of serious myelosuppression (leukopenia and thrombocytopenia).

The Stanford experience (Carde et al., 1983) reporting on 132 patients, suggests that B symptoms and rate of drug delivery, not age, significantly influenced the complete remission rate. However, survival was influenced by advanced age. Unfortunately, it is unclear from this study how many patients were in the older age category. Another review from Stanford (Austin-Seymour et al., 1984) of 52 patients over age 60 suggested that survival and drug toxicity were higher for the older group in general, although a subgroup with early disease did very well with standard treatment.

A study carried out by SWOG (Fabian et al., 1984) suggested that a group of patients older than 60 years of age did not have a significantly different complete response rate from a younger group of patients, although the trend was to a shorter complete response rate (67% for less than 40 years and 59% for greater than 60 years). Survival was also shorter for the older group of patients, although there was no significant difference in the incidence of severe life-threatening leukopenia or drug dose.

Finally, a retrospective review from France (Eghbali et al., 1984) looked at their 20-year experience of patients older than 70 years of age (mean age not stated but six were over 80 years). Although treatments were variable (single-agent pro-carbazine versus combination chemotherapy), there appeared to be an acceptable response rate (77%) and disease-free interval ("one of three cured") although toxicity may have been excessive for aggressively treated patients (five of 30 were treatment-related deaths). The major benefit was accrued by patients with early stage disease. Additional studies are obviously required in the treatment of Hodgkin's disease in the elderly to help clarify the situation because there may very well be differences in disease histology and behavior, as well as therapy.

Treatment for Non-Hodgkin's Lymphomas

Information regarding the treatment of non-Hodgkin's lymphoma in the elderly is more extensive, although clear conclusions again cannot be obtained. The group from the National Cancer Institute (Fisher et al., 1977) analyzed their early experience with combination chemotherapy in the treatment of advanced diffuse histiocytic lymphoma (DHL) analyzing for age, sex, stage, constitutional symptoms, sites of disease, and tumor mass as prognostic factors. Unfortunately, there was not a clear age breakdown (median age, 50 years; range, 20–74 years). There is also no information regarding whether there were differences in drug doses for the older group of patients. However, they concluded that there was no statistical correlation between age and response to chemotherapy or survival. Factors related to disease such as advanced stage, bone marrow involvement, gastrointestinal involvement, and a tumor mass greater than 10 cm in a single location were considered important prognostic factors. This same group also reviewed their institutional experience of non-Hodgkin's lymphoma patients treated between 1964 and 1977 (Fisher et al., 1981). They did not consider patient age an important prognostic factor in the prediction of survival. Details regarding treatment protocol changes or excessive toxicity in the older group of patients were not available.

Cabanillas et al. (1978) in a review from the M.D. Anderson Hospital analyzed their experience involving 97 patients with advanced stage non-Hodgkin's lymphoma treated with combination chemotherapy. Unfortunately, again there was no clear breakdown of whether drug doses were changed for the older group of patients or a clear breakdown of the exact ages involved. However, these investigators proposed that the response rate and survival of patients older than 60 years were similar to that of patients younger than 60 years.

Another analysis carried out by a group at the Memorial Sloan-Kettering Cancer Center looked at their experience in 65 patients with advanced stage DHL treated with combination chemotherapy with or without radiotherapy or central nervous system prophylaxis (the latter not given to the older patients) (Koziner et al., 1982). In this study there was also no mention of dose changes for the older group of patients. The patient ages ranged from 15 to 74 years (median, 55 years). There was no difference with respect to the number of complete responses or the predicted 3-year disease-free survival.

Armitage and Potter (1984) reported on 20 patients 70 years of age or older (range, 70–94 years; median 75 years) as compared to 55 younger patients 33- to 69-years-old being treated with cyclophosphamide, adriamycin, vincristine, and prednisone for DHL. There were no dose adjustments made for age. The complete remission rate was no different from the younger patients, and although the survival was somewhat shorter, it was not statistically significant. Patient death from causes other than lymphoma during the first two treatment cycles occurred significantly more often in the elderly group (25% of patients over 70 years of age compared to 2% of the younger patients). Although the authors concluded that it might be appropriate to alter drug doses in treating elderly patients and give particular attention to supportive measures, it is instructive to look at the causes of early death during treatment. Of the nine elderly patients who died while receiving their induction chemotherapy three died of sepsis and two of cardiac-related events such as congestive heart failure. Although adriamycin might be implicated in the early cardiac deaths, it is unclear what the cardiovascular status of this small group of patients was despite exclusion of patients from study who had preexisting congestive heart failure, severe coronary artery disease, or previous treatment with adriamycin. The high incidence of sepsis in this older group of patients is certainly disturbing, although again the numbers are relatively small.

Recently, SWOG has also reported on their experience in the treatment of malignant lymphoma involving a large group of patients (696 evaluable) (Jones et al., 1985). Unfortunately, despite dose reductions (50% of starting dose) being built into their protocols for patients over age 65, there were no details regarding age analysis or its effects on efficacy or toxicity. Dixon and colleagues (1986) subsequently reviewed the results of two of these SWOG clinical trials involving 307 patients being treated with combination chemotherapy based predominantly on CHOP. They noted that the complete response rate as well as the survival decreased significantly with age. However, they did note that the treatment guidelines included an initial dose reduction of 50% for patients aged 65 or older as well as for the younger patients with bone marrow disease. Despite this, 23 of the 81 patients who were 65 or older received initial full dose therapy. When these patients were analyzed separately, their complete response rate and frequency of treatment complications were no different, although their survival was inferior to younger patients. These authors have suggested that older age may be associated with a worse prognosis in advanced DHL, although they suggested that the initial dose reduction for the older patients may have contributed to their inferior outcomes. However, as pointed out by a subsequent editorial, there were some difficulties in this previous report with respect to details of what constituted the older group (Zagonel et al., 1986).

Carbone et al. (1986) carried out a retrospective review of 50 patients aged 65 or older (median, 71.5 years) with non-Hodgkin's lymphomas being treated with chemotherapy. There was a mixture of patients being treated with conservative single-agent chemotherapy as well as more aggressive combination chemotherapy. Although the review claimed that there were no significant differences in response and survival between these two forms of treatment, it is unclear what selection factors took place to guide their treatment decisions. The differences in toxicity between the two treatment approaches were not criticially analyzed, although it was claimed that for the whole group severe toxicity was seen in seven patients of which four patients died of toxicity owing to aggressive therapy.

A recent study carried out by Connors et al. (1987) reported on the efficacy and toxicity of brief chemotherapy consisting of three cycles of CHOP and involved field radiation for limited-stage histologically aggressive lymphoma. This study enrolled 78 patients ranging in age from 21 to 82 years with a median age of 64 years (20 patients over age 70). All treatments were delivered as planned resulting in a very high response rate and actuarial relapse-free survival. There were no deaths owing to toxicity, and it was concluded that toxicity from this approach was acceptable even for elderly patients. However, it needs to be emphasized that the duration of chemotherapy was limited.

Finally, a group from Italy reviewed their experience using teniposide or etoposide and predmustine in a group of elderly patients (66 patients, 70 years of age or older; median age 75 years) (Tirelli et al., 1987). They reported a reasonable objective response rate and survival with relatively mild toxicity in this group of patients.

It appears from this brief review of these reports that the correct management of elderly patients with non-Hodgkin's lymphoma is unsettled and should be evaluated in prospective randomized trials. It is also unclear what selection bias took place for inclusion of the elderly patients into these studies.

HOST–DRUG INTERACTIONS IN THE ELDERLY

The issue that must be addressed is whether advanced age is an important contributor to the toxicity of anticancer drugs. If differences in drug effects in the elderly actually occur, it is important to know whether this is a result of changes in drug disposition or changes in sensitivity of host tissues. However, for most anticancer drugs there are insufficient data to make any conclusions about whether changes in pharmacokinetics result in increased drug toxicity or altered efficacy. Changes in a drug's pharmacokinetics owing to the aging process may be more easily dealt with, for example, by dosage modification, whereas pharmacodynamic changes, for example, changes in receptor response (i.e., tumor response or bone marrow toxicity) are much more difficult to control. If these various relationships can be further clarified, then therapeutic drug monitoring may prove to have a useful role in the future in helping to individualize doses in some of the elderly and other high-risk patients (Erlichman et al. 1980; Erlichman, 1986). Among the practical difficulties that have to be overcome are the analysis of combinations of drugs (most drugs today are given by combination chemotherapy) and the interrelationship between the individual drug pharmacokinetics and their pharmacodynamic (e.g. toxicity/efficacy) relationships.

Certainly, in the noncancer literature it is clear that there are changes in drug pharmacokinetics with aging (Bender, 1974; Triggs and Nation, 1975; Ouslander, 1981; Schmucker, 1985; Mayersohn, 1986). In the cancer literature much less data are available (Kerr & Chabner, 1983; Kennedy, 1986; Kelly, 1986). The factors that have to be considered are drug absorption for orally administered drugs, drug distribution and binding, and drug metabolism and excretion.

Despite the large volume of noncancer drug literature, Schmucker (1985) has pointed out the many shortcomings and difficulties of trials describing pharmacokinetic changes of drugs in the elderly. He further stated that our understanding of the mechanisms responsible for altering drug pharmacokinetics in the elderly is incomplete. This is not surprising when one considers the multitude of factors, both genetic and environmental, that may influence drug pharmacokinetics with time. Age is but a single factor in a number of host factors, which not only have the potential to interact with each other but their interrelationships may be continuously changing (Vesell, 1982). Thus, it is surprising indeed that pharmacokinetic studies in the elderly viewing only a single point in time have been able to discern age as a contributing factor to changes in drug disposition. The very process of aging is associated with increased variability owing to differing effects of the aging process on the various end organs involved in drug elimination (Wilkinson, 1983). Vesell (1984) has recently commented on the requirement of conducting carefully controlled studies to isolate the host factors under study by maintaining other factors as constant as possible. This, it is hoped, would allow more reproducible results from the various studies. Admittedly, the nature and the toxicity of antineoplastic agents and the conditions in which these agents are administered are quite different from the ideal control subject situation discussed by Vesell (1984).

That host responsiveness to cancer chemotherapy agents in the elderly may differ is intimately linked to the physiology of aging. Aging has been described as the gradual loss of adaptive capabilities (Goldstein, 1971; Masoro, 1987). Whether this loss in adaptive capabilities, or ability to withstand stress, means that the elderly are more susceptible to drug toxicity—in this case antineoplastic drug toxicity—is not known. If one accepts the data from Begg and colleagues (1980), then it would appear that, with the exception of the hematopoietic system and the drugs methotrexate and methyl-CCNU, the aged have more than adequate reserve to withstand the stress induced by antineoplastic agents (Begg & Carbone, 1983). However, firm conclusions from these data are difficult for several reasons. The reviews were based on retrospective data, the disease sites were quite diverse, there were numerous drug combinations to be considered, and the patient selection may have been biased toward relatively healthy elderly individuals (Kelly, 1986; Kennedy, 1986). Clearly, this latter point illustrates the difficulty in distinguishing chronologic age from biologic or physiologic age. At issue is the process or normal aging, which is not uniform between individuals or for that matter between various organ systems within a given individual (Goldstein, 1971; Leventhal, 1986; Masoro, 1987).

The mammalian cells are divided into three groups in the adult according to mitotic capabilities and can be classified as continuously mitotic, intermittently mitotic, and nonmitotic (Goldstein, 1971). With respect to cancer chemotherapeutic agents, it is the continuously mitotic cells that are at greatest risk for toxicity. Are these dividing cells infinitely capable of renewal or do these cells lose their seemingly infinite proliferative capacity in responding to the stress induced by antineoplastic drug therapy? Evidence in animals and humans suggest that aging is associated with decreased hematopoietic stem cell potential (Botnick et al., 1978; Lipschitz et al., 1984; Mauch et al., 1982) particularly when the system is stressed, for example, by cytotoxic drugs (Botnick et al. 1976, 1978). However, a recent abstract suggested that the elderly may have adequate bone marrow reserve to respond to chemotherapy-induced toxicity (Panettiere, 1985). The effect of cytotoxic drugs on the hematologic reserve in the elderly is therefore unclear.

The changes seen with aging of another population of continuously dividing cells in the gastrointestinal tract has been reviewed with respect to potential influences on drug absorption (Bender, 1974; Ouslander, 1981; Schmucker, 1985). However, we were unable to find any information with respect to the consequences these changes have on tissue responsiveness to antineoplastics in the elderly (e.g., mucositis and diarrhea). Even less is known about the influence of normal aging of other organ systems and antineoplastic drug toxicity in the elderly. Data examining the effects of anthracyclines on the heart, bleomycin on the lungs, and cisplatin on the kidneys are examples of problems in analyzing the interrelationships of aging tissue and its potential responsiveness to the individual drugs and the way this may vary with changes in drug pharmacokinetics.

SPECIFIC ANTICANCER DRUGS

There is very little in the cancer literature that specifically refers to the differences in pharmacokinetics or pharmacodynamics (efficacy and/or toxicity) of individual drugs in the elderly as compared to a younger population. However, with the growth of pediatric oncology there have been some reports dealing with the differences in both the pharmacokinetics and tolerance of antineoplastic agents in children versus adults (Marsoni, 1985; Evans et al., 1987). In these studies it appears that there is variability in the pharmacokinetics of various and anticancer drugs and that there may be a trend for decreasing drug clearance with increasing age, although this relationship is only weakly positive. This appeared to be the strongest for the epipodophylotoxins (Evans et al., 1987). When the results of Phase I and Phase II studies looking at maximum tolerated doses of anticancer drugs in children versus adults are compared in general, the maximum tolerated doses were higher for children than for adults. There is no breakdown unfortunately of the very elderly as compared to younger adults. However, one report of a Phase II trial of teniposide in elderly patients with Hodgkin's disease suggests that this drug is well tolerated in patients older than 70 years of age (Tirelli et al., 1984). This is of interest with the previous comments from Evans's group regarding the epipodophylotoxins, although they studied a very limited age range (Evans et al., 1987). Certainly, the report by Panettiere (1985) suggests that older patients may not have as poor bone marrow tolerance to chemotherapy as is assumed. They suggest that changes start in middle age and appear to be much more marked in patients older than 75 years of age rather than in the 60s, which is often assumed to be an important age cut-off. Although dosage adjustment guidelines have been available for several common drugs, particularly in situations of excretory organ dysfunction, recently there have also been some questions about how reliable these guidelines are (Sulkes & Collins, 1987). Finally, there have as yet been no specific guidelines for using individual anticancer drugs in the elderly despite the common use of empiric dose reductions or the elimination of elderly patients from clinical trials.

Anthracyclines

The anthracyclines doxorubicin and daunorubicin are among the most commonly used anticancer drugs used today both in children and adults. Their use in children has been recently reviewed by Crom et al., (1987). However, the age-dependent pharmacokinetics of adriamycin in the adult population has resulted in conflicting results (Robert et al., 1982; Robert & Hoerni, 1983). Although one study has suggested that there is age dependence in early phase pharmacokinetics of doxorubicin, another report suggested that the area under the concentration time curve did not vary with age of patients. Therefore, it is unclear from a pharmacokinetic point of view that a reduction in dose is justified. However, one recent report

(Egorin et al., 1987) suggested that the clearance of daunorubicin may be decreased in patients older than 60 years of age. Although one of the major acute toxicities of the anthracyclines consists of myelosuppression, a major late toxicity of concern is that of congestive heart failure. It does appear that there is an increased risk of congestive heart failure with increasing age as well as with increasing cumulative dose (Von Hoff et al., 1979; Praga et al., 1979). However, there is one case report in the literature of a 78-year-old woman who received a total dose of 510 mg/M^2 of doxorubicin over a 4-month period without any significant toxicity (Adducci, 1976). What the critical factors are for this relationship is unclear. Whether these changes are related to changes in pharmacokinetics or changes in pharmacodynamics (increased sensitivity of cardiac tissue) are not known.

Cisplatin

Cisplatin and its analogues are commonly used drugs in the adult population. There are very little data available to suggest that there are changes in pharmacokinetics with increasing age. However, because the major dose-limiting toxicity of cisplatin consists of renal toxicity, this is a potentially important age-related toxicity to study. Although there is one report (Blom et al., 1985) that suggested there may be increased renal deterioration with increasing age, another report (Hrushesky et al., 1984) suggested that there is a lack of age-dependent renal toxicity from cisplatin in a study of 43 patients 29–77 years of age. Despite reduced renal function in the elderly (Rowe et al., 1976; Lindeman et al., 1985), these investigators (Hrushesky et al., 1984) suggested that cisplatin irreversibly diminished renal function in most patients regardless of age and that advancing age did not show an additional detrimental effect. These latter investigators suggested that cisplatin dose or schedule modification is not indicated on the basis of advancing age.

Methotrexate

Methotrexate is one of the oldest drugs being used in the anticancer drug armamentarium (Jolivet et al., 1983). Despite its broad use, there is relatively little information available regarding changes with respect to pharmacokinetics or toxicity in the elderly. Although we know that renal function decreases with age (Lindeman et al., 1985; Rowe et al., 1976) and that methotrexate is predominately excreted *via* renal mechanisms, there is not necessarily a clear relationship between renal function, as noted by creatinine clearance, and methotrexate clearance (Jolivet et al., 1983; Kerr, et al., 1983). Fortunately for moderate- or high-dose infusions the risk of toxicity can be alleviated somewhat with the appropriate use of therapeutic drug monitoring and folinic acid (leucovorin) rescue (Jolivet et al., 1983). One pharmacokinetic study involving high-dose methotrexate infusions suggested that methotrexate clearance does decline with age, but is not clearly associated with changes in creatinine clearance (Kerr, et al., 1983). Certainly, the results of this study are consistent with data from Evans et al. (1987) in children, which confirmed that although there are large interindividual variations in total body clearance of this drug, there is a trend to decreasing clearance with age. The impact of age on toxicity from this agent is even more difficult to discern. One study by Hansen and associates (1971) suggested that there was increasing toxicity with increasing patient age with single-agent methotrexate therapy. However, clear relationships between pharmacokinetics and these toxicity profiles are not available. If the results of the report by Evans et al. (1986) suggesting that there is a relationship between methotrexate concentration and effect in the treatment of acute leukemia holds up, then it may be very important by using the tools of therapeutic drug monitoring to not only try and obtain appropriate drug concentrations for maximum drug efficacy but also to try to limit drug-induced toxicity. Similar studies for solid tumors are currently underway. The various relationships between pharmacokinetics and toxicity as well as efficacy obviously need further study.

Bleomycin

Although bleomycin has a limited spectrum of activity, it is used in older patients for the treatment of various lymphomas. Because the predominant route of elimination is via the kidneys (analogous to methotrexate), one needs to recognize the fact (as mentioned above) that renal function does decrease with increasing age. It is clear that there is some relationship between decreasing bleomycin clearance and decreasing renal function. It is also apparent that advanced age is associated with a high risk of lung toxicity (which is the major dose-limiting toxicity of bleomycin). However, it is difficult to make direct associations between normal aging and bleomycin toxicity because the major risk factors for lung injury are multifactorial, consisting of cumulative dose, age, radiotherapy to the chest, and oxygen therapy (Cooper et al., 1986; Haas et al., 1976). We know that the aging lung has reduced elastic recoil and function (Anderson et al., 1986). Does this predispose elderly patients clinically to manifest lung damage earlier; is the older lung more sensitive to blemoycin itself, or can some of the increased sensitivity be due to elevated blood levels (e.g., increased drug exposure) as a result of impaired renal function and hence drug clearance? Accurate correlations between pharmacokinetics and toxicity and changes with age, however, are not available.

5-Fluorouracil

Although 5-fluorouracil has been in wide use in cancer chemotherapy since the early 1950s, there are very little data available on its specific effects in the elderly patient population. Despite this, arbitrary empiric dose reductions have been incorporated into protocols dealing with an older patient population (Gelman & Taylor, 1984).

FUTURE DIRECTIONS

As can be seen from this review, there are very little data available regarding the interaction of advanced age with the use of anticancer drugs. The hypothesis that needs to be tested is whether advanced age is an important contributor to the toxicity of anticancer drugs. The reasons for age-related differences in the effects of drugs are difficult to demonstrate because changes in drug disposition (e.g., pharmacokinetics) must first be excluded before differences in drug effects (e.g., pharmacodynamics) can be critically analyzed. If these relationships can be clarified, then therapeutic drug monitoring may prove to have a useful role in helping to individualize doses of some of the anticancer drugs in the elderly and other high-risk patients. Unfortunately, many of the reports from which conclusions regarding the elderly have been generated have been retrospective, may have had patient selection bias, and have involved diverse treatment protocols and drug combinations. Prospectively designed trials are needed to develop more rational guidelines for the use of chemotherapy in the elderly and thus avoid many of the empiric and possibly erroneous guidelines that are presently in place. In addition, careful attention needs to be paid to comparing results from the "just elderly" (e.g., over 65) to the "very elderly" (e.g. over 75) as well as functional status before generalized recommendations can be made.

REFERENCES

Adducci, J.E. (1976). Doxorubicin (Adriamycin) therapy of uterine sarcoma without surgery in an elderly patient. *Journal of the American Geriatric Society, 24*:473–474.

Anderson, W.M., Ryerson, G.G., & Wynne, J.W. (1986). Pulmonary disease in the elderly. In Rossman, I. (Ed.), *Clinical geriatrics*, Ed. 3. Philadelphia: J.B. Lippincott.

Armitage, J.O., & Potter, J.F. (1984). Aggressive chemotherapy for diffuse histiocytic lymphoma in the elderly. Increased complications with advancing age. *Journal of the American Geriatric Society, 32*:269–273.

Austin-Seymour, M.M., Hoppe, R.T., Cox, R.S., et al. (1984). Hodgkin's disease in patients over sixty years old. *Annals of Internal Medicine, 100*:13–18.

Balis, F.M., Holcenberg, J.S., & Bleyer, W.A. (1983). Clinical pharmacokinetics of commonly used anticancer drugs. *Clinical Pharmacokinetics, 8*:202–232.

Begg, C.B., Cohen, J.L., & Ellerton, J. (1980). Are the elderly predisposed to toxicity from cancer chemotherapy? *Cancer Clinical Trials, 3*:369–374.

Begg, C.B., & Carbone, P.P. (1983). Clinical trials and drug toxicity in the elderly: The experience of the Eastern Cooperative Oncology Group. *Cancer, 52*:1986–1992.

Bender, A.D. (1974). Pharmacodynamic principles of drug therapy in the aged. *Journal of the American Geriatric Society, 22*:296–303.

Bern, M.M., Wallach, S.R., Arkin, C.F., et al. (1987). Etoposide in combination with cytarabine, doxorubicin and 6-thioguanine for treatment of acute nonlymphoblastic leukemia in a protocol adjusted for age. *Cancer Treatment Reports, 71*:201–203.

Blom, J.H.M., Kurth, K.H., & Splinter, T.A.W. (1985). Renal function, serum calcium and magnesium during treatment of advanced bladder carcinoma with cis-dichlorodiamineplatinum: Impact of tumor site, patient age and magnesium suppletion. *International Urology and Nephrology, 17*:331–339.

Bonadonna, G., & Valagussa, D. (1981). Dose–response effect of adjuvant chemotherapy in breast cancer. *New England Journal of Medicine, 304*:10–15.

Botnick, L.E., Hannon, E.C., & Hellman, S. (1976). Limited proliferation of stem cells surviving alkylating agents. *Nature, 262*:68–70.

Botnick, L.E., Hannon, E.C., & Hellman, S. (1978). Multisystem stem cell failure after apparent recovery from alkylating agents. *Cancer Research, 38*:1942–1947.

Cabanillas, F., Burke, J.S., Smith, T.L., et al. (1978). Factors predicting for response and survival in adults with advanced non-Hodgkin's lymphoma. *Archives of Internal Medicine, 138*:413–418.

Carbone, A., Tirelli, U., Volpe, R., et al. (1986). Non-Hodgkin's lymphoma in the elderly: A retrospective clinicopathologic study of 50 patients. *Cancer, 57*:2185–2189.

Carde, P., MacKintosh, F.R., & Rosenberg, S.A. (1983). A dose and time response analysis of the treatment of Hodgkin's disease with MOPP chemotherapy. *Journal of Clinical Oncology, 1*:146–153.

Connors, J.M., Klimo, P., Fairey, R.N., et al. (1987). Brief chemotherapy and involved field radiation therapy for limited-stage histologically aggressive lymphoma. *Annals of Internal Medicine, 107*:25–30.

Cooper, J.A.D., White, D.A., & Matthay, R.A. (1986). Drug induced pulmonary disease. Part I: Cytotoxic drugs. *American Review of Respiratory Disease, 133*:321–340.

Crom, W.R., Glynn-Barnhart, A.M., Rodman, J.H., et al. (1987). Pharmacokinetics of anticancer drugs in children. *Clinical Pharmacokinetics, 12*:168–213.

Dembo, A.J. (1987). Time–dose factors in chemotherapy: Expanding the concept of dose–intensity. *Journal of Clinical Oncology, 5*:649–696.

DeVita, V.T. (1986). Dose response is alive and well. *Journal of Clinical Oncology, 4*:1157–1159.

Dixon, D.O., Neilan, B., Jones, S.E., et al. (1986). Effect of age on therapeutic outcome in advanced diffuse histiocytic lymphoma: The Southwest Oncology Group experience. *Journal of Clinical Oncology, 4*:295–305.

Eghbali, H., Hoerni-Simon, G., De Mascarel, I., et al. (1984). Hodgkin's disease in the elderly: A series of 30 patients aged older than 70 years. *Cancer, 53*:2191–2193.

Egorin, M.J., Zuhowski, E.G., Thompson, B., et al. (1987). Age-related alterations in daunorubicin (DNR) pharmacokinetics. *Proceedings of the American Society of Clinical Oncology, 6*:38.

Erlichman, C. (1986). Potential applications of therapeutic drug monitoring in treatment of neoplastic disease by antineoplastic agents. *Clinical Biochemistry, 19*:101–106.

Erlichman, C., Donehower, R.C., & Chabner, B.A. (1980). The practical benefits of pharmacokinetics in the use of antineoplastic agents. *Cancer Chemotherapy and Pharmacology, 4*:139–145.

Evans, W.E., Crom, W.R., Abromowitch, M., et al. (1986). Clinical pharmacodynamics of high-dose methotrexate in acute lymphocytic leukemia. *New England Journal of Medicine, 314*:471–477.

Evans, W.E., Crom, W.R., & Rodman, J.H. (1987). Age-related variability in drug disposition in children with cancer: A factor affecting dose intensity. *Proceedings of the American Society of Clinical Oncology, 6*:45.

Fabian, C., Sayre, R., Dixon, D., & Mansfield, C. (1984). Response rates as a function of age in Hodgkin's disease: A SWOG study. *Proceedings of the American Society of Clinical Oncology, 3*:240.

Fisher, R.I., De Vita, V.T., Johnson, B.L., et al. Prognostic factors for advanced diffuse histiocytic lymphoma following treatment with combination chemotherapy. *American Journal of Medicine, 63*:177–182.

Fisher, R.I., Hubbard, S.M., Devita, V.T., et al. (1981). Factors predicting long-term survival in diffuse mixed histiocytic or undifferentiated lymphoma. *Blood, 58*:45–51.

Frei, E., & Canellos, G.P. (1980). Dose: A critical factor in cancer chemotherapy. *American Journal of Medicine, 69*:585–594.

Gale, R.P., Foon, K.A., Cline, M.J., et al. (1981). Intensive chemotherapy for acute myelogenous leukemia. *Annals of Internal Medicine, 94*:753–757.

Gehan, E.A. (1984). Dose–response relationship in clinical oncology. *Cancer, 54*:1204–1207.

Gelman, R.S., & Taylor, S.G. (1984). Cyclophosphamide, methotrexate and 5-FU chemotherapy in women more than 65 years old with advanced breast cancer: The elimination of age trends in toxicity by using doses based on creatinine clearance. *Journal of Clinical Oncology, 2*:1404–1413.

Goldstein, S. (1971). The biology of aging. *New England Journal of Medicine, 285*:1120–1129.

Grygiel, J.J., Kerr, I.G., & Myers, C.E. (1983). Antineoplastics. In Chernow, B., & Lake, C.R. (Eds.), *The pharmacologic approach to the critically ill patient.* New York: Raven Press.

Haas, C.D., Coltman, C.A., Gottlieb, J.A., et al. (1976). Phase II evaluation of bleomycin: A southwest oncology group study. *Cancer, 38*:8–12.

Hansen, H.H., Selawry, O.S., Holland, J.F., et al. (1971). The variability of individual tolerance to methotrexate in cancer patients. *British Journal of Cancer, 25*:298–305.

Hrushesky, W.J.M., Shimp, W., & Kennedy, B.J. (1984). Lack of age-dependent cisplatin nephrotoxicity. *American Journal of Medicine, 76*:579–584.

Hryniuk, W., & Bush, J. (1984). The importance of dose intensity in chemotherapy of metastatic breast cancer. *Journal of Clinical Oncology, 2*:1281–1288.

Hryniuk, W., & Levine, M.N. (1986). Analysis of dose intensity of adjuvant chemotherapy trials in stage II breast cancer. *Journal of Clinical Oncology, 4*:1162–1170.

Jones, S.E., Grozea, P.N., Miller, T.P., et al. (1985). Chemotherapy with cyclophosphamide, doxorubicin, vincristine and prednisone alone or with levamisole or with levamisole plus BCG for malignant lymphoma: A Southwest Oncology Group study. *Journal of Clinical Oncology, 3*:1318–1324.

Jolivet, J., Cowan, K.H., Curt, G.A., et al. (1983). The pharmacology and clinical use of methotrexate. *New England Journal of Medicine, 390*:1094–1104.

Kahn, S.B., Begg, C.B., Mazza, J.J., et al. (1984). Full dose versus attenuated dose daunorubicin, cytosine arabinoside and 6-thioguanine in the treatment of acute nonlymphocytic leukemia in the elderly. *Journal of Clinical Oncology, 2*:865–870.

Kelly, J.F. (1986). Clinical pharmacology of chemotherapeutic agents in old age. *Frontiers of Radiation Therapy and Oncology, 20*:101–111.

Kennedy, B.J. (1986). Chemical and hormonal therapies in the elderly. *Frontiers of Radiation Therapy and Oncology, 20*:93–100.

Kerr, I.G., & Chabner, B.A. (1983). The effect of age on the clinical pharmacology of anticancer drugs. In Yancik, R., Carbone, P.P., Patterson, W.B., et al. (Eds.), *Perspectives on prevention and treatment of cancer in the elderly.* New York: Raven Press.

Kerr, I.G., Jolivet, J., Collins, J.M., et al. (1983). Test dose for predicting high-dose methotrexate infusions. *Clinical Pharmacology and Therapeutics, 33*:44–51.

Koziner, B., Little, C., Passe, S., et al. (1982). Treatment of advanced diffuse histiocytic lymphoma: An analysis of prognostic variables. *Cancer, 49*:1571–1579.

Leventhal, E.A. (1986). The dilemma of cancer in the elderly. *Frontiers of Radiation Therapy and Oncology, 20*:1–13.

Levin, L., & Hryniuk, W.M. (1987). Dose intensity analysis of chemotherapy regimens in ovarian carcinoma. *Journal of Clinical Oncology, 5*:756–767.

Lindeman, R.D., Tobin, J., & Shock, N.W. (1985). Longitudinal studies on the rate of decline in renal function with age. *Journal of the American Geriatric Society, 33*:278–285.

Lipschitz, D.A., Udupa, K.B., Milton, K.Y., et al. (1984). Effect of age on hematopoiesis in man. *Blood, 63*:502–509.

Lokich, J.J., Pinkus, G.S., & Moloney, W.C. (1974). Hodgkin's disease in the elderly. *Oncology, 29*:484–500.

MacMahon, B. (1957). Epidemiologic evidence on the nature of Hodgkin's disease. *Cancer, 10*:1045–1054.

Marsoni, S., Underleider, R.S., Hurson, S.B., et al. (1985). Tolerance to antineoplastic agents in children and adults. *Cancer Treatment Reports, 69*:1263–1269.

Masoro, E.J. (1987). Biology of aging: Current state of knowledge. *Archives of Internal Medicine, 147*:166–169.

Mauch, P., Botnick, L.E., Hannon, E.C., et al. (1982). Decline in bone marrow proliferative capacity as a function of age. *Blood, 60*:245–252.

Mayersohn, M. (1986). Special pharmacokinetic considerations in the elderly. In Evans, W.E., Schentag, J.J., & Jusko, W.J. (Eds.), *Applied therapeutics: Prinicples of therapeutic drug monitoring.* Spokane, WA: Applied Therapeutics.

Mor, V., Masterson-Allen, S., Goldberg, R.J., et al. (1985). Relationship between age at diagnosis and treatment received by cancer patients. *Journal of the American Geriatric Society, 33*:585–589.

Newell, G.R., Cole, S.R., Miettinsen, O.S., et al. (1970). Age differences in the histology of Hodgkins' disease. *Journal of the National Cancer Institute, 45*:311–317.

Ouslander, J.G. (1981). Drug therapy in the elderly. *Annals of Internal Medicine, 95*:711–722.

Panettiere, F.J. (1985). Age and chemotherapy myelosuppression: Data from a SWOG adjuvant study. *Proceedings of the American Association of Cancer Research, 26*:188.

Peterson, B.A., Pajak, T.F., Cooper, M.R., et al. (1982). Effect of age on therapeutic response and survival in advanced Hodgkin's disease. *Cancer Treatment Reports, 66*:889–898.

Praga, C., Beretta, G., Vigo, P.L., et al. (1979). Adriamycin cardiotoxicity: A study of 1273 patients. *Cancer Treatment Reports, 63*:827–834.

Reiffers, J., Raynal, F., & Broustet, A. (1980). Acute myeloblastic leukemia in elderly patients: Treatment and prognostic factors. *Cancer, 45*:2816–2820.

Robert J., & Goerni, B. (1983). Age dependence of the early-phase pharmacokinetics of doxorubicin. *Cancer Research, 43*:4467–4469.

Robert, J., Illiadis, A., Hoerni, B., et al. (1983). Pharmacokinetics of adriamycin in patients with breast cancer: Correlation between pharmacokinetic parameters and clinical short-term response. *European Journal of Cancer and Clinical Oncology, 18*:739–745.

Rowe, J.W., Andres, R., Tobin, J.D., et al. (1976). The effect of age on creatinine clearance in man: A cross-sectional and longitudinal study. *Journal of Gerontology, 31*:155–163.

Schmucker, D.L. (1985). Aging and drug disposition: An update. *Pharmacological Reviews, 37*:133–148.

Stoll, B.A. (1973). Hypothesis: Breast cancer regression under oestrogen therapy. *British Medical Journal, 3*:446–450.

Sulkes, A., & Collins, J.M. (1987). Reappraisal of some dosage adjustment guidelines. *Cancer Treatment Reports, 71*:229–233.

Tirelli, U., Carbone, A., Crivellari, D., et al. (1984). A phase II trial of teniposide (VM 26) in advanced non-Hodgkin's lymphoma with emphasis on the treatment of elderly patients. *Cancer, 54*:393–396.

Tirelli, U., Carbone, A., Zagonel, V., et al. (1987). Non-hodgkin's lymphomas in the elderly: Prospective studies with specifically devised chemotherapy regimens in 66 patients. *European Journal of Cancer and Clinical Oncology, 23*:535–540.

Triggs, E.J. & Nation, R.L. (1975). Pharmacokinetics in the aged: A review. *Journal of Pharmacokinetics and Biopharmaceutics, 3*:387–418.

Von Hoff, D.D., Layard, M.W., Basa, P., et al. (1979). Risk factors for doxorubicin-induced congestive heart failure. *Annals of Internal Medicine, 91*:710–717.

Vesell, E.S. (1982). On the significance of host factors that affect drug disposition. *Clinical Pharmacology and Therapeutics, 31*:1–7.

Vesell, E.S. (1984). Selection of subjects for investigation of host factors affecting drug response: A method to identify new pharmacogenetic conditions. *Clinical Pharmacology and Therapeutics, 35*:1–11.

Wilkinson, G.R. (1983). Drug distribution and renal excretion in the elderly. *Journal of Chronic Diseases, 36*:91–102.

Winograd, C.H. (1986). Geriatric medicine and the cancer patient. *Frontiers of Radiation Therapy and Oncology, 20*:27–37.

Yancik, R., (1983). Frame of reference: Old age as the context for the prevention and treatment of cancer. In Yancik, R., Carbone, P.P., Patterson, W.B., et al. (Eds.), *Perspectives on prevention and treatment of cancer in the elderly*. New York: Raven Press.

Zagonel, V., Tirelli, U., & Carbone, A. (1986). Treatment of non-Hodgkin's lymphoma in the elderly. *Journal of Clinical Oncology, 4*:1866–1867.

10

Multidrug Resistance in Human Cancer Cells: Changes in Protein Phosphorylation and Protein Kinase C

Robert L. Fine, Jitendra Patel, James Carmichael, and Bruce A. Chabner

DRUG RESISTANCE AND AGING

Drug resistance in human cancer cells is one, if not the most important factor preventing the successful treatment of cancer in patients. At the time of diagnosis many tumors are not curable and often not responsive to cancer chemotherapy drugs. The majority of tumors that are curable with chemotherapy tend to occur in younger patients and include acute lymphocytic leukemia, Burkitt's lymphoma, Hodgkin's disease, choriocarcinoma, and aggressive lymphomas with diffuse histology. The tumors that occur predominately in older patients, such as colorectal, lung, breast, and prostate, tend to be less responsive and curable with chemotherapy alone. The etiology of these tumors may be related to long-term carcinogen exposure which may explain their predominance in older patients. It is also known that these carcinogen-related tumors are drug-resistant *de novo* to many of the agents available to the clinical oncologist. The mechanisms underlying this form of resistance are not completely understood, but work by Fairchild et al.

158

(1987) shows remarkable similarities between the biochemical characteristics of *de novo* drug resistance in carcinogen-induced rat liver cancer and multidrug resistance (MDR) found in human breast cancer cells. Thus, there may be similar mechanisms between carcinogen-induced drug resistance that occurs more commonly in the elderly and MDR in mammalian cancer cells.

OVERVIEW OF MULTIDRUG RESISTANCE

MDR develops as a broad pattern of drug resistance in cancer cells exposed to agents derived from natural products. MDR can be induced by exposure to a single agent from natural products such as the anthracyclines, vinca alkaloids, dactinomycin, or colchicine (Rogan et al., 1984). A common feature of MDR cells is a net decreased intracellular accumulation of drug that has been ascribed to an increased efflux pump mechanism. This defect in drug accumulation is partially or fully reversible by calcium channel blockers such as verapamil and by calmodulin antagonists such as trifluoperazine (Tsuruo et al., 1983). Increased concentrations of membrane (Kartner et al., 1983) and cytoplasmic proteins (Myers & Biedler, 1981) have been identified in animal and human MDR cells. A specific membrane protein, P-170 glycoprotein, has been shown by photoaffinity labeling to bind vinca alkaloids, and this binding is competitively inhibited by verapamil, an agent that can reverse the MDR phenotype (Cornwell et al., 1986; Safa et al., 1986). The P-170 protein, which has significant amino acid sequence homology to a bacterial transport protein, may function as a carrier protein in the efflux mechanism, but its activation or modulation is still unknown. However, protein kinases modulate many cellular proteins by phosphorylation.

Certain features of the MDR phenotype suggest a possible role of calcium-dependent cellular events. Calmodulin antagonists inhibit not only MDR but Ca^{++}-dependent protein kinases such as protein kinase C and calmodulin-associated kinases (Mori et al., 1980). Thus, we investigated protein phosphorylation profiles in 19 human breast cancer and 17 human small-cell lung cancer lines (SCLC). An increased phosphorylation of a 20-kD protein was associated with MDR in these lines (Fine et al., 1985, 1986a). Increased activity of protein kinase C was found in our MDR cells, and activation of this enzyme increased the MDR phenotype. MDR induced by protein kinase C activation was inhibited by calcium channel blockers and calmodulin antagonists (Fine et al., 1988).

HUMAN BREAST CANCER LINES

Human breast cancer lines were examined simultaneously for MDR by clonogenic assay and for associated phosphorylation changes. These included MCF-7 drug-sensitive (KC/control) and drug-resistant mutants that were selected by serial passage in adriamycin or antimetabolites such as methotrexate (MTX) (Cowan et al., 1982), N-phosphonacetyl-L-aspartic acid (PALA), or pyrazofurin (Karle et al., 1986). The adriamycin-resistant lines were selected by continuous exposure to drug: KC/ADR_1 and KC/ADR_{10}. lines capable of growth in 1 μM and 10 μM adriamycin, respectively, after 1 year of exposure to increasing concentrations of adriamycin, and MCF-7 RO/ADR, a line exposed to 1 μM adriamycin for 3 days every 2 weeks for 1 year. All of these lines were cross-resistant in clonogenic assays to continuous exposure of colchicine, vincristine, and vinblastine.

Phosphorylation Changes in the 20-Kilodalton Region

Cell homogenates or membranes were tested in an *in vitro* phosphorylation assay using ^{32}P-ATP by a previously published method (Patel et al., 1983). Phosphorylated samples, each with 17 μg protein, were separated on a 10% SDS-PAGE and exposed to film for 18 hours. Phosphorylation changes were quantitated by densitometry. The density of the 20-kD region was expressed as the phosphorylation intensity in this region divided by the total phosphorylation intensity of the whole lane. This fraction was then normalized by comparison with the fractional phosphorylation intensity of the 20-kD region in the parent MCF-7 KC/control cell line. Thus, a density of 3 units signifies a threefold greater intensity of the 20-kD phosphorylation in the subject line as compared to the MCF-7 KC/control.

Clonogenic IC_{50}s (concentration required to inhibit the number of tumor colonies formed to 50% of control during continuous exposure assays) to adriamycin (ADR) and vinblastine (VBT) were done for all lines. Two main differences were noted between the drug-sensitive ($IC_{50} \leq 10$ nM for ADR and VBT) and drug-resistant ($IC_{50} \geq 20$ nM for ADR and VBT) cell lines. We observed a general marked increase in the phosphorylation of many proteins from the drug-resistant lines and a specific increase in phosphorylation of the 20-kD region that was barely detectable in the drug-sensitive parent lines. There was no detectable staining of a 20-kD protein in sensitive or resistant lines by Coomassie blue or silver staining techniques (data not shown).

MCF-7 cell lines resistant to the antimetabolites methotrexate, PALA, and pyrazofuran did not have increased phosphorylation of the 20-kD region and were not resistant to ADR or VBT in clonogenic assay (Figure 10.1). In contrast, the MDR MCF-7 KC/ADR_1 line has a band in the 20-kD region with intense phosphorylation, whereas the sensitive MCF-7 KC/control lacks a 20-kD region phosphorylation. Thus, the increased phosphorylation of the 20-kD region occurred only in the MDR MCF-7 cells. We tested other human breast cancer lines that were not of MCF-7 origin: ZR-75, ZR-75 resistant to MTX, ZR-75 resistant to PALA, T47D, and Hs578t (Figure 10.2). These lines were established from patient specimens prior to chemotherapy with ADR or VBT, and all were shown to be sensitive to these agents by clonogenic assay. There was no increase in the phosphorylation of the 20-kD region in any of these sensitive lines (Figure 10.2) (Fine et al., 1985).

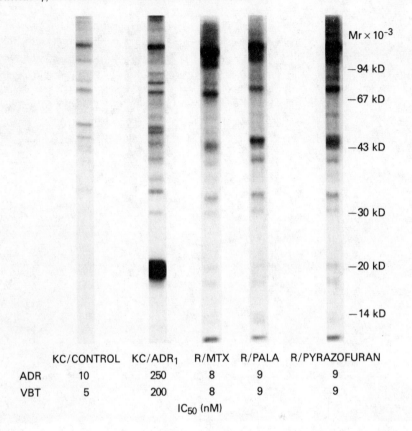

	KC/CONTROL	KC/ADR$_1$	R/MTX	R/PALA	R/PYRAZOFURAN
ADR	10	250	8	9	9
VBT	5	200	8	9	9

IC$_{50}$ (nM)

FIGURE 10.1 Autoradiogram of homogenates from KC/control and KC/ADR$_1$ lines and lines resistant to methotrexate (R/MTX), PALA (R/PALA), and pyrazofurin (R/pyrazofurin). Beneath each line is the clonogenic IC$_{50}$ in nanomolar (nM) concentrations for adriamycin (ADR) and vinblastine (VBT) after continuous exposure to drug. Lines with an IC$_{50}$ less than or equal to 10 nM were considered sensitive, and lines with an IC$_{50}$ greater than or equal to 20 nM were considered resistant. All *in vitro* phosphorylations were performed as described (Patel et al., 1983) in the presence of free 10 mM Mg^{++}. Briefly, cells were scraped from plates in cold buffer A containing 50 mM Tris-HC1 (pH 7.4), 5 mM EGTA, 5 mM dithiothreitol, 2 mM phenylmethylsulfonylfluoride, and 125 μM leupeptine. Cells were then disrupted by sonication of 4°C in buffer A. Aliquots of 60 μl containing 75 μg of protein in buffer A were incubated in a final volume of 0.1 ml with 50 mM Tris-HC1 (pH 7.4) and 10 mM MgCl$_2$. Phosphorylation was initiated with the addition of 5 μM [^{32}P] (2.5 μCi) in 10 μl and terminated 30 seconds later with 25 μl Laemmli's stopping solution. Samples, 35 μl, containing 17 μg protein were run on a discontinuous 10% SDS polyacrylamide gel electrophoresis (SDS-PAGE).

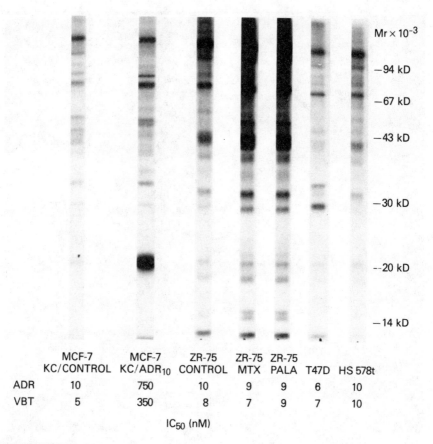

	MCF-7 KC/CONTROL	MCF-7 KC/ADR$_{10}$	ZR-75 CONTROL	ZR-75 MTX	ZR-75 PALA	T47D	HS 578t
ADR	10	750	10	9	9	6	10
VBT	5	350	8	7	9	7	10

IC$_{50}$ (nM)

FIGURE 10.2 Autoradiogram of homogenates from the MCF-7 lines KC/control, KC/ADR$_{10}$ and from nonMCF-7 lines ZR-75 control, ZR-75 MTX (resistant to methotrexate), ZR-75 PALA (resistant to PALA), T47D and Hs 578t. Beneath each lane of these human breast cancer lines is the clonogenic IC$_{50}$ in nanomolar (nM) concentrations for adriamycin (ADR) and vinblastine (VBT) after continuous exposure to drug. The *in vitro* phosphorylations were performed as described (Patel et al., 1983) in the presence of 10 mM free Mg^{2+}. The procedure is described briefly in Figure 10.1. This figure illustrates the intense phosphorylation of the 20-kD region for the KC/ADR$_{10}$ line as compared to the other lines; this correlates with the MDR state in KC/ADR$_{10}$ and its absence in the other lines.

Biochemical Characteristics of the 20-Kilodalton Phosphoprotein

The kinetics of the phosphorylation were examined in a timed experiment from 5 to 480 seconds in KC/control and KC/ADR_{10} cells. In the presence of 10 mM Mg^{++} the homogenate or membrane fraction of KC/ADR_{10} promoted rapid phosphorylation to a maximum at 30–40 seconds; phosphorylation decreased after 120 seconds. However, no significant phosphorylation in the 20-kD region occurred from homogenate or particulate fraction in the sensitive KC/control cells during the same time period (Fine et al., 1985). When 10 mM NaF, a phosphatase inhibitor, was added to the reaction mixture from both cell lines, the marked 20-kD phosphorylation in the KC/ADR_{10} cells was unaffected as before, but no appreciable phosphorylation occurred in the KC/control cells. These findings suggest that increased phosphatase activity in the KC/control cells could not account for the minimal phosphorylation in those cells.

Various kinase stimulators were tested to investigate which kinase may be involved in the 20-kD phosphorylation in KC/control and KC/ADR_{10} cell lines. These included Mg^{++} alone and Mg^{++} with the following: 0.4 mM free Ca^{++}; 0.025 mg/ml calmodulin with 0.4 mM free Ca^{++}; 40 μg/ml phosphatidylserine with 0.8 mg/ml diolene (a diacylglycerol analog) and 0.4 mM free Ca^{++}; 50 μM cAMP; and 100 μM cyclic GMP. The cyclic nucleotides did not simulate *in vitro* phosphorylation over Mg^{++} alone in both cell lines. An enhancement of 20% was produced by Ca^{++} alone in the MDR cell line KC/ADR_{10} (Figure 10.3). Calcium with calmodulin or phosphatidylserine and diolene were the same as Ca^{++} alone in both cell lines (Fine et al., 1985). These data are consistent either with a new kinase or possibly protein kinase C. Protein kinase C is normally stimulated with Mg^{++}, Ca^{++}, phosphatidylserine, and diolene. Although we could not demonstrate these requirements, it is consistent with the catalytically cleaved subunit of protein kinase C known as the M kinase (Kishimoto et al., 1983), which requires only Mg^{++} for stimulation. This possibility has yet to be proven in our laboratory.

Particulate and soluble fractions were assayed to determine the presence of the 20-kD phosphoprotein. The 20-kD phosphoprotein was not detected in either the particulate or soluble fraction from KC/control cells. However, it was found to reside solely in the particulate fraction of the KC/ADR_{10} cells (Fine et al., 1985). 2-D gel electrophoresis of phosphorylated samples demonstrated that the pI of the 20-kD protein lies between 8.2 and 8.5. Myers and Biedler (1981) have described a 19-kD protein that is associated with MDR in Chinese hamster fibroblasts. It is unlikely to be the same protein because it is found only in the soluble fractions and its pI is approximately 5.7.

We further considered the possibility that the 20-kD phosphorylation band was myosin light chain. Immunoprecipitation of myosin with polyclonal antibody failed to remove the 20-kD protein from either the solubilized particulate or homogenate

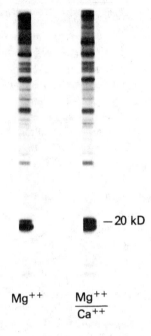

$$Mg^{++} \qquad \frac{Mg^{++}}{Ca^{++}}$$

FIGURE 10.3 Autoradiogram of the homogenate from the MCF-7 KC/ ADR$_{10}$ line with Mg^{2+} ± Ca^{2+} stimulation, demonstrating a modest (20%) increase in phosphorylation. The *in vitro* assay was performed as described before in the legend of Figure 10.1.

fractions from KC/ADR$_{10}$ cells, suggesting that the 20-kD protein is not myosin light chain. Also, the pI of myosin light chain is less than 6. Marsh and Center (1985) have identified a number of phosphoprotein changes in Chinese hamster lung cells resistant to adriamycin. One of these is a 20-kD particulate bound phosphoprotein that is identified only in the MDR cells, and its phosphorylation requires Mg^{2+}. Whether it is the same protein as found in our breast cancer cells is unknown at this time.

HUMAN SMALL-CELL LUNG CANCER LINES

We assayed 17 human SCLC lines to assess whether the 20-kD phosphoprotein is found in cells other than breast carcinomas and whether it develops in lines derived from treated patients. These lines were not exposed to drugs after they were established from patient samples.

Correlation of the 20-Kilodalton to Clinical Status

Seven lines from untreated patients were tested in the aforementioned *in vitro* phosphorylation assay. Six of these had 20-kD phosphoprotein values ranging from 0.9 to 1.7, with a mean of 1.4 (Fine et al., 1986a). All of these patients had objective responses to combination chemotherapy containing ADR and vincristine. One of the seven untreated patients had a 20-kD phosphoprotein of 3.9 and did not respond to chemotherapy. Ten lines from relapsed or postchemotherapy treated patients were tested and had 20-kD phosphoproteins ranging from 3.0 to 15.4, with a mean of 6.4 (Fine et al., 1986a). All of these patients who were treated with reinduction chemotherapy failed to respond. Thus, presence of the 20-kD phosphoprotein correlated with the clinical status of patients with SCLC.

Correlation of the 20-Kilodalton Phosphoprotein to Drug Sensitivity Assays

Drug sensitivity testing to ADR and vinca alkaloids (VBT and vincristine) by the Weisenthal dye-exclusion method (Weisenthal et al., 1983) showed that six of seven pretreated patient lines that had low 20-kD phosphoprotein values were sensitive to adriamycin and vinca alkaloids. All of the ten post-treated or relapsed patient lines had higher 20-kD phosphoprotein values, all were resistant to ADR, and 80% were resistant to vinca alkaloids. These findings suggest that the level of 20-kD phosphoprotein correlates with clinical status and with *in vivo*-induced MDR because none of these lines was exposed to drugs after they were established in culture from patient biopsy samples.

PROTEIN KINASE C

Increased Activity in Multidrug-Resistant Cells

Certain features of the work presented suggest a role for protein kinase C, such as (1) association of the 20-kD phosphoprotein with MDR in human breast and SCLC lines, (2) biochemical characteristics of the phosphorylation (3) reversibility of the MDR phenotype by calmodulin antagonists that also inhibit protein kinase C (PKC), (4) a common characteristic of MDR cells is increased efflux of drug leading to a net decreased intracellular accumulation, and (5) PKC activation is associated with increased exocytosis of certain chemical moieties in various cell systems. These features led us to examine PKC activity in the KC/control and KC/ADR$_{10}$ cells.

Baseline PKC activity was sevenfold higher in the KC/ADR$_{10}$ line compared to KC/control (the percent ratio of activity in both lines is 40:60, soluble to particulate) (Fine et al., 1988). After activation of PKC by 200 nM phorbol-12, 13-

dibutyrate (PDBu) exposure to cells *in vitro*, this difference was further increased over ninefold. PKC activity in the KC/control cells increased twofold and increased 2.5-fold in the KC/ADR$_{10}$ cells (Fine et al., 1988). Exposure of cells *in vitro* to phorbol-13,20-diacetate (PDA), a relatively inactive phorbol ester, did not activate PKC. These experiments were done with a 2.5-hour phorbol exposure to intact cells, and PKC activity was assessed with histone III as substrate according to a previously described method (Rebois & Patel, 1985).

Phosphoprotein Changes

Phosphorylation of cellular homogenate protein after a 2.5-hour exposure of cells to phorbol ester was investigated. *In vivo* labeling with $^{32}PO_4$ revealed that the baseline 20-kD phosphoprotein was approximately fourfold higher in KC/ADR$_{10}$ cells compared to KC/control. PDBu (200 nM) exposure increased the 20-kD phosphoprotein labeling in KC/control approximately 3.5-fold, and in KC/ADR$_{10}$ cells it increased approximately 1.4-fold (Fine et al., 1988). Experiments with PDA showed no change in the phosphoprotein patterns. When 10 μM trifluoperazine (TFPZ) was added to PDBu during the 2.5-hour exposure, phosphorylation was inhibited more in the resistant than sensitive cell line. TFPZ alone had no effect on the 20-kD phosphoprotein in KC/control cells, and in the KC/ADR$_{10}$ cells it decreased phosphorylation to 34% of baseline phosphorylation in this cell line (Figure 10.4). These findings suggest that TFPZ, which can reverse the MDR phenotype, also inhibits the baseline 20-kD phosphorylation in resistant cells as well as the increased phosphorylation induced by phorbol esters, presumably owing to PKC activation.

Drug Sensitivity Changes

We examined the effects of phorbol esters on drug sensitivity of the KC/control and KC/ADR$_{10}$ cells to determine if the increased 20-kD phosphorylation is associated with increased resistance, as we have shown with MDR human breast and SCLC lines. Results of clonogenic experiments in which PDBu ± TFPZ and PDA were added for a 2.5-hour period to vincristine (VCR) or ADR showed the following: (1) baseline IC$_{50}$ to VCR and ADR were 100-fold higher in the KC ADR$_{10}$ cells compared to the parent-sensitive KC/control; (2) the addition of the inactive phorbol ester PDA did not change the IC$_{50}$ to VCR or ADR in either cell lines; and (3) PDBu increased the IC$_{50}$ for both drugs in the KC/control line approximately fourfold and in the KC/ADR$_{10}$ line approximately 1.5-fold (Fine et al., 1988). The addition of 10 μM TFPZ to PDBu for the same time period blunted the increased IC$_{50}$ for KC/controls and completely abrogated the effects of PDBu in KC/ADR$_{10}$ by decreasing the IC$_{50}$ below the baseline IC$_{50}$. When TFPZ was added alone, the IC$_{50}$ to both drugs did not change in the KC/control cells and further decreased in

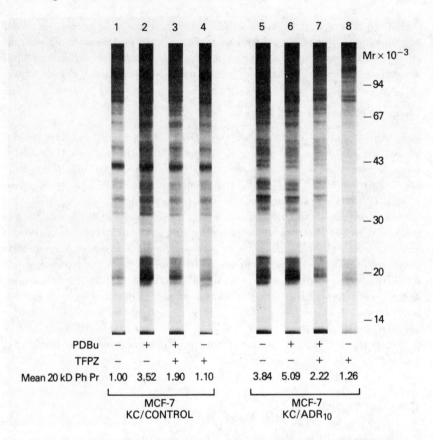

FIGURE 10.4 Autoradiogram of the homogenates from the MCF-7 lines KC/control and KC/ADR$_{10}$ with ^{32}PO$_4$ orthophosphate labeling done *in vivo*. Beneath each lane are the conditions used in the assay with the phorbol ester PDBu and the calmodulin antagonist TFPZ and the mean densitometry value for the intensity of the phosphorylation in the 20-kD phosphoprotein (20 kD Ph Pr) region. The procedure was done as previously described (Fine et al., 1988). Briefly, the cells were exposed to 1 ml of phosphate-depleted media *in vivo* for 1 hour. Then they were exposed to [^{32}PO$_4$] in the same media for 2 hours and solubilized in buffer A containing 1% Triton X-100 and separated by one-dimensional 10% SDS-PAGE.

the KC/ADR_{10} cells (Fine et al., 1986b, 1988). These data suggest that PKC activation by PDBu leads to increased resistance, an effect correlated with increased phosphorylation of protein(s) in the 20-kD region; these effects are most obvious in sensitive cells and are at least partially blocked by TFPZ.

Drug Accumulation Changes

Because a common characteristic of MDR cells is decreased intracellular accumulation owing to increased efflux of drug and that PKC activation is known to increase exocytosis of many chemicals (Nishizuka, 1986), we investigated drug accumulation changes. $[^3H]$-VCR intracellular accumulation in KC/control and KC/ADR_{10} cells was assessed in 2.5-hour exposure experiments by methods that have been previously published (Louie et al., 1986). Basal VCR accumulation in the KC/control cells was over sixfold higher than in the KC/ADR_{10} cells (Fine et al., 1988). PDA (200 nM) did not alter accumulation in either line; 200 nM PDBu decreased net intracellular accumulation 40% and 10% in the KC/control and KC/ADR_{10} cells, respectively (Fine et al., 1988). When 10 μM TFPZ was added at the same time as PDBu, the inhibitory effects of PDBu on drug accumulation were reversed. The effect of TFPZ was increased in resistance compared to sensitive cells. The addition of TFPZ had no effect on sensitive cell drug accumulation but further increased drug accumulation above the baseline in KC/ADR_{10} cells (Fine et al., 1988).

CONCLUSIONS

The data presented here demonstrate a correlation between the MDR phenotype and increased phosphorylation of the 20-kD protein in human breast and SCLC lines. This correlation exists whether MDR was induced *in vitro* (breast cancer lines) or in *in vivo* clinical situations (SCLC lines). Biochemical characteristics suggest that PKC or a similar serine-threonine kinase is involved in the increased phosphorylation of the 20-kD protein. Experiments with PDBu further support this concept because activation of PKC activity by PDBu increases the phosphorylation of the 20-kD protein and decreases intracellular drug accumulation. The general increase in protein phosphorylation in MDR cells and in PDBu-treated sensitive cells suggests that other kinases may be activated as well in these cells. The identity of the 20-kD protein is unknown, but experiments suggest that it is not myosin light chain. The increased MDR associated with PKC activation suggests that this enzyme may play a role in the MDR phenotype. Increased exocytosis of histamine and arachidonate in platelets, amylase and insulin secretion in pancreatic cells, dopamine release from neurons, aldosterone secretion from adrenal cortical cells, and lysosomal enzyme release from neutrophils occur with PKC activation. Also, many membrane transport proteins are proposed substrates for

PKC and may be regulated by phosphorylation (Nishizuka, 1986). It is possible that decreased drug accumulation in MDR cells may be from PKC modulation by phosphorylation of the P-170 glycoprotein transport protein and/or the 20-kD phosphoprotein.

REFERENCES

Cornwell, M.M., Safa, A.R., Felsted, R.L., Gottesman, M.M., & Pastan, I. (1986). Membrane vesicles from multidrug-resistant human cancer cells contain a specific 150- to 170 kDa protein detected by photoaffinity labeling. *Proceedings of the National Academy of Sciences USA, 83*:3847–3850.

Cowan, K. H., Goldsmith, M. E., Levine, R.M., Aitken, S.C., Douglass, E., Clendeninn, N. et al. (1982). Dihydrofolate reductase gene amplification and possible rearrangement in estrogen-responsive methotrexate-resistant human breast cancer cell lines. *Journal of Biological Chemistry, 257*:15079–15086.

Fairchild, C.R., Ivy, S.P., Rushmore, T., Lee, G., Koo, P., Goldsmith, M.E., et al. (1987). Carcinogen-induced MDR overexpression is associated with xenobiotic resistance in rat preneoplastic liver nodules and hepatocellular carcinomas. *Proceedings of the National Academy of Sciences USA, 84*:7701–7705.

Fine, R.L., Carmichael, J., Patel, J., Carney, D.N., Gazdar, A., Curt, G.A., et al. (1986a). Increased phosphorylation of a 20-kD protein is associated with pleiotropic drug resistance (PDR) in human small-cell lung cancer (SCLC) lines. *American Society of Clinical Oncology, 5*:17.

Fine, R.L., Patel, J., Allegra, C.J., Curt, G.A., Cowan, K.H., Ozols, R.F., et al. (1985). Increased phosphorylation of a 20-KD new protein in pleiotropic drug-resistant MCF-7 human breast cancer cell lines. *Proceedings of the American Association of Cancer Research, 26*:345.

Fine, R.L., Patel, J., Carmichael, J., Cowan, K., Curt, G.A., & Chabner, B.A. (1986b). Phosphoprotein markers and protein kinase C changes in human drug-resistant cancer cells. *In Vitro, 22*:56A.

Fine, R.L., Patel, J., & Chabner, B.A. (1988). Phorbol esters induce multidrug resistance in human breast cancer cells. *Proceedings of the National Academy of Sciences USA 85*:582–586.

Karle, J., Dowan, K.H., & Cysyk, R. (1986). Uracil nucleotide synthesis in a human breast cancer line (MCF-7) and in two drug-resistant sublines that contain increased levels of enzymes of the de novo pyrimidine pathway. *Molecular Pharmacology, 30*:136–141.

Kartner, N., Riordan, J. R., & Ling, V. (1983). Cell surface P-glycoprotein associated with multidrug resistance in mammalian cell lines. *Science, 221*:1285–1288.

Kishimoto, A., Kajikawa, N., Shiota, M., & Nishizuka, Y. (1983). Proteolytic activation of calcium-activated phospholipid-dependent protein kinase by calcium-dependent neutral protease. *Journal of Biological Chemistry, 258*:1156–1164.

Louie, K.G., Hamilton, T.C., Winkler, M.A., Behrens, B.C., Tsuruo, T., Klecker, R.W., et al. (1986). Adriamycin accumulation and metabolism in adriamycin sensitive and resistant human ovarian cancer cell lines. *Biochemical Pharmacology, 35*:467–472.

Marsh, W., & Center, M.S. (1985). In vitro phosphorylation and the identification of multiple protein changes in membranes of Chinese hamster lung cells resistant to adriamycin. *Biochemical Pharmacology, 34*:4180–4184.

Mori, T., Tokai, Y., Minakuchi, R., Yu, B., & Nishizuka, Y. (1980). Inhibitory action of chlorpromazine, dibucaine, and other phospholipid interacting drugs on calcium-activated, phospholipid-dependent protein kinase. *Journal of Biological Chemistry, 255*:8378–8380.

Myers, M.B., & Biedler, J.L. (1981). Increased synthesis of a low molecular weight protein in vincristine-resistant cells. *Biochemical and Biophysical Research Communications, 99*:228–235.

Nishizuka, Y. (1986). Studies and perspectives of protein kinase C. *Science, 233*:305–312.

Patel, J., Marango, P.J., Heydorn, W.E., Chang, B., Verma, A., & Jacobowitz, D. (1983). S-100 mediated inhibition of brain phosphorylation. *Journal of Neurochemistry, 41*:1040–1045.

Rebois, R.V., & Patel, J. (1985). Phorbol ester causes desensitization of gonadotropin-responsive adenylate cyclase in a murine Leydig tumor cell line. *Journal of Biological Chemistry, 260*:8026–8931.

Rogan, A.M., Hamilton, T.C., Young, R.C., Klecker, R.W., & Ozols, R.F. (1984). Reversal of adriamycin resistance by verapamil in human ovarian cancer. *Science, 224*:994–996.

Safa, A.R., Glover, C.J., Myers, M.B., Biedler, J.L., & Felsted, R.L. (1986). Vinblastine photoaffinity labeling of a high molecular weight surface membrane glycoprotein specific for multidrug-resistant cells. *Journal of Biological Chemistry, 261*:6137–6140.

Tsuruo, T., Iida, H., Tsukagoshi, S., & Sakurai, Y. (1983). Potentiation of vincristine and adriamycin effects in human hemopoietic tumor cell lines by calcium antagonists and calmodulin inhibitors. *Cancer Research, 43*:2267–2272.

Weisenthal, L.M., Dill, P., Kurnick, N., & Lippman, M.E. (1983). Comparison of dye exclusion on assays with a clonogenic assay in the determination of drug-induced cytotoxicity. *Cancer Research, 43*:258–264.

11

Control of Oncogene Expression: A Novel Approach for the Treatment of Cancer

Jose A. Fernandez-Pol

The cancerous cell is generally speculated to be the final result of a series of genetic lesions (Spandidos, 1985). The link between these genotypic changes and the expression of the neoplastic phenotype has been extensively studied, and a number of general conclusions were established (Heldin & Westermark, 1984; Weinberg, 1985). Oncogenes that induce transformation *in vitro* and are responsible for the development of tumors *in vivo* have been identified, and the functional properties of their gene products have been partially elucidated (Weinberg, 1985). These studies, when connected to recent information on the structure and function of polypeptide growth factors (PGF), have produced a unifying concept of the molecular mechanisms of malignant transformation and normal mitogenesis (Heldin & Westermark, 1984; Spandidos, 1985; Weinberg, 1985).

Generally, PGF have been identified through their mitogenic effects on cells in culture (Heldin & Westermark, 1984). It was discovered that serum contains specific growth-promoting substances with key regulatory functions in cell division. These observations were subsequently expanded by the findings that certain malignant cells have relaxed serum requirements and are able to proliferate in a medium containing reduced serum concentrations. These observations led to the proposal of an autocrine mechanism of growth control (Heldin & Westermark, 1984), i.e., transformed cells produce and respond to their own growth factors

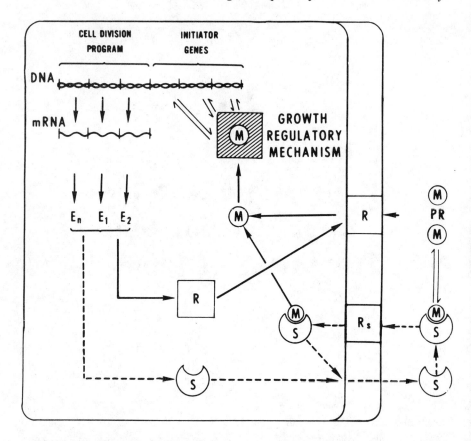

FIGURE 11.1. Mechanism of growth in normal and transformed cells. Schematic representation of exogenous growth factor that transmits the growth-promoting signal from the receptor to the nucleus, activating the cell division program. In this example, PR represents transferrin loaded with iron (M), the transferrin receptor (R) on the cell surface, and the intracellular system that delivers iron to the nucleus. E: enzymes. (Fernandez-Pol, 1978, 1981a). Schematic representation of endogenous production of growth factor that stimulates growth of the transformed cell in an autocrine fashion. The endogenously produced growth factor (S) may be secreted and interacts with growth factor receptors (Rs) at the cell surface. In this example transformed cells produce siderophore-like (S) or transferrin-like polypetides as their own growth factors, which may stimulate cell growth and may be a part of the cell iron transport system. The autocrine production of transferrin-like activity may play a crucial role for proliferation of certain cell types (Fernandez-Pol, 1978, 1981a; Kitada and Hays, 1985).

(Figure 11.1). Later a considerable number of PGF were identified and characterized biologically and structurally (Heldin & Westermark, 1984). In this review we will focus our attention on two of these factors, epidermal growth factor (EGF) and transforming growth factor β (TGFβ), which may be regarded as paradigms of growth stimulatory and inhibitory factors, respectively. These are well-characterized molecules that have been found to be active on numerous cells, including human epithelial normal and malignant cells (Carpenter & Cohen, 1979; Sporn et al., 1986; Fernandez-Pol et al., 1986).

Dominant cancer producing genes (oncogenes) were first identified in the genomes of a variety of spontaneous and chemically induced tumors by gene transfer (transfection) experiments (Weinberg, 1985; Spandidos, 1985). When the protein products of the oncogenes were characterized, they were found to be homologous to known substances that are normally involved in the control of the cell cycle (Weinberg, 1985). Studies on platelet-derived growth factor and EGF have been of particular importance for the elucidation of the links among growth factors, growth factor receptors, and oncogenes (Waterfield, 1985). In addition to providing new insights in the molecular biology of cancer, the discovery of oncogenes suggests new approaches to the prevention and treatment of cancer.

The focus of this book is aging. Many of the changes that occur in our body as we age are well recognized and are universal phenomena. Statistics clearly show that there is an increased prevalence of cancer in the aged population. The statistics present an undeniable reality to the prevalence of cancer in the elderly: 62% of all cancers occur past age 60 years and 36% past 70 years of age (Schrier, 1982). Almost nothing is known about the mechanisms by which aging leads to alterations of cell–cycle genes (proto-oncogenes). Thus, in this review speculation will center on the possible connection between proto-oncogene activation and aging.

GROWTH STIMULATORY AND INHIBITORY FACTORS: THEIR RECEPTORS AND SIGNAL TRANSDUCTION IN MITOGENESIS AND GROWTH INHIBITION

Epidermal Growth Factor

The EGF, a 53-amino-acid-long single chain polypeptide, is a potent mitogen that plays a major role in regulation of growth of numerous normal and malignant cells (Carpenter & Cohen, 1979). The initial step in the mechanism of action of EGF is its binding to specific cell–surface receptors (Carpenter, 1984). The receptor for EGF, like other receptors, functions as signal transducer and originates a series of intracellular events, which ultimately leads to the initiation of DNA synthesis and cell division (Carpenter, 1984) (Figure 11.2). The receptor for EGF is an integral membrane glycoprotein of Mr = 170 kD with an extracellular EGF binding regulatory domain, a transmembrane portion, and an intracellular catalytic domain

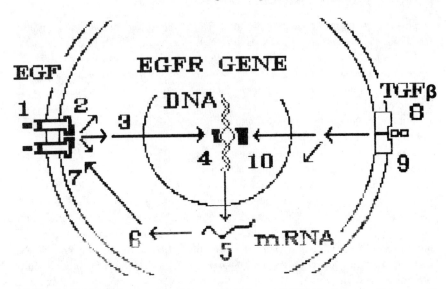

FIGURE 11.2. The molecular mechanism of EGF-induced mitogenesis
and TGFβ-induced growth inhibition in human breast carcinoma cells.
Specific high affinity cell surface receptors are indicated as transmembrane rectangles; subunit receptor structure is depicted. EGF (1) binds to
the external regulatory domain of EGF receptors. The internal functional
domain of the receptor (2) is activated and triggers the postreceptor
pathway (3). The EGF receptor gene transcription is activated (4), mRNA
is synthesized (5), the EGF receptor protein is produced (6), and inserted
in the cell membrane. Thus, EGF receptor internalization and degradation induced by EGF is counterbalanced by an increase in EGF receptor
synthesis. No attempt is made to depict the process of receptor internalization and/or degradation. TGFβ (8) binds to the external domain
of the TGFβ receptor (9) and triggers the postreceptor pathway, which in
turn enhances transcription (10) of the EGF receptor gene. This paradoxical model may well be adequate to explain growth inhibition induced
by TGFβ in certain human breast carcinoma cells.

(Waterfield, 1985). The latter functions as a protein kinase that catalyzes the
phosphorylation of tyrosine residues (Cohen et al., 1982). Activation of the EGF
receptor tyrosine kinase is thought to initiate the mitogenic signal(s) (Hunter &
Cooper, 1981). The observation that other growth factor receptors also display
tyrosine kinase activity indicates that tyrosine-phosphorylated proteins have a key
role in the transmission of the mitogenic signal from the activated receptors to the
nucleus (Heldin & Westermark, 1984).

The mechanism of action of EGF is beginning to be elucidated (Figure 11.2). Numerous studies have demonstrated the existence of two classes of EGF receptors, of low and high affinity, on a number of different cell lines (Fanger et al., 1986a; Fernandez-Pol, 1985; Yarden and Schlessinger, 1987). Several lines of evidence suggest that the high affinity sites are responsible for the mitogenic response. Studies indicate that EGF receptor clustering is also a required step for mitosis to occur as suggested by the reports that (a) antibody-induced clustering of receptors can substitute for EGF in the stimulation of cellular proliferation (Yarden & Schlessinger, 1987); and (b) the initial stages of EGF-induced receptor clustering involves transient formation of receptor complexes of Mr ~360,000 (Fanger et al., 1986b).

Our laboratory has characterized the properties of a unique type of monoclonal anti-EGF receptor antibody, which was used as a tool to further understand the mechanism of action of EGF receptors (Fernandez-Pol, 1985). This antibody, denoted 2D1-IgM, stimulates the binding of ^{125}I-EGF to EGF receptors and mimics the biologic actions of EGF in human A431 carcinoma cells. We have found that 2D1-IgM, which binds to a carbohydrate determinant at a site distinct from the EGF binding site, (a) enhances the affinity of the EGF receptors of intact cells without changing their total number, (b) stimulates the EGF receptor tyrosine kinase activity, (c) induces clustering and internalization of EGF receptors, (d) as in the case of EGF, induces a biphasic growth response with stimulation of DNA synthesis at low and inhibition at high concentrations of 2D1-IgM in A431 cells, and (e) the intrinsic EGF-like bioactivity of 2D1-IgM is enhanced by the presence of EGF. These studies support the notion that the binding of 2D1-IgM to the EGF receptor at a different site from that to which EGF binds can inititiate an effective EGF-like biologic response and that high affinity EGF receptors and EGF receptor clustering are involved in the control of cellular growth.

Following the steps delineated above, the ligand–receptor complex is internalized and degraded in lysosomes (Merlino et al., 1985). This results in rapid removal of both ligand and receptor from the cell surface (Merlino et al., 1985; Fernandez-Pol, 1981b, 1982). Recently, several investigators have reported that exposure of cultured cells to EGF results in elevated levels of EGF receptor mRNA and that the synthesis of new EGF receptor follows the increase in EGF receptor mRNA (Clark et al., 1985; Earp et al., 1986; Kudlow et al., 1986; Fernandez-Pol et al., 1987b). How these events shown in Figure 11.2, lead to stimulation of DNA synthesis and cellular proliferation is unknown.

Transforming Growth Factor β

TGFβ, a multifunctional growth factor that controls cell proliferation, differentiation, and other functions in many cell types has emerged as a paradigm of potent growth inhibitor for human epithelial normal and cancerous cells (Fernandez-Pol et al., 1986; Massague, 1987; Moses et al., 1985; Sporn et al., 1986). Type β TGF is a 25-kD disulfide-linked homodimer, which binds to specific high affinity cell surface receptors of high molecular weight ($\geq$ 180- to 360-kD) present on numerous normal and transformed cell types (Fernandez-Pol et al., 1986; Fanger et al., 1986b). One of the properties of TGFβ is its capacity to stimulate mitosis of fibroblastic cells under certain culture conditions (Assoian, 1985). Although the initial studies with TGFβ focused on its ability to stimulate proliferation of fibroblasts (Moses et al. 1985), subsequent studies demonstrated that TGFβ is a potent growth inhibitor for many normal and malignant epithelial cells in culture (Fernandez-Pol et al., 1986; Moses et al., 1985; Roberts et al., 1985). The molecular mode of action of TGFβ remains poorly understood, but it is considered to be a modulator protein (Sporn et al., 1985).

Studies indicate that EGF receptors are not only modulated by its respective ligand but also by other growth factors (Fernandez-Pol, 1982; Collins et al., 1983), including TGFβ. Experiments indicate that in certain fibroblasts TGFβ regulates the number and affinity of cell surface receptors for EGF (Assoian, 1985). Regulation of growth of epithelial cells by ligands with antiproliferative activities such as interferons may also involve modulation of the EGF receptor system (Zoon et al., 1986). Recent experiments suggest that TGFβ inhibits growth of certain malignant epithelial cells, at least in part, by regulating the expression of EGF receptors (Fernandez-Pol, 1987b).

ONCOGENES, GROWTH FACTORS, GROWTH FACTOR RECEPTORS, AND TRANSFORMATION: A UNIFYING THEORY

Proto-oncogenes and Oncogenes

All cells possess genes, termed proto-oncogenes, with potential transforming activity (Spandidos, 1985; Weinberg, 1985). A proto-oncogene may modify its activity and turn into a transforming gene (oncogene) by specific genetic mechanism such as mutation, amplification, rearrangement, or transduction by retroviruses. The activated oncogene controls the synthesis of qualitatively or quantitatively abnormal proteins that are the molecules responsible for the transformed state. Proto-oncogenes have important roles in cell growth, development, and differentiation (Weinberg, 1985). This concept is supported by the findings that proto-oncogenes encode proteins with known functions at various steps of the normal cell cycle (Waterfield, 1985). Thus, the corresponding oncogenes produce their transforming effect by encoding analogous proteins with equivalent functions in the mitogenic pathway. Figure 11.3 summarizes the relationship between proto-oncogenes and oncogenes.

The finding of a direct connection between oncogenes and growth factor receptors may be regarded as a major breakthrough in recent cancer research because it provides a unifying view of the molecular mechanisms of transformation (Waterfield, 1985). Direct evidence that an oncogene may code for a growth factor

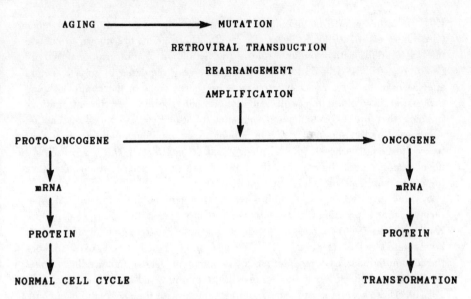

FIGURE 11.3. Transmutation of proto-oncogenes into oncogenes. Proto-tooncogenes are normal cellular genes that control the synthesis of proteins with normal functions in cell growth, development, and differentiation. A proto-oncogene may be transformed into an oncogene by a number of genetic mechanisms such as mutation, retroviral transduction, amplification, or rearrangement. The oncogene controls the synthesis of qualitatively and quantitatively abnormal proteins, which are the effector molecules in transformation. Aging most likely affects proto-oncogenes by inducing progressive mutations.

receptor was derived from the amino acid sequence of the EGF receptor, which showed sequence homology with the v-erbB gene product of the avian erythroblastosis (erb) virus (Downward et al., 1984). It is thus apparent that the erb virus has obtained transforming capacity by acquiring cellular EGF receptor gene sequences. The transforming gene product, gp65^{erbB}, represents a truncated EGF receptor that has lost its extracellular EGF-binding regulatory domain and a portion of the intracellular C-terminus (Waterfield, 1985). It is possible then that the loss of these sequences results in the permanent activation of the v-erbB protein, which emulates the action of an activated EGF receptor, which in turn activates substrates in an unregulated manner.

Expression and Suppression of Oncogenes Induced by Growth Stimulatory and Inhibitory Factors

A new area of molecular biology is the study of the expression of proto-oncogenes/oncogenes in response to growth factors. Particularly important findings are that

EGF and other growth factors stimulate the expression of c-*fos* and c-*myc* genes (Greenberg et al., 1986; Kelly et al., 1983). These genes are known to encode nuclear proteins with a putative role in the regulation of transcriptional activity (Weinberg, 1985). The finding that these genes are regulated by growth factors suggest that the c-*fos* and c-*myc* proteins are key factors in the control of gene expression in conjunction with initiation of cell replication. Recent findings indicate that the EGF-dependent induction of c-*myc* gene expression can be suppressed by the action of TGFβ in human breast carcinoma cells under serum-free conditions (Fernandez-Pol et al., 1987a). This effect of TGFβ represents a novel action of this hormone at the level of gene expression, which may have important implications in growth control.

Several investigators have addressed the problem of the regulation of EGF receptor gene expression in mammalian cells (Clark et al., 1985; Earp et al., 1986; Kudlow et al., 1986). Experiments indicate that EGF receptor gene expression can be regulated by EGF (Figure 11.2). We have found that EGF progressively induces the accumulation of EGF receptor mRNA in human breast carcinoma cells to levels fivefold to tenfold greater than are present in the uninduced state (Fernandez-Pol, 1987b). These results are in substantial agreement with the observations of Clark et al. (1985) with human KB carcinoma cells. These studies support the contention that the action of EGF that leads to receptor degradation is counterbalanced by an increase in receptor synthesis.

We have found that EGF-receptor gene expression is enhanced by TGFβ, indicating that EGF receptors are involved in the process that controls growth inhibition induced by TGFβ in human breast carcinoma cells (Fernandez-Pol et al., 1987b). It may be inferred from published reports that there is a relationship between cell surface EGF receptors and growth response, and when an optimum quantity of EGF receptors is surpassed, growth inhibition results on exposure to EGF (Kawamoto et al., 1984; Fernandez-Pol, 1985; Filmus et al., 1985). Thus, it is conceivable that an increase in the level of EGF receptors induced by TGFβ in the presence of EGF contributes to the paradoxical inhibition of growth of certain human mammary carcinoma cells (Fernandez-Pol et al., 1987a) (Figure 11.2).

AGING AND PROTO-ONCOGENES

The general theory that deals with the mutagenic effect of external agents impinging randomly upon a system has been previously formalized by Bunge (1979). In this model the system contains m components (targets) sensitive to certain discrete transmuting agents (bullets). The sensitive components must be a critical part of the whole system even if they are only a small part; they may be cellular nuclei, organelles, etc. The disrupting agents can be ionizing particles, radiation, etc. Every hit or collision of a bullet with a target is assumed to either mutate or destroy the latter. One should also assume that the effects are mutually independent, so that only their cumulative effect is of importance (Bunge, 1979). Thus, the problem of aging is to compute the probability that n random bullets will produce a change (or transmutation) in a system with m sensitive components. Then, the probability that the bullets will be ineffectual decreases exponentially as the number of bullets increases, while the probability that the system undergoes a radical transmutation increases monotonically with the number of bullets (Bunge, 1979).

Every cell system is subjected to some mutagenic or other type of pernicious agent such as fast charged particles, hard radiation, and toxic environmental substances. Furthermore, the agents are likely to have some effects—not necessarily destructive but in any case transmuting. Therefore, every cellular system is subject to random actions that eventually elicit its breakdown or mutation. In the cells the mutagenic agents may be external to its sensitive components or internal. Damage from external factors may lead to defects. Toxic and other factors within the cell environment (chemical and thermal actions of the surrounding cytoplasm) may also lead to progressive damage of the cells. Mechanisms certaintly exist within the cell to repair such damage. However, with time the effects accumulate and the repair mechanisms also age, becoming ineffective. A primary effect of such damage may be on the DNA. As internal and external damages compound, they eventually form the error catastrophe that would result in the transmutation or death of the cells. Thus, it may be concluded that aging will have a major effect in the activation of specific proto-oncogenes into oncogenes (Figure 11.4). According to this contention, all that we have to do is to wait for the transmutations to occur.

The general hypothesis of aging and cancer formulated above is in accordance with the multistep origin of cancer (Klein and Klein, 1985). It is widely accepted that human cancer originates as a multistep process. This concept is based on

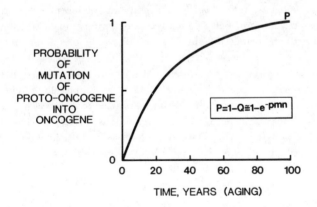

FIGURE 11.4. **Probable effects of aging in the conversion of proto-oncogenes into oncogenes. Probability P, that all m sensitive components of a proto-oncogene system will be hit and mutate; n, transmuting agents. Thus, proto-oncogenes are subjected to the random actions of aging that eventually will elicit its mutation or its breakdown.**

numerous lines of evidence. The most convincing evidence includes the long time course of oncogenesis described by oncologists and documented by pathologists. The statistical analysis of age–incidence cancer data suggest that several independent events are required for the emergence of human epithelial cancers (Peto, 1977). The presence of multiple chromosome abnormalities in most tumor cells and the increasingly aberrant chromosome structures that arise during tumor growth and progression (German, 1983) also provide evidence for a role of cellular damage in the etiology of cancer. Furthermore, the localization of oncogenes at translocation breakpoints in specific forms of cancer (Rowley, 1984) greatly strengthens the evidence that chromosomal damage plays a causal role in the transmutations of proto-oncogenes to oncogenes. The high probability of cancer developing in patients with genetic diseases that promote chromosomal instability (German, 1983) also provides very convincing evidence for the causal role of DNA damage in cancer etiology.

CANCER TREATMENT AND ONCOGENES

Undoubtedly, future attempts to develop new cancer therapeutic methods will include pharmacologic intervention in some of the steps in the mechanism of action of specific oncogenes delineated in this review. Possible avenues for *ex vivo* or *in vivo* cancer therapy may include the following: (1) development of antagonists of growth stimulatory factors; (2) toxic substances linked to specific growth factors; (3) monoclonal antireceptor antibodies, e.g., anti-EGF receptor antibodies; (4) drug or toxin conjugates of monoclonal antireceptor antibodies; and (5) growth inhibitory factors or analogues, e.g., TGFβs. Furthermore, in recent years, recombinant DNA technology has provided a radically new opportunity to control abnormal gene expression. By reversing the direction of the gene of interest relative to its promoter, the opposite (noncoding) strand of DNA can be transcribed, producing a complementary antisense RNA (Hunts et al., 1986). This antisense RNA can then be hybridized with the sense RNA to inhibit its translation into protein. Therefore, it is conceivable that antisense RNA may be utilized to suppress the expression of the EGF receptor oncogene in malignant cells (Hunts, 1986). Thus, the level of EGF receptor protein activity should be suppressed in the cancerous cells, leading to a more normal phenotype. This approach may have clinical value in modulating the course of neoplastic transformation.

CONCLUSION

It is becoming increasingly evident that the malignant character is not the result of the expression of one single oncogene (Spandidos, 1985). The development of the fully transformed phenotype most likely requires the expression of several complementary oncogenes; thus, aging will have a major role in the promotion of such events. Because aging most likely affects critical components of the mitogenic pathway, it may be proposed that the conversion of proto-oncogenes to oncogenes induced by aging will have a limited number of specific mechanisms. Thus, this contention is therapeutically optimistic as it renews interest in the possibility of preventing the effects of aging on proto-oncogenes or restoring growth control to cancerous cells by intervention in specific steps of oncogene expression. It is conceivable that as knowledge of the transmutation of proto-oncogenes into oncogenes increases, the specific relationship with aging will be found.

REFERENCES

Assoian, R.K. (1985). Biphasic effects of type β transforming growth factor on epidermal growth factor receptors in NRK fibroblasts. *Journal of Biological Chemistry*, *260*:9613–9617.

Bunge, M. (1979). Treatise on basic philosophy. Vol. 4. *Ontology II: a word of systems*, (pp. 273–291). Publishing Company. D. Reidel: Dordrecht, Holland.

Carpenter, G. (1984). Properties of the receptor for epidermal growth factor. *Cell*, 37:357–358.

Carpenter, G., & Cohen, S. (1979). Epidermal growth factor. *Annual Review of Biochemistry*, *48*:193–216.

Clark, A.J.L., Ishii, S., Richert, N., Merlino, G.T., & Pastan, I. (1985). Epidermal growth factor regulates the expression of its own receptor. *Proceedings of the National Academy of Sciences USA*, *82*:8374–8378.

Cohen, S., Ushiro, H., Stoscheck, C., & Chinkers, M.A. (1982). Native 170,000 epidermal growth factor receptor-kinase complex from shed plasma membrane vesicles. *Journal of Biological Chemistry*, *257*:1523–1531.

Collins, M.K.L., Sinnett-Smith, J.W., & Rozengurt, E. (1983). Platelet-derived growth factor treatment decreases the affinity of the epidermal growth factor receptors of Swiss 3T3 cells. *Journal of Biological Chemistry*, *258*:11689–11693.

Downward, J., Yarden, Y., Mayes, E., Scrace, G., Totty, N., Stockwell, P., et al. (1984). Close similarity of epidermal growth factor receptor and v-erb-B oncogene protein sequences. *Nature*, *307*:521–527.

Earp, H.S., Austin, K.S., Blaisdell, J., Rubin, R.A., Nelson, K.G., Lee, L.W., et al. (1986). Epidermal growth factor (EGF) stimulates EGF receptor synthesis. *Journal of Biological Chemistry*, *261*:4777–4780.

Fanger, B.O., Austin, K.S., Earp, S.H., & Cidlowski, J.A. (1986a). Cross-linking of epidermal growth factor receptors in intact cells: Detection of the initial stages of receptor clustering and determination of molecular weight of high-affinity receptors. *Biochemistry*, *25*:6414–6420.

Fanger, B.O., Wakefield, L.M., & Sporn, M.B. (1986b). Structure and properties of the cellular receptor for transforming growth factor Type β. *Biochemistry*, *25*:3083–3091.

Fernandez-Pol, J.A. (1978). Isolation and characterization of a siderophore-like growth factor from mutants of SV40-transformed cells adapted to picolinic acid. *Cell*, *14*:489–499.

Fernandez-Pol, J.A. (1981a). Peptide and protein complexes of transition metals as modulators of cellular replication. *International Journal of Nuclear Medicine and Biology*, *8*:231–235.

Fernandez-Pol, J.A. (1981b). Epidermal growth factor: Relationship between receptor down regulation in cultured NRK cells and epidermal growth factor enhancement of phosphorylation of a 170,000 molecular weight membrane protein in vitro. *Biochemistry, 20*:3907–3912.

Fernandez-Pol, J.A. (1982). Modulation of epidermal growth factor-dependent protein phosphorylation in cell membrane preparations by receptor down regulation. *Journal of Cellular Biochemistry, 19*:205–222.

Fernandez-Pol, J.A. (1985). Epidermal growth factor receptor of A431 cells: Characterization of a monoclonal anti-receptor antibody noncompetitive agonist of epidermal growth factor action. *Journal of Biological Chemistry, 260*:5003–5011.

Fernandez-Pol, J.A., Klos, D.J., & Grant, G.A. (1986). Purification and biological properties of type β transforming growth factor from mouse transformed cells. *Cancer Research, 46*:5153–5161.

Fernandez-Pol, J.A., Talkad, V.D., Klos, D.J., & Hamilton, P.D. (1987a). Supression of the EGF-dependent induction of c-myc proto-oncogene expression by transforming growth factor β in a human breast carcinoma cell line. *Biochemical and Biophysical Research Communications, 144*:1197–1205.

Fernandez-Pol, J.A., Klos, D.J., Hamilton, P.D., & Talkad, V.D. (1987b). Modulation of epidermal growth factor receptor gene expression by transforming growth factor-β in a human breast carcinoma cell line. *Cancer Research, 47*:4260–4265.

Filmus, J., Pollak, M.N., Cailleau, R., & Buick, R.N. (1985). MDA-468, a human breast cancer cell line with a high number of epidermal growth factor receptors, has an amplified EGF receptor gene and is growth inhibited by EGF. *Biochemical and Biophysical Research Communications, 128*:898–905.

German, J. (Ed.). (1983). *Chromosome mutation and neoplasia.* New York: Alan R. Liss.

Greenberg, M.E., Hermanowski, A.L., & Ziff, E.B. (1986). Effect of protein synthesis inhibitors on growth factor activation of c-fos, c-myc and actin gene transcription. *Molecular and Cellular Biology, 6*:1050–1057.

Heldin, C.-H., & Westermark, B. (1984). Growth factors: Mechanism of action and relation to oncogenes. *Cell, 37*:9–20.

Hunter, T., & Cooper, J.A. (1981). Epidermal growth factor induces rapid tyrosine phosphorylation of proteins in A431 human tumor cells. *Cell, 24*:741–752.

Hunts, J., Merlino, G., Pastan, I., & Shimizu, N. (1986). Reduction of EGF receptor synthesis by antisense RNA vectors. *FEBS Letters, 206*:319–322.

Kawamoto, T., Mendelsohn, J., Le, A., Sato, G.H., Lazar, C.S., & Gill, G.N. (1984). Relation of epidermal growth factor receptor concentration to growth of human epidermoid carcinoma A431 cells. *Journal of Biological Chemistry, 259*:7761–7766.

Kelly, K., Cochran, B.H., Stiles, C.K., & Leder, P.D. (1983). Cell-specific regulation of the c-myc gene by lymphocyte mitogens and platelet-derived growth factor. *Cell, 35*:603–610.

Kitada, S., & Hays, E.F. (1985). Transferrin-like activity produced by murine malignant T-lymphoma cell lines. *Cancer Research, 45*:3537–3540.

Klein, G., & Klein, E. (1985). Evolution of tumors and the impact of molecular oncology. *Nature, 315*:190–195.

Kudlow, J.E., Cheung, C.-Y.M., & Bjorge, J.D. (1986). Epidermal growth factor stimulates the synthesis of its own receptor in a human breast cancer cell line. *Journal of Biological Chemistry, 261*:4134–4138.

Massague, J. (1987). The TGFβ family of growth and differentiation factors. *Cell, 49*:437–438.

Merlino, G.T., Xu, Y., Richert, N., Ishii, S., Clark, A.J.L., Stratton, R.H., et al. (1985). Cloning and characterization of human epidermal growth factor-receptor gene sequences in A431 carcinoma cells. In Feremisco, J., Ozanne, B., & Stiles, C. (Eds.), *Cancer cells 3/ Growth factors and transformation.* (pp. 19–24). Cold Spring Harbor, NY: Cold Spring Harbor Laboratory.

Moses, H.L., Tucker, R.F., Leof, E.B., Coffey, R.J., Jr., Halper, J., & Shipley, G.D. (1985). Type β transforming growth factor is a growth stimulator and a growth inhibitor. In Feremisco, J., Ozanne, B., & Stiles, C. (Eds.), *Cancer cells 3/ Growth factors and transformation,* (pp. 65–71). Cold Spring Harbor, NY: Cold Spring Harbor Laboratory.

Peto, R. (1977). Epidemiology, multistage models, and short-term mutagenicity tests. In Hiatt, H.H., Watson, J.D., & Winsten, J.A. (Eds.), *Origins of human cancer* (pp. 1403–1428). Cold Spring Harbor, NY: Cold Spring Harbor Laboratory.

Roberts, A.B., Anzano, M.A., Wakefield, L.M., Roche, N. S., Stern, D.F., & Sporn, M.B. (1985). Type β transforming growth factor: A bifunctional regulator of cellular growth. *Proceedings of the National Academy of Sciences USA, 82*:119–123.

Rowley, J.D. (1984). Biological implications of consistent chromosome rearrangements in leukemia and lymphoma. *Cancer Research, 44*:3159–3168.

Schrier, R.W. (1982). *Clinical internal medicine in the aged.* Philadelphia: W.B. Saunders.

Spandidos, D. (1985). Mechanism of carcinogenesis: The role of oncogenes, transcriptional enhancers and growth factors. *Anticancer Research, 5*:485–498.

Sporn, M.B., Roberts, A.B., Wakefield, L.M., & Assoian, R.K. (1986). Transforming growth factor-β: Biological function and chemical structure. *Science, 233*:532–534.

Waterfield, M.D. (1985). Two distinct mechanisms involving growth factors employed in subversion of growth regulation by oncogenes. *Progress in Medical Virology, 32*:129–141.

Weinberg, R.A. (1985). The action of oncogenes in the cytoplasm and nucleus. *Science, 230*:770–776.

Yarden, Y., & Schlessinger, J. (1987). Self-phosphorylation of epidermal growth factor receptor: Evidence for a model of intermolecular allosteric activation. *Biochemistry, 26*:1434–1442.

Zoon, K.C., Karasaki, Y., Nedden, D.K., Hu, R., & Arnheiter, H. (1986). Modulation of epidermal growth factor receptors by human α interferon. *Proceedings of the National Academy of Sciences USA, 83*:8226–8230.

PART IV

Special Issues in the Care of the Elderly Cancer Patient

12

Prevention of Cancer in the Elderly

David D. Celentano

The goal of public health is the eradication of preventable disease and the reduction in human suffering engendered by unnecessary morbidity. The fundamental public health approach is to apply preventive strategies to maximize human performance and well-being and to minimize deterioration, symptom expression, or disease progression to the extent feasible. In contrast, clinical medicine's focus is upon applying known technologies to the needs of individual patients, with the goal of eliminating or attenuating the disease process. The public health perspective is largely preventive, leading to a quite different orientation (Last, 1980).

Prevention focuses on the population, not individuals, and emphasizes intervening upon risk factors identified as prevalent in the population. This approach also recognizes that risks are not universal and that interventions and treatment will not help all persons at risk for the disease. Attention is focused where the greatest good can come to the most people. Given these caveats, in assessing the health needs of a population, a conscious decision is made as to where to place relatively scarce resources; the social, economic and political benefits that would accrue are thus evaluated (Miller, 1985a).

The prevention of cancer has been widely advocated because as a group of diseases it constitutes the second leading cause of death in the United States (Silverburg & Lubera, 1987). Further, the risk factors for many cancers are viewed to be functions of lifestyle, behaviors including alcohol and tobacco use, sunlight exposure, use of estrogens and other drugs, diets, as well as exposure to carcinogenic agents, primarily in the workplace (Lilienfeld, 1980; National Research Council, 1982). It is generally acknowledged that a large proportion of cancer risks are avoidable; as such, their sequelae are considered preventable (Somers, 1980). The preventive approach is either to alter the behavior of the individual at risk or to modify the environment in such a way as to reduce the risk of exposure in the population (Kegeles & Grady, 1982).

When we address the notion of prevention of disease, a continuum of opportunities for application is presented. Traditionally, preventive interventions are described within three stages: primary, secondary, and tertiary (Last, 1980). Primary prevention refers to the elimination of exposure to the risk factors or agents themselves. For example, health education interventions with primary school children concerning the dangers of cigarette smoking have as their goal preventing the initiation of this carcinogenic behavior. Secondary prevention refers to the early detection of disease, where treatment may be far more successful and the disease more amenable to cure. The widespread use of mammography for the early detection of breast cancer among middle-aged and elderly women is one form of secondary prevention (Howard, 1987b). Tertiary prevention refers to aggressive and comprehensive medical treatment, with the aim of extending life, improving the quality of life, and potentially curing the disease. Rehabilitation and aftercare services for the cancer patient as well as various treatment modalities including radiotherapy and chemotherapy, are examples of such activities (Greenwald et al., 1985).

In addressing the issues surrounding the prevention of cancer, trade-offs have traditionally been made as to which type of preventive intervention should be used. These reflect our knowledge of the disease process, the technologies we have available to effectively intervene, the acceptability of our intervention activities in the population at risk, and the societal evaluation of the importance of the disease (Howard 1987a). To date, activities for disease prevention in general have received significantly less attention than curative approaches as reflected by level of financial expenditures. The emphasis on cure over prevention has emerged from a variety of factors, including the emphasis on a medical model of the disease process and associated interventions over the public health approach, desires for rapid solutions to health problems, as well as historical emphases on individual responsibility for health status and disease risks and risk reduction behavior.

When focusing on the issues of the prevention of cancer in the elderly, it may be questioned as to the needs for prevention and the true social benefit of such expenditures. An assessment of expenditures on medical care demonstrates that almost one-half of the health care bill is accounted for by the elderly, who comprise only 12% of the population (Yancik, 1983). Clearly, any successful prevention program that could have an impact on reducing this level of expenditures would be welcomed if only from a financial perspective. Yet it seems clear that primary prevention strategies might well be lost on the elderly, for maximal effectiveness requires a long lead time for the prevention of most cancers. Because the majority of primary prevention strategies are focused at eliminating initial exposures to cancer risks (smoking, dietary components, workplace exposures), which would be anticipated to have their effect demonstrated years later, the introduction of such programs to the elderly does not appear particularly warranted. Thus, secondary and tertiary approaches for prevention remain. These are desirable only if available treatment exists that is documented effective in prolonging life or improving the quality of life remaining. A review by Sorenson et al. (1983) suggests that little empirical research has been conducted on this issue to date.

Each cancer has its own etiology, risk factors, course, and treatment. Cancers differ widely in their incidence by age, survivorship, and preventability. Rather than address all prevention strategies that impinge upon the elderly, we focus here on one cancer site for which there is a known and effective prevention strategy: cervical cancer and its early detection through cervical cytology. With consistent routine screening of women by the Pap test, cervical cancer, in large part, should be eradicated. Although the death rate has dramatically declined in recent decades, the fact remains that thousands of women die from this preventable cause of death each year. This cancer serves as an example of the special needs and problems of cancer prevention for the elderly, for it demonstrates the behavioral, biologic, and medical care issues involved in prevention.

CERVICAL CANCER

Clinical Features

Cervical cancer has been recognized as an important clinical disease for centures (Hulka, 1982). It is a relatively slow-growing cancer with several defined stages. Early (precancerous) cellular changes have been cytologically defined: morphologic transitions of normal squamous cells of the cervix into mild, moderate, and severe dysplastic cells. Although the progression of the disease is not always direct, with reversion to normal cells being seen in many cases, it passes from severe dysplasia into carcinoma in situ, which is clinically recognized and aggressively treated (primarily by surgical ablation or cryosurgery) (Peterson, 1956; Koss et al., 1963). Although carcinoma in situ of the uterine cervix may not progress, in many cases it proliferates and develops in a number of years, resulting in invasive cancer. Even at this stage, with appropriate treatment, nearly two-thirds of cases survive for 5 years. If untreated, death will ensue (Green, 1977).

The typical symptomatology of clinically apparent squamous cervical cancer is the occurrence of a thin, blood-tinged discharge from the vagina; later, more obvious intermittent intermenstrual bleeding occurs, often recognized postcoitally. If untreated, tumor enlargement leads to heavier and more frequent bleeding. Among the elderly, frequent bleeding episodes lead to seeking medical attention because postmenopausal bleeding is widely recognized as abnormal (Arneson & Kao, 1987).

Epidemiology of Cervical Cancer

There are approximately 7000 deaths from cervical cancer expected in the United States in 1987, with the mortality rate being nearly 50% higher among nonwhite women as whites. Information from the Surveillance, Epidemiology and End Results (SEER) cancer registry enumeration system, which collects incidence (new cases of disease) data for ten geographical areas in the United States (cities and entire states), shows that approximately 12.4 new cases of invasive cervical cancer per 100,000 population of women occurred during the period 1973–77. In addition, 36.5 cases of *in situ* cancer of the uterine cervix were reported for the same time period (Young et al., 1982). The SEER data show that the disease is more common in blacks than whites, and is also high for women of Hispanic heritage (Malone et al., 1986). With respect to mortality, there is lower survivorship among elderly and poorer women (Milner and Watts, 1987).

There is considerable evidence in the epidemiologic literature that there are a number of biologic and behavioral risk factors for the disease (Celentano et al., 1988; Hulka, 1982). Chief among these are older age (Celentano et al., 1982), reproductive behaviors (Cramer, 1982), most notably early menarche and early and frequent intercourse with many partners (Boyd & Doll, 1964), history of sexually transmitted disease (Li et al., 1982), and cigarette smoking (Winkelstein et al., 1984). Interestingly, some risk factors formerly reported to lead to higher rates of disease, such as oral contraceptives and the use of barrier methods of contraception (diaphragm and condom), are now found to be protective of cervical cancer (Celentano et al., 1987). The physical barrier afforded by such contraceptives and the virucidal effects of spermicides appears to be the important factor (Singh et al., 1976). A principal behavioral risk factor identified is frequency of obtaining Pap tests (Clarke & Anderson, 1979; LaVecchia et al., 1984).

Early Detection of Cervical Cancer

The diagnostic screening technique for cervical cancer is the Papanicolaou test, exfoliative cytology, in which cellular abnormalities can be detected. Results that show moderate dysplasia or more substantial alterations are then subjected to additional tests for the purpose of making a definitive diagnosis (biopsy and tissue section). Although there has never been a randomized clinical trial of the efficacy of cervical cytology as an early detection technique, it has enjoyed widespread international acclaim for that purpose. In countries where universal detection programs have been implemented, death rates have declined and the stage of disease at the time detected has been reduced (Miller, 1985b). Thus, cervical cancer screening is a recommended component of the routine health care of women (Greenwald & Sondik, 1986).

Issues with respect to cervical cancer screening are as follows: who should be screened (age at initiation of screening), how often screening should be performed (periodicity), and at what age screening can be safely stopped without risk of a cancer developing later (age at discontinuation). Despite some controversy over these recommendations (Weisman et al., 1986), the American Cancer Society criteria seems a middle ground. It recommends (American Cancer Society, 1980) the following: Pap testing should be initiated at age 20 or at the onset of sexual activity; after two annual negative smears, it should be performed every three years; and cervical screening can be discontinued at age 65.

Miller (1982, 1985a) has evaluated the factors governing successful implementation of screening programs; they can be used as guidelines for indicating issues regarding cervical cancer screening for the elderly. The first principal is that the disease must be important (both in terms of its prevalence and lethality). Although cervical cancer is not a major cause of death, its unique nature in terms of almost universal preventability suggests its relevance. Further, the majority of deaths occur among middle-aged and elderly women. The second principal is that the natural history of the disease must be known in order to detemine a reasonable screening schedule. Clearly, cancer of the cervix and its early detection using exfoliative cytology adequately meet this requirement. Third, there must be adequate treatment of the the disease. Again, confirmation of diagnosis and treatment for cervical cancer is well accepted. Finally, the screening test must be acceptable to the population and be safe. Despite initial concerns that cervical cancer screening might be rejected by women, especially older women, this has not occurred in most populations. As such, screening for the disease is viewed as warranted and efficacious.

Despite recent progress in improving accessibility of screening and detection services and in reducing the mortality owing to cervical cancer nationally, especially among blacks, there remain subgroups of women at high risk for the disease. There is a widespread belief in the clinical literature that many women, especially the poor and elderly, either have significant gaps in their history of receiving Pap tests or have never received such screening (Celentano et al., 1988; Weisman et al., 1987). This assertion has rarely been documented in a rigorous fashion. Given the caveat that screening is effective in detecting cervical cancer at an early stage, which then decreases the risk of death and increases survivorship, routine Pap testing is currently recommended for most women.

Pap testing requires an encounter with the medical care system. It has been widely documented that women at highest risk for cervical cancer are disproportionately found to not participate in mass screening programs or to have regular Pap tests even if they have a regular source of care (Celentano et al., 1982, 1988; Eardley et al., 1985; Mettlin et al., 1985) Warneke et al., (1983) suggest three approaches to understanding the factors related to awareness and use of screening programs. First are economic and sociodemographic explanations; here, lack of insurance coverage and poverty are seen as general barriers to obtaining routine cytologic examinations. Second are what Warneke et al. refer to as behavioral factors, principally comprising patient health attitudes and beliefs as well as knowledge of symptoms and signs. One should also consider actual behavior (smoking, reproductive history, and contraceptive use) here as well. Third are structural factors that are implicit in mass screening programs and either encourage utilization by appeals to the hard to reach or high-risk patient or decrease barriers to utilization through decreased cost or improved access. Clearly, all three approaches must be considered when investigating a disease such as cervical cancer, which can best be seen as a "failure" of the medical care system (a failure in the sense that early detection could have led to a less severe form of the disease or to increased survivorship). The analysis of the etiology of cervical cancer from a sociobehavioral perspective requires consideration of the socioeconomic, behavioral, and medical care system components, for each makes a unique contribution to utilization behavior that is associated with opportunities to receive (or miss) a routine Pap test (Shapiro, 1986).

Cervical Cancer Screening Among the Elderly

In general, the elderly have disproportionately not either been offered or availed themselves of opportunities for screening for cancer of the uterine cervix (Celentano et al., 1982). The evidence comes from national surveys, local investigations, case–control studies, and other epidemiologic studies. Although only rarely have studies directly focused on the cervical cancer screening needs of the elderly, inferences can frequently be made from the published data. A brief review of these findings suggests a number of avenues for investigating needs for and utilization of cancer prevention among the elderly.

The 1985 Health Promotion and Disease Prevention study interviewed 33,630 U.S. citizens and included information on cervical cancer screening (National Center for Health Statistics, 1986). Those under 65 years of age are over four times as likely as women 65 and over to have had a Pap test (15% vs. approximately 3% to 4%), and only 50% of the latter have been screened within the prior 3 years. In a random sample of upstate New York residents, Howe and Bzduch (1987) showed that elderly women were the least likely to obtain an annual or triennial smear in comparison with younger women. Warneke and Graham (1976) conducted a random household survey of blacks living in Buffalo, New York. They report that the frequency of receiving Pap smears is directly related to age, with those over 65 years being regularly screened only 3% of the time, with 61% reporting never having received such screening. Finally, Celentano et al. (1982) demonstrated a direct negative relationship between lifetime screening for cervical cancer and age in a sample of Maryland women.

Case–control studies provide similar evidence. For example, Clarke and Anderson (1979) conducted an investigation of 212 cases of invasive cervical cancer and a control group of 1060 age-matched neighborhood controls. Their estimate of the relative risk of disease increased significantly with age, with the women aged 60 years and older having the least frequency of Pap smear screening. This finding has been replicated in diverse settings, for example, among Hispanic and Anglo women in Los Angeles (Peters et al., 1986), Cali, Columbia (Aristizabal et al., 1984), and in Thailand (Wangsuphachart et al., 1987). Older women have been universally less likely to have ever been screened or have had less consistent screening over their lifetimes.

Turkel et al. (1969) conducted one of the first investigations of the gynecologic health of the elderly. From a hospitalized population, they reported that "the proportion of abnormal findings [on Pap test] is much higher than the average, as might be expected in our population sample [of the elderly]." This statement presaged significant scientific documentation on population bases. Oster (1980) conducted a survey of two nursing homes in New York and reported detecting three cases of cancer in women who had no knowledge of ever having been screened for cervical cancer. Mandelblatt and Hammond (1985) found a strong association ($r = 0.93$) between age and interval since prior Pap test in a pilot study of patients in an urban ambulatory care clinic with a large elderly population. They found a rate of positive Pap smears of 27/1000 which reflected low prior use of screening. More recent findings (Mandelblatt et al., 1986) show that one-fourth of 1542 elderly patients reported having no prior screening, most had only sporadic screening, and the prevalence rate of positive Pap smears was 13.5 per 1000. Wheat et al. (1987) found a reverse trend in a sample of elderly women in two San Francisco hospitals, a low rate of cervical dysplasia and carcinoma, which may reflect a high rate of prior screening. However, these women were not likely to seek care from gynecologists and were more likely to have recently refused a Pap smear. Clearly, differences in samples, risk status, and designs are important.

Given these findings, we have recently completed several studies on the factors associated with cervical cancer from a behavioral epidemiologic approach. The data demonstrate the special issues and concerns in secondary prevention efforts for the elderly and offer some suggestions on methods for mounting preventive interventions for the elderly.

METHODS

The data to be presented are from two related studies on cervical cancer, which together provide information on the cancer prevention needs of the elderly population. The first study focused on the identification of risk factors for cervical cancer; we interviewed 153 cervical cancer cases and 153 matched controls in 1985. The second component was a survey of the middle-aged and elderly population of Maryland. A telephone survey conducted in 1986 with 1200 women 45 years of age and older focused on detailing the prevalence of risk factors for cervical cancer in the larger population. Together, these studies provide useful evidence for assessing the state of prevention needs for the elderly.

The purpose of our case–control study was to identify prior health care utilization patterns of cervical cancer patients and compare them to a matched control group of women free of the disease, as well as to ascertain other risk factors, both behavioral and biologic, for the disease. The general hypothesis was that these cases would have been less likely over the course of their lives to have received regular Pap testing (what has been deemed missed opportunities), primarily owing to differences in their medical care utilization patterns. Sasco et al. (1986) demonstrated that the case–control design is useful for monitoring the effectiveness of existing screening programs.

Women, especially those who are less affluent and those who are elderly, have medical care utilization patterns that place them at greater risk of not receiving routine Pap testing and gynecologic care. The review above has shown that the elderly are less likely than younger women to have ever had a routine cytologic examination and to have received them routinely over the course of their lives. Further, these same women are less likely to have developed medical care utilization patterns that included care from an obstetrician–gynecologist, the specialty most likely to provide Pap testing routinely. Thus, it is anticipated that cervical cancer cases would (1) be less likely than normal controls to have ever received a Pap test (prior to the examination that was diagnostic of their condition); (2) have had fewer Pap tests over the course of their lives than matched controls; and (3) have been more likely to have had more missed opportunities for routine Pap tests (visits to a medical care provider where a Pap test was not given). These utilization risks are considered of sufficient magnitude that they are expected to remain significant even after adjustment for other documented risk factors.

In the population survey the aim was to assess how prevalent these factors were. Case–control findings give suggestions as to etiologic mechanisms or risk factors, but estimates of the frequency of these characteristics in the general population cannot be made. Hence, our second study addressed these issues and "oversampled" the elderly to focus on their needs and attendant knowledge, attitudes, and practices regarding cervical cancer screening.

Case–Control Study Methods

We have presented the methodology of this study elsewhere in detail (Celentano et al., 1987). We briefly describe the study here; 153 pairs of cases and matched controls were interviewed during the spring of 1985. All cases were women with pathologically documented invasive cervical cancer who were referred for evaluation or treatment to the Johns Hopkins Hospital during 1982 to 1984. Controls were selected based upon a case nomination procedure or neighborhood canvassing to locate and interview a woman of similar age (plus or minus 5 years), race, and area of residence. A final criterion for control selection was that she had to have an intact uterus at the time of the interview.

The 153 cases we interviewed were those patients who were alive at the time of the interview, representing a response rate of 85% of eligible cases. A personal interview was conducted in the subjects' homes by trained female interviewers.

The interview lasted approximately 90 minutes. The women were questioned about their reproductive histories, risk factors for cervical cancer, and history was obtained of their medical care use. We used a diary method in which we ascertained a series of events (marriage, residential moves, childbirth, etc.) from the present (1985) back in time to 1955. For women whose age at menarche occurred after 1955, we obtained information back to that date. This history was used to identify gaps in routine Pap testing and medical care factors associated with not receiving regular screening. We also determined medical care utilization for obstetrician–gynecologists, general/family practitioners, and internists as well as hospital visits. For each year in which a visit occurred, we determined whether the woman had received a Pap test. From these histories a number of variables were constructed: number of years in which visits to any provider occurred (provider visit-years); extent of obstetrician–gynecologist utilization (measured as visit-years); a measure of missed opportunities for Pap testing (visit years with no Pap test), as well as a measure of gaps in Pap testing.

We also inquired about the more traditional cervical cancer risk factors in our interview: reproductive history, age at menarche, first intercourse, childbirth and other reproductive events, menopausal status, and history of contraceptive techniques. Finally, we included questions on smoking, sociodemographic characteristics, as well as knowledge, attitudes, and beliefs about cancer in general, cervical cancer in particular, and access to medical care.

Results of the Case–Control Study

Table 12.1 shows the demographic distributions of the cervical cancer cases and healthy controls. Approximately three-eighths of the sample was young (under 45) and an equal number middle-aged (45–59 years); about one-fourth were elderly, age 60 years and older. One-fourth of the sample was black, a proportion equivalent to the black population in the state of Maryland, but a seemingly underrepresented patient population given the overrepresentation of blacks in both incidence and mortality figures. This finding may be indicative of a referral bias in these data. Cases were slightly less likely to have ever been married, and had less education and income than their matched controls. None of these factors, however, attained statistical significance.

Figure 12.1 shows the proportion of cases and controls in the three age groups who reported never having had a Pap test (prior to the Pap test that was associated with the diagnostic sequence leading to identification). There is a direct association of never receiving cervical cancer screening and increasing age; this association holds for both cases and controls. However, the case–control ratio increases with advancing age to the point where the majority of the elderly women (55%) reported never having received a Pap test during their lifetimes.

There is also a systematic differential in the time interval since the last Pap test received and the date at interview for cases and controls, with control subjects

**TABLE 12.1 Distribution of Cervical Cancer Cases and Controls
According to Age, Race, Residence, Marital Status, Education,
and Income, Maryland, 1985**

Characteristic	Cases		Controls	
	No.	Percentage	No.	Percentage
Age (years)				
22–44	57	37.3	57	37.3
45–59	56	36.6	56	36.6
60–85	40	26.1	40	26.1
Total	153	100.0	153	100.0
Race				
White	116	75.8	116	75.8
Nonwhite	37	24.2	37	24.2
Residence				
Baltimore	61	39.9	61	39.9
Other area in Maryland	92	60.1	92	60.1
Marital status				
Never married	18	11.8	12	7.8
Married	55	36.0	49	32.0
Other	80	52.2	92	60.1
Education				
< High school	70	45.8	52	34.0
High school graduate	48	31.4	60	39.2
> High school	35	22.9	41	26.8
Household income				
< $15,000	73	47.7	54	35.3
$15–40,000	55	36.0	61	39.9
> $40,000	14	9.2	23	15.0
Refused, do not know	11	7.2	15	9.8

Percentage distributions are based on unmatched comparisons within cases and controls.

reporting more recent Pap tests (Celentano et al., 1988). If the time period is constrained to the interval recommended by the American Cancer Society, we find cases of each age group less likely to be screened as compared to their matched controls. Controls were, on average, three times more likely than cases to have been appropriately screened in the recent past. This discrepancy held for women of all ages including the elderly.

Our analysis has demonstrated that there are a number of risk factors for cervical cancer that proved to be significant in the analysis (Celentano et al., 1987). Chief among these were age at first sexual intercourse, a shorter interval between menarche and first intercourse, and years having smoked. However, we also found that use of barrier contraceptives (diaphragm, condom use by a partner, and vaginal spermicides) was protective of cervical cancer.

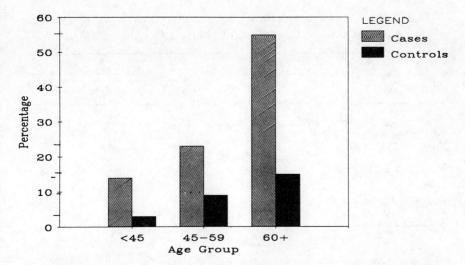

FIGURE 12.1. Percentage of women who have never received a Pap test.

The health care utilization patterns reported by the women in our study demonstrate major differences for cases and controls. As shown in Table 12.2, middleaged and elderly cases are significantly less likely to report ever having seen an obstetrician–gynecologist (although the odds ratio is quite high and in the same direction among the younger women, the small numbers of cases and controls who have never been to an obstetrician–gynecologist limits the significance). Because obstetrician–gynecologists are the most likely health care provider to perform Pap tests, using other types of health care providers does not lead to as high chances of being adequately screened (Weisman et al., 1986, 1987).

Table 12.2 also demonstrates that older cases are less likely to seek any medical care as compared to their matched controls, for significantly fewer cases over the age of 45 years report any physician visit in the 3 years prior to cancer being detected and diagnosed. Overall, however, there were no significant differences in hospitalization rates, emergency department visits, or visits to an internist in the 3 years preceding case diagnosis for cases and controls. Rather, the lack of recent examinations and not receiving care from an obstetrician–gynecologist appear the most important utilization factors.

Table 12.3 presents the results of a logistic regression analysis in which we model the risk of disease while simultaneously controlling for a number of significant risk factors. The results show that after adjusting for use of oral and barrier contraceptives and age at first cervical cancer screening, the utilization risk factors found in the bivariate case continue to be significant. The odds ratio for ever having had an obstetrician–gynecologist visit of 0.40 demonstrates that having such a visit leads to a diminished risk of cancer of 2.5 times. A similar (and

TABLE 12.2 Utilization-Related Behaviors by Age in the Maryland Cervical Cancer Case—Control Study, 1985 Odds Ratios

Risk behavior	Total	Age (years)		
		Under 45	45–59	60+
Never seen an obstetrician–gynecologist	3.40 (1.01–5.79)*	6.00	2.25	3.80
Never told to have regular Pap test	4.00 (1.66–6.34)	2.80	4.60	4.75
Never had Pap test before onset	1.60 (0.53–2.67)	4.00	0.88	2.60
>5 years difference in age first Pap test	2.94 (1.27–4.61)	4.00	2.83	2.57

*95% Confidence intervals.

slightly stronger) result is found for any outpatient utilization in the past 3 years. Finally, Pap testing within this interval is seen to provide a high level of protection from cervical cancer, with equivalent results found for women of all ages; hence, the elderly appear to be protected as much as younger women.

Table 12.4 provides summary statistics on patterns of medical care over the lifetimes of cases and controls. In these analyses we compare cases and their matched controls on overall numbers of visits to any provider, to obstetrician–gynecologists, and to missed opportunities for cytologic examination. A summary statistic, the Wilcoxon sign-rank test, indicates differences in utilization over time between cases and their matched controls. Cases are significantly less likely to report medical care visits to any type of provider during the preceding 30 years

TABLE 12.3 Odds Ratio Estimates and 95% Confidence Intervals from Conditional Logistic Analysis: Utilization Risk Factors and Age, Maryland Cervical Cancer Case—Control Study, 1985

Risk factor	OR*	95% CI
Ever had obstetrician–gynecologist visit	0.40	0.17–0.94
Any outpatient physician visit in past 3 years	0.28	0.10–0.78
Any Pap test within 3 years		
Ages 18–44	0.30	0.10–0.92
Ages 45–59	0.29	0.10–0.84
Ages 60+	0.28	0.08–1.02

*Adjusted for lifetime history of oral and barrier contraceptive use and older age at first cervical cancer screening.

TABLE 12.4 Utilization Behavior Risk Factors in the Maryland
Cervical Cancer Case–Control Study (Wilcoxon Matched Pairs
Signed–Ranks Tests by Age)

	Age (years)		
Utilization risk factor	Under 45	45–59	60+
Any provider visit-years	–3.04	–2.78	–2.85
	$p < 0.01$	$p < 0.01$	$p < 0.01$
Obstetrician-gynecologist visit-years	–2.58	–1.84	–2.91
	$p < 0.01$	$p < 0.10$	$p < 0.01$
Visit-years with no Pap test	–2.84	–1.18	–0.27
	$p < 0.01$	NS	NS
Years with Pap test	–3.04	–2.78	–2.85
	$p < 0.01$	$p < 0.01$	$p < 0.01$
N of pairs	57	56	40

Note: Pairs with case age less than 45 years enter the utilization chart at the age of menarche. A minus sign indicates that cases had less frequent visits than controls. Statistical significance is based upon a Z statistic.

than controls, as is evidenced by their lower Wilcoxon test value for "any provider" visit-years. Looking specifically at obstetrician–gynecologist utilization, cases are also less likely to have obstetrician–gynecologist visit–years than controls (i.e., they consistently have fewer years in which a visit is made to an obstetrician–gynecologist.

When we restrict the analysis to looking at years when a medical care encounter took place, cases were less likely than controls to receive a Pap test during the course of a physician visit (or during an inpatient stay). Thus, there are significantly more missed opportunities for Pap testing in cases as compared to controls. This is borne out when we look at years in which Pap testing took place; cases are less likely than controls to have regular Pap tests across time prior to their diagnosis. Table 12.4 demonstrates that utilization risk factors hold for almost all of the age groups observed. Thus, these utilization risk factors are not merely a function of age; rather, we find consistent patterns of gaps for younger as well as older women.

Figure 12.2 graphically displays the differences in lifetime utilization patterns of elderly cases and controls. As is evident, the average annual rate of visits to any provider (office-based and in the hospital) is consistently higher among controls than cases, with both groups reporting more frequent visits as they aged. Figure 12.3 shows the average annual rates of Pap testing reported by the older women in this study. As shown, controls consistently reported a rate of 0.2 pap tests per year, or an average of one Pap test every 5 years. This rate is quite steady and shows remarkably little interyear variation. For cases a similarly flat distribution is seen,

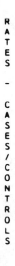
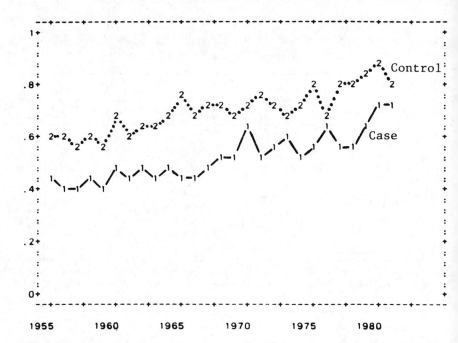

FIGURE 12.2. Average annual rate of visits to any provider for women 60 years of age and older.

with an average annual rate less than 0.1 or an average of one Pap test every 12 years. Only in the very recent period is there a convergence in the lines, perhaps reflecting Pap tests first performed because of some symptom, which was later determined to be associated with their diagnosis of cancer. The difference between the two utilization patterns presented for each group (cases and controls) is often explained as the missed opportunities. As shown in Table 12.4, although there was no significant difference in the overall rate of missed opportunities for the elderly, the direction was in favor of controls having fewer overall visits that can be so classified. The lack of statistical difference in this comparison is in part attributable to the overall high rate of missed opportunities seen overall (i.e., it was consistent for both cases and controls).

Finally, Figure 12.4 demonstrates the significant lifetime difference in utilization of obstetrician–gynecologists among older cases and controls. On average, cases had one visit to such a specialist every 5 years, whereas controls reported a rate of visits nearly once every 2.5 years. The consistent pattern that emerges probably overcomes any potential reporting biases that might be operating. In this respect the bias would have been for cases to be more likely to remember visits and/or report them more reliably than controls because they had given a full medical history at least twice prior to our interview.

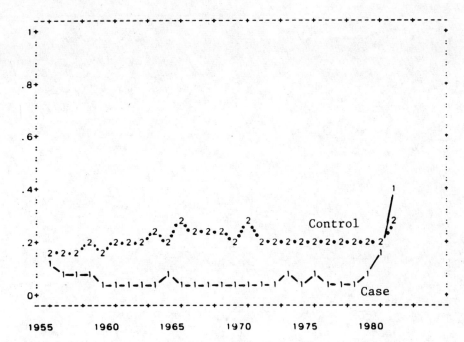

FIGURE 12.3. Average annual rate of Pap tests reported by women 60 years of age and older.

Population Survey Methods

A telephone survey of the middle-aged and elderly female population of Maryland was conducted in 1986. Using the Waksberg method of random digit dialing, from a sample of 13,299 telephone numbers we obtained a sample of 1200 completed interviews. A disproportionate sampling schema was used to provide 400 interviews in each of the following three age strata: 45–54, 55–64, and 65 years and older. These strata were selected based in part on initial results from the case–control study and because we wished to ascertain whether there were significant shifts in behaviors and screening practices during the transition from middle-to older-age. The use of the Waksberg method provides a sample that is geographically balanced and directly represents the telephone exchanges proportionately to their listings (i.e., the method produces a "self-weighting" sample).

The sample of telephone listings was screened for eligible respondents (i.e., a female Maryland resident 45 years of age and older); numbers were randomly preassigned to one of the sample strata. If no woman of the preselected age lived in the household, a second stratum (preassigned) was tried; again, if no eligible respondent lived there, the final stratum was used. Using this method households in which more than one woman over the age of 45 years lived were randomly selected. We obtained a completed interview with 73% of the eligible women

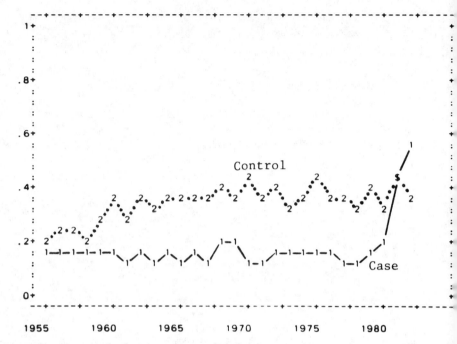

FIGURE 12.4. Average annual rate of obstetrician–gynecologist visits for 60 years of age and older.

contacted. In the analyses presented below, we report on only the 723 women who had not undergone a hysterectomy to allow direct comparisons of risk with the data collected in the invasive cancer analysis.

The structured interview was conducted by telephone with the selected respondent. The interview, which lasted approximately 30 minutes, collected information on sexual history, lifetime and current contraceptive techniques, reproductive history, smoking, and health care utilization. We also inquired about age at first Pap test, as well as the history of all Pap tests received during the prior 10 years. We selected this interval because it appeared optimal based on the results of the case–control study.

Results of the Population Survey

Table 12.5 displays the percentage distributions by age for the recency of the last Pap test. There is a significant difference by age in the proportions of women who report never having had a Pap test, with nearly one of five elderly women reporting never having been screened for cervical cancer. Virtually all of the women in the youngest age group (45–54 years) had received a Pap test in the past 5 years; three-fourths of women 55–64 years reported being screened, as had 58% of the

TABLE 12.5 Reported Recency of Last Pap Test by Maryland Women*
(Percentage Distributions) by Age, 1986

| | Age (years) | | |
Reported recency of last Pap test	45–54	55–64	65+
Never	2.3%	7.1%	18.3%
> 10 Years	2.7	8.9	8.5
5–10 Years	5.8	8.5	10.0
< 5 Years	89.2	75.4	57.9
N	259	224	240

*Includes only those women who have not had a hysterectomy.

elderly. Figure 12.5 shows the percentages of women reporting Pap tests in accordance with the American Cancer Society recommendations on periodicity. There is a direct linear relationship between age (5-year intervals) and the percentage reporting being screened. Interestingly, over one-half of the women 65–74 years of age report being screened on at least a triennial basis, with nearly three-eighths of the oldest women (75 years and older) reporting at least one Pap test in the preceding 3 years. These findings are important; a large proportion of the elderly are continuing to be screened even though they are past the recommended age of discontinuance, reflecting the fact the obstetrician–gynecologists

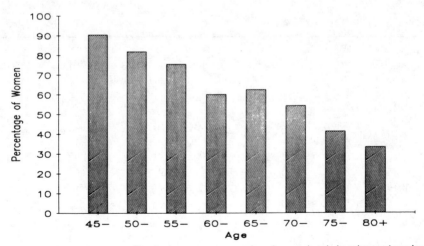

FIGURE 12.5. Percentage of Maryland women reporting a Pap test in the past 3 years.

and other specialists believe that the elderly should continue to be screened for cancer of the cervix (Weisman et al., 1986, 1987).

Table 12.6 shows the demographic factors associated with self-reports of receipt of a Pap test within the past 5 years (the interval representing a conservative estimate of risk). There are no racial differences overall in screening, a finding that substantiates the finding of no racial difference in the case–control results. Urban dwellers are systematically less likely to report a recent Pap test, although it is slightly more pronounced among the elderly. Married women are found to receive screening more frequently, as are the better educated. The latter finding is especially significant among the elderly, where women who have not completed high school are significantly less likely to have had a recent Pap test compared to those with more education. No consistent finding is seen for screening by employment status, although the elderly who are employed are more likely to have been recently screened as compared to those who do not work. This may reflect better health status, a greater likelihood of having supplemental health insurance, more income, or greater mobility, all factors that make it easier to obtain preventive health services.

Table 12.7 displays the usual source of care reported by the sample of Maryland

TABLE 12.6 Demographic Characteristics of Maryland Women* Reporting a Pap Test Within the Past 5 Years (Percentage Distributions), by Age, 1986

Demographic Characteristic	Age (years)		
	45–54	55–64	65+
Race			
Black	87.3	60.4	55.9
White	89.8	79.5	58.3
Area density			
Urban	84.6	71.1	51.9
Suburban	89.1	74.5	60.9
Rural	93.5	83.3	60.6
Currently married			
Yes	89.3	81.4	65.7
No	88.7	65.5	52.5
Education			
< High school	73.8	72.2	48.4
High school graduate	89.1	73.6	64.4
> High school	94.4	79.5	64.4
Currently employed			
Yes	87.4	70.7	69.2
No	92.9	78.2	57.3

*Includes only those women who have not had a hysterectomy.

**TABLE 12.7 Usual Source of Care Reported by Maryland Women*
(Percentage Distributions), by Age, 1986**

Reported usual source of care	Age (years)		
	45–54	55–64	65+
Internist	21.6%	25.9%	21.3%
General/family practitioner	38.2	35.7	50.0
Obstetrician/gynecologist	12.4	6.7	1.7
Other	8.5	12.9	12.9
No usual source	19.3	18.8	14.2
N	259	224	240

*Includes only those women who have not had a hysterectomy.

women. The elderly are more likely to report a general practitioner or family practitioner as their usual source of care than younger women, and the elderly are least likely to report an obstetrician–gynecologist as the usual care provider. Nearly equal proportions by age report no usual source of care. Table 12.8 gives the percentages of women who report a Pap test in the past 5 years by age and usual source of care. These data demonstrate that there is a strong relationship between specialty or location of usual source of care with cervical cancer screening. This is especially true among the elderly; nearly all of the women who use an internist or obstetrician–gynecologist report a recent cervical smear, whereas only about one-half of those who use general or family practitioners report this test. Those with no usual source of care are least likely to be screened, reflecting the importance of provider characteristics for screening.

**TABLE 12.8 Percentage of Maryland Women* Reporting a Recent
(<5 Years) Pap Test According to Usual Source of Medical Care,
by Age, 1986**

Reported usual source of care	Age (years)		
	45–54	55–64	65+
Internist	98.2%	91.4%	86.3%
General/family practitioner	91.9	72.5	56.7
Obstetrician/gynecologist	100.0	100.0	100.0
Other	95.5	86.2	45.2
No usual source	54.0	42.9	26.5
N	259	224	240

*Includes only those women who have not had a hysterectomy.

DISCUSSION

These data suggest that past utilization and paths to medical care are significantly associated with cervical cancer, primarily through missed opportunities for Pap testing. All of the women with cervical cancer we interviewed had many encounters with the medical care system; in most instances Pap tests were not offered to cases or were not taken advantage of. The finding that virtually all of the traditional biologic risk factors failed to attain significance in the case–control analyses underscores the renewed attention that needs to be paid to screening as the primary defense against cervical cancer. This assertion is underscored by the findings of the population survey. Although the picture drawn from those findings suggests that the problem may not be as large as once thought, the fact that a sizable proportion of the elderly have never been screened warrants attention. Further, there remains a moderate number of middle-aged women who are not receiving routine screening despite the fact that they have utilization practices which lead them into the health care system where presumably a Pap test could be performed.

Clearly, there are barriers to performing Pap tests for older women. The elderly may not avail themselves of opportunities for screening for a variety of reasons (Chao et al., 1987): they may never have had a Pap test and therefore have only limited chances of having one when older; they may alter their health care utilization patterns, such as switching from an obstetrician–gynecologist to a family practitioner after menopause, which would lessen their chances of being routinely screened; or they may refuse Pap testing, misassociating its need with reproduction.

The medical care system itself may be partially responsible for the large numbers of women not receiving Pap testing at the recommended intervals (Shapiro, 1986). First, there is confusion in the field about the conflicting cervical cytology recommendations (Weisman et al., 1986, 1987). Second, there are specialty differences in reputed responsibility for gynecologic care, with specialists other than obstetrician–gynecologists less likely to want to do Pap tests, to be less qualified to perform adequate tests, or to see cervical cancer screening as falling within their domain (Teitelbaum et al., 1988). Finally, there are structural barriers to obtaining Pap tests. However, even when structural barriers are removed, success is not immediately obvious (Warneke et al., 1983). Lurie et al., (1987) have demonstrated that cost-sharing is associated with decreased utilization of preventive care in the Health Insurance Experiment. Although cost-sharing was associated with less frequent rates of obtaining Pap smears than a free plan, especially among women over the age of 45 years, approximately one-third of women in the free plan did not receive a Pap smear in compliance with preventive care recommendations.

It is apparent that alteration of the health care system, provider's perceptions, and the knowledge and attitudes of the elderly concerning Pap testing must all be addressed if cervical cancer is to be reduced in both incidence and mortality. As one of the few cancers in which avoidable mortality should be possible to demonstrate a significant impact of organized prevention programs, significant additional efforts will need to be made.

REFERENCES

American Cancer Society (1980). Guidelines for the cancer-related checkup: Recommendations and rationale. *CA: A Cancer Journal for Clinicians, 30*:193–240.

Aristizabel, N., Cuello, C., Correa, P., Collazoa, T., & Haenszel, W. (1984). The impact of vaginal cytology on cervical cancer risks in Cali, Colombia. *International Journal of Cancer, 34*:5–9.

Arneson, A.N., & Kao, M.S. (1987). Long-term observations of cervical cancer. *American Journal of Obstetrics and Gynecology, 156*:614–625.

Boyd, J.T., & Doll, R., (1964). A study of the aetiology of carcinoma of the cervix. *British Journal of Cancer, 18*:419–434.

Celentano, D.D., Klassen, A.C., Weisman, C.S., & Rosenshein, N.B. (1988). Cervical cancer screening practices among older women: Results from the Maryland Cervical Cancer Case–Control Study. *Journal of Clinical Epidemiology, 41*:531–541.

Celentano, D.D., Klassen, A.C., Weisman, C.S., & Rosenshein, N.B. (1987). The role of contraceptive use in cervical cancer: The Maryland Cervical Cancer Case–Control Study. *American Journal of Epidemiology, 126*:592–604.

Celentano, D.D., Shapiro, S., & Weisman, C.S. (1982). Cancer preventive screening behavior among elderly women. *Preventive Medicine, 11*:454–463.

Chao, A., Paganini-Hill, A., Ross, R.K., & Henderson, B.E. (1987). Use of preventive care by the elderly. *Preventive Medicine, 16*:710–722.

Clarke, E.A., & Anderson, T.W. (1979). Does screening by "Pap" smears help prevent cervical cancer? *Lancet, 1*:1–4.

Cramer, D.W. (1982). Uterine cervix. In Schottenfeld, D. & Fraumeni, J.F., Jr., (Eds.), *Cancer epidemiology and prevention.* Philadelphia: W.B. Saunders.

Eardley, A., Elkind, K., Spencer, B., Hobbs, P., Pendleton, L.L., & Haran, D. (1985). Attendance for cervical screening—whose problem? *Social Science and Medicine, 20*:955–962.

Green, T.H. (1971). *Gynecology; essentials of clinical practice.* Boston: Little, Brown.

Greenwald, P., & Sondik, E.J. (Eds.) (1986). *Cancer control objectives for the nation: 1985–1990.* NIH Publication No. 86-2880, Number 2. Bethesda, MD: U.S. Department of Health and Human Services.

Greenwald, P., Costlow, R., Prorok, P., & Sondik, E.J. (1985). Screening in the context of cancer control. In Miller, A.B. (Ed.), *Screening for cancer.* San Diego: Academic Press.

Howard, J. (1987a). "Avoidable mortality" from cervical cancer: Exploring the concept. *Social Science and Medicine, 24*:507–514

Howard, J. (1987b). Using mammography for cancer control: An unrealized potential. *CA: A Cancer Journal for Clinicians, 37*:33–48.

Howe, H.L., & Bzduch, H. (1987). Recency of Pap smear screening: A multivariate model. *Public Health Reports, 102*:295–301.

Hulka, B.S. (1982). Risk factors for cervical cancer. *Journal of Chronic Diseases, 35*:3–11.

Kegeles, S.S., & Grady, K.E. (1982). Behavioral dimensions. In Schottenfeld, D., & Fraumeni, J.F., (Eds.). *Cancer epidemiology and prevention.* Philadelphia: W.B. Saunders.

Koss, L.G., Steward, K.W., Foote, F. W., et al. (1983). Some histological aspects of epidermoid carcinoma in situ and related lesions of the uterine cervix: a long-term prospective study. *Cancer, 16*:1160–1211.

Last, J.M. (1980). Scope and methods of prevention. In Last, J.M. (Ed.), *Public health and preventive medicine*, Ed. 11. New York: Appleton-Century-Crofts.

LaVecchia, C., DeCarli, A., Gentile, A., et al. (1984). Pap smear and the risk of cervical neoplasia: Quantitative estimates from a case–control study. *Lancet, 2*:779–782.

Li, J.Y., Li, F.P., Blot, W.J., et al. (1982). Correlation between cancers of the uterine cervix and penis in China. *Journal of the National Cancer Institute, 69*:1063–1064.

Lilienfeld, A. (1980). Cancer. In Last, J.M. (Ed.), *Public health and preventive medicine*, Ed. 11. New York: Appleton-Century-Crofts.

Lurie, N., Manning, W.G., Peterson, C., Goldberg, G.A., Phelps, C.A., & Lillard, L. (1987). Preventive care: Do we practice what we preach? *American Journal of Public Health, 77*:801–804.

Malone, T.E., & Johnson, K.W. (1986). *Report of the Secretary's Task Force on Black and Minority Health*. Washington, D.C.: U.S. Government Printing Office.

Mandelblatt, J., Gopaul, I., & Wistreich, M. (1986). Gynecological care of elderly women; another look at Papanicolaou smear testing. *Journal of the American Medical Association, 256*:367–371.

Mandelblatt, J., & Hammond, D.B. (1985). Primary care of elderly women: Is Pap smear screening necessary? *Mount Sinai Journal of Medicine, 52*:284–290.

Mettlin, C., Cummings, M., & Walsh, D. (1985). Risk factor and behavioral correlates of willingness to participate in cancer prevention trials. *Nutrition and Cancer, 7*:189–198.

Miller, A.B. (1982). Fundamental issues in screening. In Schottenfeld, D., & Fraumeni, J. F., Jr. (Eds.), *Cancer epidemiology and prevention*. Philadelphia: W.B. Saunders.

Miller, A.B. (1985a). Principles of screening and of the evaluation of screening programs. In Miller, A.B. (Ed.), *Screening for cancer*. San Diego: Academic Press.

Miller, A.B. (1985b). Screening for cancer of the cervix. In Miller, A.B. (Ed.), *Screening for cancer*. San Diego: Academic Press.

Milner, P.C., & Watts, M. (1987). Effect of socioeconomic status on survival from cervical cancer in Sheffield. *Journal of Epidemiology and Community Health, 41*:200–203.

National Center for Health Statistics (1986). Health promotion data for the 1990 objectives: Estimates from the National Health Interview Survey of Health Promotion and Disease Prevention, United States, 1985. *Advance data from vital and health statistics*. No. 126. DHHS Publication No. (PHS) 86–1250. Hyattsville, MD: Public Health Service.

National Research Council (1982). Assembly of Life Sciences, Committee on Diet Nutrition, and Cancer: *Diet, nutrition, and cancer*. Washington, D.C.: National Academy Press.

Oster, S. (1980). Cervical vaginal screening in the over 65 female. *Mount Sinai Journal of Medicine, 47*:192–193.

Peters, R.K., Thomas D., Hagan, D.G., Mack, T.M., & Henderson, B.E. (1986). Risk factors for invasive cervical cancer among Latinas and non-Latinas in Los Angeles County. *Journal of the National Cancer Institute, 77*:1063–1077.

Peterson, O. (1956). Spontaneous course of cervical precancerous conditions. *American Journal of Obstetrics and Gynecology, 72*:1063.

Sasco, A.J., Day, N.E., & Walter, S.D. (1986). Case–control studies for the evaluation of screening. *Journal of Chronic Diseases, 39*:399–405.

Shapiro, S. (1986). Cancer control and the health-care system. *Preventive Medicine, 15*:321–329.

Silverberg, E., & Lubera, J. (1987). Cancer statistics, 1987. *CA: A Cancer Journal for Clinicians, 37*:2–19.

Singh, B., Postic, B., & Cutler, J., (1976). Virucidal effect of certain chemical contraceptives on type 2 herpesvirus. *American Journal of Obstetrics and Gynecology, 125*: 442–445.

Somers, A.R. (1980). Life-style and health. In Last, J.M. (Ed.), *Public health and preventive medicine*, Ed. 11. New York: Appleton-Century-Crofts.

Sorenson, A.W., Seltser, R., & Sundwall, D. (1983). Primary cancer prevention as an attainable objective for the elderly. In Yancik, R., Carbone, P.P., Patterson, W.B., Steel, K., & Terry, W.D. (Eds.), *Perspectives on prevention and treatment of cancer in the elderly*. New York: Raven Press.

Teitelbaum, M.A., Weisman, C.S., Klassen, A.C. & Celentano, D.D. (1988). Pap testing intervals: Specialty differences in physicians' recommendations in relation to women's Pap testing behavior. *Medical Care, 26*:607–618.

Turkel, W.V., Stone, M.L., & Napp, E.E. (1969). A geriatric gynecological survey. *Journal of the American Geriatric Society, 17*:191–197.

Wangsuphachart, V., Thomas, D.B., Koetsawang, A., & Riotton, G. (1987). Risk factors for invasive cervical cancer and reduction of risk by "Pap" smears in Thai women. *International Journal of Epidemiology, 16*:362–366.

Warneke, R.B., & Graham S. (1976). Characteristics of blacks obtaining Papanicolaou smears. *Cancer, 37*:2015–2015.

Weisman, C.S., Celentano, D.D., Hill, M.N., & Teitelbaum, M.A. (1986). Pap testing: opinion and practice among young obstetrician-gynecologists. *Preventive Medicine, 15*:342–351.

Weisman, C.S., Celentano, D.D., Klassen, A.C., & Rosenshein, N.B. (1987). Utilization of obstetrician–gynecologists and prevention of cervical cancer. Obstetrics and Gynecology, 70:373–377.

Wheat, M.E., Mandelblatt, J., & Kunitz, G. (1987). Pap smear screening in women aged 65 and over. Presented at the Annual Meeting of the American Public Health Association, New Orleans, LA.

Winkelstein, W., Jr., Shillitoe, E.J., Rand, R., et al. (1984). Further comments on cancer of the uterine cervix, smoking, and herpesvirus infection. *American Journal of Epidemiology, 119*:1–9.

Yancik, R. (1983). Frame of reference: Old age as the context for the prevention of cancer. In Yancik, R., Carbone, P.P., Patterson, W.B., Steel, D., & Terry, W.D. (Eds.), *Perspectives on prevention and treatment of cancer in the elderly*. New York: Raven Press.

Young, J.L., Percy, C.L., & Asire, A.J. (Eds.) (1981). *Surveillance, Epidemiology, and End Results: Incidence and Mortality Data, 1973–77*. National Cancer Institute Monograph No. 57, NIH Publication No. 81–2330. Washington, D.C.: U.S. Government Business Office.

13

Surgical Management of the Elderly Cancer Patient

Bernard S. Linn

Surgical management of the elderly cancer patient raises two questions. One is whether or not older and younger patients differ in operative risk. The other is whether or not decisions regarding cancer surgery differ from other types of surgery, and if so, whether age plays a significant role there.

AGE AND OPERATIVE RISK

Regarding the first questions, i.e., of age and operative risk, the elderly have usually been found to have comparable postoperative morbidity and mortality rates to that of younger patients when surgery is performed electively. However, emergency surgery, which always is more of a risk than elective surgery, carries an even greater risk in the elderly. In a review of 108 studies of surgery in the elderly, Linn et al. (1982a) found the risk of emergency surgery to be about three times that of elective surgery in the elderly. What often happens is that surgery may be delayed in the elderly until it becomes an emergency because of a reluctance by some surgeons to operate on the older individual in the belief that age itself produces an increased risk. Operative risk in the elderly is complex. As indicated, emergency surgery should be avoided if at all possible. Coexisting morbidity must always be taken into account because risk factor and chronic diseases increase with age. Thus, any increased surgical risk in the elderly can be attributed in part to multiple pathology, more advanced diseases, and more frequent emergency operations.

Biologic variability also increases with age. Some elderly persons may be frail while others are durable. In physical reserve and experience with illness, many individuals who live into extreme old age appear to be more biologically sound and resistant to illnesses (Linn et al., 1969; Linn et al., 1972). They are, therefore, by virtue of their age, survivors who have outlived most of their birth cohorts and by virtue of the fact that they did survive, physically "tougher" than their birth cohorts. A positive aspect of surgery in the elderly is often the age of the patient. Survival into advanced years predicts more survival. It is reported that Wangensteen, an accomplished surgeon and educator, often said no patient who needed a lifesaving operation should be permitted to die simply because of chronologic age. The trends in surgery, documented by numerous studies, suggest that good results can be obtained in operating on the elderly when they are properly managed.

Although many of the old are strong physiologically, a number of body functions do change with normal aging and need to be considered in evaluating patients for surgery. Some of these, such as renal function, glucose tolerance, cardiac output, vital capacity of the lungs, lean muscle mass, and cell-mediated immunity, could influence surgical outcomes. Many other values and functions, however, do not change in any important ways clinically. For example, levels for hematocrit and serum electrolytes, or results of urinalysis, are not influenced much by age, and a treatable disease may be overlooked if an abnormal finding on such a test is simply attributed to old age. Principles of good surgical care are not specific to the elderly. Assessment of surgical risk involves the same criteria regardless of age, but the age-related changes and the possibility of more coexisting illness must be considered.

Surgical management can be divided into preoperative, operative, and postoperative periods. Preoperative assessment is the most important of the three, with careful assessment and planning in this stage leading to avoidance of future problems. Comprehensive preoperative assessment (Table 13.1) means treating systems that can be improved before surgery to optimize their function, within any limitations that might be imposed by one's estimate of the risk involved by

TABLE 13.1 Preoperative Management Considerations

Assess patient's operability
Assess indication for cancer surgery
Assess urgency for surgery
Assess patient attitudes
Evaluate nutritional status
Evaluate co-morbidity
Optimize improvable systems
Maximize mobility
Provide patient education
Offer emotional support

whatever delay might be required for such preoperative management. This perspective is necessary to avoid the possible deterioration of the need for elective surgery to the need for an emergency operation. Keeping the patient mobile and out of bed as much as possible and preparing the patient for postoperative events are also part of the preoperative management. In the operative management stage (Table 13.2) there is less to do that is influenced by age of the patient. The surgeon needs to work closely with the anesthesiologist to plan the operation so that possible problems can be avoided. During surgery care in the handling of tissue is always important but even more so in older patients who may have reduced vascular supply and diminished ability to heal and regenerate after surgery. The postoperative period is also a time of increased risk. During the postoperative stage (Table 13.3) vital signs of older patients need to be followed frequently, extremes of therapy avoided, signs of mental confusion monitored, and activity and rehabilitation initiated as early as possible. Therefore, in answer to the first question raised, older patients usually can do as well as younger ones if operated on electively and if carefully assessed and managed.

CANCER SURGERY VERSUS OTHER SURGERY

Turning to the second question, the technical aspects of cancer surgery are not that different from the technical aspects of other types of surgery. There are more often the questions of resectability and of curative versus palliative surgery to consider. Probably the greatest difference between cancer surgery and other forms of surgery rests with the attitudes of the patients and to a lesser degree the hospital staff. For surgery in general, even minor procedures can result in anxiety for patients concerning degree of pain and discomfort while fear of outcome and unfamiliarity with surgical procedures lead to fears of being anesthetized and possibly dying. In addition to these usual problems associated with any surgery, however, patients with cancer also have more psychologic distress and feelings of helplessness (Lewis et al., 1979; Gottesman and Lewis, 1982). The patient with cancer not only faces

TABLE 13.2 Operative Management Considerations

Integrate with anesthesiology
Minimize preoperative medications
Use lightest feasible anesthesia
Avoid anoxia
Assess resectability
Determine curative versus palliative procedure
Minimize blood loss
Handle tissue gently

TABLE 13.3 Postoperative Management Considerations

Monitor vital signs frequently
Monitor mental status
Avoid anoxia
Avoid extremes of treatment
Minimize analgesics
Initiate early activity
Begin rehabilitation
Discuss surgical findings
Continue patient education
Provide emotional support

concern about unknown surgery but also about the possiblity of mutilation or alteration of body functions, as well as social and economic consequences of cancer.

Staff may also have some attitudes that play a role in operating on the elderly cancer patient. One is reluctant to operate because the person is old and nearer to death than a younger individual. Cancer is seen as a disease of aging or a condition that may be on schedule in regard to the life cycle, whereas cancer in the younger patient is seen as an untimely event. At the same time that surgeons should not be reluctant to operate on the elderly when surgery is indicated, the use of heroic measures for the sole purpose of simply extending life through surgery for patients who are really terminally ill is a different matter. Sometimes this is done without enough thought as to whether the result will enhance the quality of survival that is left. Surgery can make the remaining time even less rewarding. When considering operations that postpone inevitable death, the chance of improving quality of life should be evaluated carefully and is frequently a very sensitive and complicated issue. The fact that a lesion is operable or resectable is not a sufficient indication, in and of itself, for operating. Although the technical aspects of surgery for cancer do not differ so much from those involved in other types of major surgery, attitudes of the staff about aging and cancer and attitudes of the patients with cancer are both factors that are known to be able to interact with each other and with sugery in affecting surgical outcomes.

INFLUENCE OF AGE ON PHYSICIANS' DECISIONS

The influence of physicians' attitudes about operating on the elderly cancer patient can be demonstrated by a recently completed study of old and young patients with head and neck cancer hospitalized for evaluation for surgery. Malnutrition is known to be high in head and neck cancer patients. Nutritional and immune status are interrelated, and both can influence postoperative complications (Buzby et al., 1980; Linn and Jensen, 1983). Men (N = 120) were evaluated for nutritional and immune status after admission to a surgical ward. They were evaluated with the 21-item Protein Energy Malnutrition Scale (PEMS) (Linn et al., 1968), which measures degree of malnutrition based on clinical history, physical examination, anthropometrics, and seven laboratory tests (such as serum albumin, retinol-binding proteins, and transferrin). Nitrogen balance and creatinine-height index were also calculated. Immune function was assessed by delayed hypersensitivity skin testing, using seven antigens and one control, by lymphocyte responses to three mitogens in culture, and by neutrophil chemotaxis. Nutritional and immune assessments were repeated 5 and 30 days after surgery. Patients were monitored daily after surgery by a research nurse for postoperative complication for 30 days or until discharge or death. Patients were also followed for 2 years regarding mortality.

Data were analyzed by multivariate analysis of variance and covariance in a 2 × 2 factorial design in which one factor was age (under 60 years or 60 years and older), and the other factor was nutritional status (malnourished or well-nourished as determined by the PEMS). Average age of the old patients was 64 years and of the young was 44 years. Table 13.4 characterizes the clinical characteristics of operated and nonoperated patients. The first finding was that 75% of the young and 58% of the old actually underwent surgery. Furthermore, only the old with significantly lower average preoperative clinical stages of cancer were selected for surgery. Slightly more of the young than the old who were not operated upon were considered unresectable after biopsy. Severity of illness, nutritional status, and number of coexisting illnesses did not discriminate between those who did and those did not have surgery.

Table 13.5 describes the characteristics of nonoperated patients by age. It shows that although a significantly larger proportion of the old were not operated, they were not significantly different in regard to the reasons why they were not operated (if anything, there were less old who were found to be unresectable). In summary,

TABLE 13.4 Surgery in Old and Young Patients

Variables	Old		Young	
	Surgery	No Surgery	Surgery	No Surgery
Percent of age group*	58	42	75	25
Preoperative clinical stage*	2.7	3.3	3.3	2.8
PEMS Score	7.4	9.7	8.6	8.5
Coexisting illness	5.2	4.2	2.8	1.9
Severity illness score	10.3	11.2	9.6	11.1

*Statistically significant interaction with age.

TABLE 13.5 Old and Young Patients Without Surgery

Variables	Older (%)	Younger (%)
Percent of age group*	42	25
Unresectable	22	33
Death before surgery	5	8
Referred for radiation/chemotherapy	73	59

*Statistically significant.

there was no clear reason as to why fewer of the old than young did not have surgery.

In regard to nutritional status of those who had surgery, 58% of the young and 55% of the old were malnourished. Demographic variables, location of the cancer, and symptoms were similar between age groups. The older patients tended to come in sooner after onset of cancer than younger patients. Sixty percent of the old malnourished as compared with only 20% of the young malnourished were anergic on skin testing and had lower lymphocyte responses to concanavalin A and pokeweed mitogens than younger patients. The older malnourished patients also had poorer surgical outcomes than any other group in regard to nutritional status and immune function after surgery. Table 13.6 shows the surgical outcomes by age. Although the old malnourished had significantly more postoperative complications and higher mortality within 1 year, the outcomes of the well-nourished old did not differ significantly from the young. In trying to answer why the malnourished old had worse outcomes than the malnourished young, preoperative treatments were examined. Findings showed that 60% of the young and only 20% of the old malnourished received enteral or parenteral nutritional support.

The study then suggests age bias in physician selection of patients for surgery that may need to be explored further. If chronologic age, rather than physiologic age, is the determinant of medical care, then the elderly may be deprived of care that can prevent premature morbidity and mortality (Berg and Robbins, 1961).

TABLE 13.6 Surgical Outcomes

Variables	Old		Young	
	Mal-nourished	Well-nourished	Mal-nourished	Well-nourished
Complications*	7.6	4.0	4.4	2.5
Death (1 year)* (%)	50	11	17	15

Complication score = 0 to 12.
*Statistically significant interaction with age.

There are suggestions of this from other studies. One study (Samet et al., 1986) found that elderly patients with cancer received less curative treatments than younger patients with cancer even after taking stage of the disease into account. Likewise, a study (Chu et al., 1987) of 1680 women with breast cancer treated in 17 hospitals showed a linear trend for older patients to receive fewer services such as biopsies, number of lymph nodes examined, chemotherapy, and radiation therapy even though stage of cancer and estrogen receptor status was not associated with age. Another recent study (Greenfield et al., 1987) controlled for co-morbidity, functional status, and tumor stage as well as for type and size of seven hospitals from which 374 cancer patients were selected for study. They found that even after controlling for all of these factors, age itself affected medical care in that physicians provided less than optimal care for older patients even with mild or no co-morbid disease. Wetle (1987) concluded that the lack of data about treatment effectiveness and side effects for older patients made clinicians reluctant to use new treatments with the elderly or overly cautious by using less than optimal dosages. In turn, this leads to a self-fulfilling prophecy in which older patients treated for cancer "do not do well" because appropriate treatment was not provided.

Table 13.7 summarizes some of the physician and patient attitudes that have been found to adversely influence surgical outcomes in the elderly. Linn and Zeppa (1987) have found that medical student attitudes about operating on the elderly could be changed positively by more information about aging and the need to individualize elderly patients in regard to biologic variability. Perhaps emphasis on attitudes about aging in continuing medical education or through quality assurance programs might have a beneficial impact on hospital staff. There was also further evidence of age bias, and that was in regard to the selection of patients for nutritional support. Although there are questions about the value of total parenteral nutrition in prolonging survival (and even some suggestion that it could possibly stimulate tumor growth), malnutrition is still a known factor in postoperative complications. At this stage in our knowledge, therefore, nutritional support

**TABLE 13.7 Adverse Influences on Surgical Outcome
in Elderly Cancer Patients**

Physician attitudes
    Reluctance to operate when indicated
    Operating without considering quality of survival
    Failure to prepare patient physically or emotionally

Patient attitudes
    Fear
    Depression
    Anxiety/stress

should not be withheld from a patient who is to have surgery and is obviously malnourished.

Providing preoperative nutritional support, however, has become a problem. The current structure of DRG reimbursement does not cover nutritional support. In another study of cancer patients, Linn and Robinson (1987) found that those admitted since institution of diagnostic related groups (DRGs) were more mal-nourished at the time of surgery than those before DRGs. In addition, those admitted after DRGs had significantly more postoperative complications than those admitted before DRGs. The average time in the hospital before surgery was only 3 days since institution of DRGs as compared to 12 days before. It would seem that delivery of nutritional support preoperatively may need to be shifted from hospital to home if these patients are to be treated adequately. The emphasis on cost containment itself endangers elective surgery for elderly patients. Questions have been raised about the necessity of operations in the old with suggestions made that second opinions be mandatory when older patients are operated upon (Geelhoed, 1985). If second opinions are deemed important, age alone should not be a factor. Coupled with cost-containment zeal, this type of attitude, no matter how well-intentioned at the outset, could all too easily take a dangerous turn, with less care advocated for the elderly, and perhaps the ultimate economy being death. There-fore, it would seem that attitudes of the surgeons and hospital staff can influence decisions about surgery in older cancer patients.

IMPACT OF PATIENT ATTITUDES ON SURGICAL OUTCOMES

Another factor impacting on surgical outcomes is attitudes of the patients them-selves. Such attitudes need to be recognized, especially in preoperative surgical management. In even relatively simple surgical procedures such as hernia repair, Linn et al., (1987a) found that recent life stress and anxiety about the surgery were associated with lower lymphocyte response to mitogens preoperatively and to more postoperative complications. Similarly, in patients undergoing cancer surgery they also found that effects of stress and anxiety about surgery were even more pro-nounced on immune function and surgical outcomes (Linn et al., 1987b). Others (Janis, 1958) have also reported that patients experiencing extreme anxiety before surgery have more postoperative complications. Feelings of helplessness are prom-inent in cancer patients. Depression is also present in cancer patients (Bergman et al., 1984) and in the elderly (Blazer, 1982). Short-term crisis intervention may be considered as a part of preoperative planning for some patients. Helping the patient take part in decisions about treatments can also increase some feelings of control over the environment. Much of the emotional stress before surgery is related to a fear of the unknown. Providing information about what can be expected following surgery and during convalescence can help. Many cancer patients who undergo curative surgery have the idea that they will be permanently impaired.

Providing information about postoperative routines and return to normal activities should be included in communication with the patient. Studies have shown that groups receiving preoperative information and emotional support have better recovery and shorter hospital stays after surgery than control groups (Johnson et al., 1978; Webb, 1983).

INCURABLE CANCER AND THE SURGEON'S ROLE

Unfortunately, not all surgery in cancer patients is curative. The surgeon's role in management does not end at the operative table for the terminally ill patient. The surgeon, no matter how busy with other patients, should not abandon his patient once he or she is not longer operable. The surgeon should continue to play a prominent role in caring for his dying patient during the postoperative management stage. It is difficult, if not impossible, to estimate the amount of time a terminally ill patient may live. It is a common observation that among cancer patients with approximately identical lesions, degree of dissemination, and treatment, some seem to survive far longer than others. Weisman and Worden (1975) have shown that longer than expected survival tended to occur in patients who had good relationships with others, accepted the reality of their illness, and refused to let others pull away from them. However, those with shorter survivals had poor social relationships, were very much more depressed and sometimes suicidal, and often wanted to die.

Traditionally, it used to be the family doctor who helped the patient make the transition between life and death while offering support and comfort to the patient's family as well, but the technologic advances in medicine, including the development of hospitals and nursing homes (as well as changes in the family structure over the past quarter century) have resulted in patients sometimes being isolated from others in their last weeks of life. Patients are now more likely to die in hospitals than at home, and the practice of medicine in our specialized hospitals tends to focus more on curing than caring.

The majority of physicians in practice today have unfortunately received little or no education in the art of meeting the needs of the dying and their families (Dickinson, 1981). In general, they are concerned more with bodily functions than with the whole person (Neale, 1973), and they are not educated to ease the distress of dying (Hackett, 1976). Some physicians even perceive death of a patient as a personal failure and professional defeat. Recently, the medical profession has shown renewed interest in quality of life as an issue in treatment, instead of aiming at extending life at all costs. The shift is reflected in such measures as the "living will." Surgeons are frequently involved in medical ethics such as determining guidelines for the terminally ill. Machines are capable of keeping hearts and respiratory functions going after destruction of the brain. Death can now be defined. Deliberate decisions can be made about death. This has generated interest in the patients' desires about dying and control of their own destiny. Death with dignity is frequently mentioned, but the law regarding death and dying has failed to provide the answers. Ethical issues about limiting treatment often focus on technical interventions, such as mechanical ventilation. Many less dramatic therapies are considered routine and ethical aspects of their use may be less closely examined. Nutritional support can be important in frail elderly patients. Yet appropriate use of nutritional therapy must consider the circumstances of the patient. Where severe underlying illness cannot be reversed, technical means of providing nutrition can represent extraordinary rather than ordinary means of prolonging life. It is important to discuss treatment choices that may arise in an illness with patients at the outset of treatment while they can understand and communicate a choice. If there is a question of a patient's capacity to make an informed decision, a psychiatric consult may be needed. All discussion with patients regarding their treatment should be recorded. If the patient is not competent to make decisions, the family can assist in arriving at consensus about treatment. The use of cost containment criteria for health policies may push decisions that are economically attractive but ethically unacceptable. Two major reasons are often given for do-not-resuscitate (DNR) orders. One is futility and the other is the patient's wishes. There may also be another underlying economic and unacceptable reason that implies that certain patients or classes of patients may not be worth the cost. Resuscitation usually means efforts to save an individual from death. It carries some uncertainty about its success. Some consideration must be given, e. g., about attempting resuscitation of a patient with advanced Stage IV cancer who has had a massive cardiovascular arrest. Some guidelines can be set. The wishes of the patient should be respected and sought out ahead of time if possible. Economics cannot be the basis for a decision. Age or other demographics should not be the determining factor. The wishes of the patient and the possibility of successful outcome should guide decisions.

General considerations in regard to management of patients with terminal malignancies include how much to tell the patient, providing counseling, and making decisions concerning life support measures. The common negative reactions aroused by cancer are anxiety, anger, and depression, and are all major points to consider in the management of dying patients. Patients usually want to talk and have a part in management of their illness. Specific measures to help the dying must be tailored to meet the patient's needs. The physician must decide whether or not to tell the patient about suspected impending death. Even when the dying person suspects that death might occur shortly, the pronouncement itself is unsettling. There are no definitive rules regarding what all patients should be told. Some want to know, others do not. The clue generally comes from the patient. Does the patient ask about what is expected? Does the patient keep questioning the physician about what is going to happen? If so, the patient probably wants to know. Some uncertainty about the time of death and some hope for life can be maintained even in the face of dying. Just because the patient may not ask about impending death does not mean that he or she is unaware of what is happening.

For the busy physician, listening to the patient with empathy may be all that is required. When dying is likely to take place over a period of time, the physician may wish to refer patients who are at high risk for developing emotional problems to a counselor. We have demonstrated earlier in a controlled study (Linn et al., 1982b) of 160 terminally ill cancer patients that counseling improved the quality of survival and that age of the patient was not an important factor. Older patients benefited the same as younger ones (Linn and Linn, 1981) from counseling. The importance of the doctor in caring for the dying patient was recognized long ago by Osler. The physician plays a central role in the emotional as well as the physical care of the dying. Worcester in an elegant little book that sadly, is now out of print, called *The Care of the Aged, the Dying, and the Dead* (Worcester, 1940) wrote that "one of my medical school professors was Oliver Wendell Holmes. I have not forgotten his insistence that, while one of the physician's functions is to assist the coming in, another is to assist at the going out." Cancer in the elderly provides a continuum for intervention for the surgeon that ranges from curative surgery to palliative surgery with the opportunity to help all along the way.

REFERENCES

Berg, J.W., & Robbins, G.F. (1961). Modified mastectomy for older, poor risk patients. *Surgery, Gynecology and Obstetrics, 113:*631–634.

Blazer, D. (1982). The epidemiology of late life depression. *Journal of the American Geriatric Society, 30:*587–592.

Bukberg, J., Perman, D., & Holland, J.C. (1984). Depression in hospitalized cancer patients. *Psychosomatic Medicine, 46:*199–212.

Buzby, G.P., Mullen, J.L., Matthews, D.C., Hobbs, C.L., & Rosato, E.F. (1980). Prognostic nutritional index in gastrointestinal surgery. *American Journal of Surgery, 139:*160–167.

Chu, J., Diehr, P., Feigl, P., Glaetke, G., Begg, C., Clicksman, A., et al. (1987). The effect of age on care of women with breast cancer in community hospitals. *Journal of Gerontology, 42:*185–189.

Dickinson, G.E. (1981). Death education in U.S. medical schools: 1975–1980. *Journal of Medical Education, 56:*111–114.

Geelhoed, G.W. (1985). Access to care in a changing practice environment. *American Collagen Surgery Bulletin. 70:*11–15.

Gottesman, D.H., & Lewis, M.S. (1982). Differences in crisis reactions among cancer and surgery patients. *Journal of Consulting and Clinical Psychology, 50:*381–388.

Greenfield, S., Blanco, D.M., Elashoff, R., & Ganz, P.A. (1987). Patterns of care related to age of breast cancer patients. *Journal of the American Medical Association, 257:*2766–2770.

Hackett, T.P. (1976). Psychological assistance for the dying patient and his family. *Annual Review of Medicine, 5:*371–378.

Janis, I.L. (1958). Cited in *Stress in Hospital* (1979) Wilson-Barnett, J. (Ed.). Edinburgh, Churchill Livingstone.

Johnson, J.W., Rice, W.H., Fuller, S.S., & Endress, M.P. (1978). Sensory information; instruction in coping strategy and recovery from surgery. *Research in Nursing and Health, 1:*4–17.

Lewis, M.S., Gottesman, D., & Gutstein, S. (1979). The course and duration of crisis. *Journal of Consulting and Clinical Psychology, 47*:128–134.

Linn, B.S., & Jensen, J. (1983). Age and immune response to a surgical outcome. *Archives of Surgery, 118*:405–409.

Linn, B.S., & Linn, M.W. (1981). Late stage cancer patients: Age difference in their psychophysical status and response to counseling. *Journal of Gerontology, 36*:689–692.

Linn, B.S., & Robinson, D.S. (1987). DRG impact on patient nutritional status at surgery. Presented at the 20th Annual Meeting of the Association of Veterans Administration Surgeons, Portland, OR, May 7–9.

Linn, B.S., & Zeppa R. (1987). Student attitudes about surgery in older patients before and after the surgical clerkship. *Annals of Surgery, 205*:324–328.

Linn, B.S., Linn, M.W., & Gurel, L. (1968). Cumulative illness rating scale. *Journal of the American Geriatric Society, 16*:622–626.

Linn, M.W., Linn, B.S., & Gurel, L. (1972). Patterns of illness in persons who lived to extreme old age. *Geriatrics, 27*:67–70.

Linn, B.S., Linn, M.W., & Gurel, L. (1969). Physical resistance and longevity. *Gerontology Clinics, 11*:362–370.

Linn, M.W., Linn, B.S., & Harris, R. (1982b). Effects of counseling for late stage cancer patients. *Cancer, 49*:1048–1055.

Linn, B.S., Linn, M.W., & Wallen, N. (1982a). Evaluation of results of surgical procedures in the elderly. *Annals of Surgery, 195*:90–96.

Linn, B.S., Linn, M.W., & Klimas, N. (1987a). The effects of psychophysical stress on surgical outcomes. Presented at the 44th Annual Meeting of the American Psychosomatic Society, Philadelphia, March 27.

Linn, B.S., Linn, M.W., & Klimas, N. (1987b). Stress, immune function and surgical outcome. Presented at 40th Annual Meeting of the Gerontological Society of America. Washington, D.C., November 20.

Neale, R.E. (1973). *The art of dying.* New York, Harper & Row.

Samet, J., Hunt, W.C., Key, C., Humble, C.G., & Goodwin, J.S. (1986). Choice of cancer therapy varies with age of patient. *Journal of the American Medical Association, 255*:3385–3390.

Webb, C. (1983). Teaching for recovery from surgery. In Wilson-Barnett, J. (Ed.), *Patient teaching.* Edinburgh: Churchill Livingstone.

Weisman, A.D., & Worden, J.S. (1975). Psychosocial analysis of cancer deaths. *Omega, 6*:61–75.

Wetle, T. (1987). Age as a risk factor for inadequate treatment. *Journal of the American Medical Association, 258*:516, 1987.

Worcester, A. (1940). *The care of the aged, the dying and the dead.* Springfield, IL: Charles C Thomas.

14

Management of Common Psychiatric Syndromes in Elderly Patients with Cancer

Mary Jane Massie, Jimmie C. Holland, and Lynna M. Lesko

Because over 50% of all cancers occur in 11% of the population over 65 years of age (Cohen, 1987a), there is a need to understand both the management of specific neoplasms common in the elderly and their psychosocial aspects. Both of these topics have been given attention in recent reviews (Cohen, 1987a, 1987b; Holland & Massie, 1987).

Although several studies comparing older and younger patients on psychosocial variables reveal that older cancer patients adjust as well or better than younger patients (Ganz et al., 1985; Maisiak et al., 1983; Plumb & Holland, 1981), a significant proportion of older patients will have distress that exceeds what is arbitrarily defined as "normal." The presence of an intolerable level of distress, which prohibits usual function of the patient, requires evaluation, diagnosis, and management. This review outlines factors that contribute to the delay of reporting symptoms by the elderly, management of the psychiatric complications commonly seen in the elderly cancer patient (depression and delirium), the special problem of compliance with treatment, and issues associated with palliative care.

DELAY OF CANCER TREATMENT BY THE ELDERLY

Early diagnosis and treatment of cancers of older age individuals produce the best prognoses. Unfortunately, older individuals more often neglect an early symptom of cancer for a longer period than do younger individuals. Pain, melena, hemoptysis, weakness, and fatigue are likely to be ignored or attributed to minor problems. Procrastination results from fear of the financial burden of treatment, lack of knowledge, less education, or pessimistic and fatalistic attitudes (Rimer et al., 1983). "If I have cancer, I will die of it anyway, so why bother to be treated?" is an attitude that persists from the early years of cancer treatment when this was more nearly the case. Lack of awareness of community health care services (Snider, 1980) and absence of an existing relationship to a physician also contribute to delay in seeking care by the elderly. It is more difficult for an older individual to identify a new doctor at the time symptoms develop. Other factors that cause delay in the elderly are lack of available family or friends to schedule appointments for the older patient or provide transportation to the oncologist's office, (Antonucci et al., 1988), lower socioeconomic status, and other chronic physical disabilities.

PSYCHIATRIC DISORDERS AND CANCER

Few studies have focused on the particular psychiatric problems as compared to psychosocial problems in the elderly. Popkin et al. (1984) reported results of a review of psychiatric consultations to elderly medically ill patients. Older patients were referred significantly less often for psychiatric consultation. Approximately one-half of the referrals were requests for assistance with managing confusional states (organic mental disorders). We have reported our analysis of data collected during an 18-month period (1980–81) from the psychiatric consultations in older versus younger patients seen by the Psychiatry Service at Memorial Sloan-Kettering Cancer Center (Holland & Massie, 1987). Fifty-four percent of the 546 patients for whom a consultation was requested were 50 years of age or older; 143 (26%) were over 60 years of age. Most patients were white (97%), married, (60%), and lived with their family (70%). In patients over 50 years of age the sites of cancer represented the common tumor types seen in this age group: colorectal, lung, prostate, ovaries, uterus, breast, along with leukemia and lymphoma. A comparison of the psychiatric (DSM-III) diagnoses for the two groups of patients (patients <50 years old and ≥50 years old) showed that the most marked difference between older versus younger groups was the increased frequency of organic mental disorders (26% versus 12%), which was seen in patients 60 years of age and older (Table 14.1). In addition, there was a lower frequency of adjustment disorder diagnosed in the 60 and older group, although major depression was higher in the 70 and older group. These data suggest few differences except the expected increase in organic mental disorders in older patients.

Although a large percentage of psychotropic medications are prescribed for the elderly, one study of patients with advanced stages of cancer found that older patients were prescribed fewer psychotropic drugs, particularly antidepressants and antianxiety drugs, than younger patients. Older groups received relatively

TABLE 14.1. Psychiatric (DSM-III) Diagnosis Among 546 Patients Referred for Evaluation at the Memorial Sloan-Kettering Cancer Center Psychiatry Service (%)

Diagnosis	Age 50+ (N = 294)	Age < 50 N = 252)	All ages (N = 546)
Adjustment disorder	50	59	54
Organic mental disorder	26	12	20
Depression	10	14	9
Major psychiatric disorders	5	7	5
Anxiety disorders	3	4	4
Other	4	4	4
None	3	4	4
Totals	100	100	100

more antipsychotics, which were used to control symptoms of confusion (Jaeger, et al., 1985).

NORMAL REACTIONS TO STRESS

The diagnosis of cancer is stressful for all patients. The elderly patient's ability to manage this stress depends on medical factors (site and stage of cancer, treatment required, and other medical problems), the presence of emotionally supportive persons in the environment, the presence of a relationship with a trusted physician, and the number of intercurrent stressors such as financial burdens, recent losses, and bereavement.

When an elderly individual is diagnosed as having cancer, the normal reaction may vary from a minimal to major disruption of emotional state and physical activities. Some elderly patients accept the diagnosis as yet another struggle near the end of a good life; however, most worry about becoming a burden to their children and about financial aspects of illness. Some experience symptoms of shock and disbelief, followed by a period of turmoil with anxiety and depressive symptoms including sadness, crying, and disruption of appetite and sleep. The ability to concentrate and carry out the usual activities of life may be impaired. These symptoms of stress often resolve in 7–10 days as treatment plans are made and as family or friends provide support and caring.

Intervention beyond that provided by empathic physicians, nurses, and social workers usually is not required. However, if symptoms interfere with function or are prolonged or intolerable, then pharmacologic intervention or psychiatric consultation should be considered (Massie & Holland, 1987a). Prescribing a hypnotic to permit normal sleep and a daytime sedative (a benzodiazepine) to reduce anxiety can help the elderly patient through the crisis period. The short-acting benzodiazepines (alprazolam, triazolam, lorazepam) are best tolerated by the elderly. The clinician should always start with low doses of benzodiazepines (i.e., alprazolam 0.25 mg or triazolam 0.125 mg); doses can be titrated up as necessary.

MANAGEMENT OF DEPRESSION

Depression has been studied in cancer patients using range of assessment methods. Several studies have reported that approximately one-fourth of hospitalized cancer patients have major depression (Bukberg et al., 1984; Evans et al., 1986; Plumb & Holland, 1977). Bukberg and colleagues (1984) did not find that elderly cancer patients are at increased risk of developing depression. Factors associated with greater prevalence of depression are a higher level of physical disability, more severe illness, the presence of pain, and advanced cancer, particularly pancreatic cancer (Holland et al., 1986).

Differentiating between adjustment disorder with depressed mood (previously called reactive depression), which responds to psychologic support, and a major depression, which usually requires pharmacologic intervention in addition to counseling, is often a diagnostic challenge in the elderly cancer patient because these diagnoses represent a continuum of severity of symptoms. The diagnosis of depression in the physically healthy elderly patient depends heavily on the presence of somatic symptoms of anorexia, fatigue, and weight loss. These are of little value as diagnostic criteria for depression in a cancer patient because they are common to both cancer and depression. In cancer patients the diagnosis must depend on psychologic symptoms such as dysphoric mood, feelings of helplessness, loss of self-esteem, feelings of worthlessness or guilt, and thoughts of suicide of "wishing for death." The presence of suicidal ideation in the elderly patient requires careful assessment. If a patient is suicidal, we arrange for a 24-hour companion to provide constant observation, to monitor the suicidal risk, and to provide reassurance to the patient (Massie & Holland, 1987a). Impulsive suicide attempts often occur when a patient has uncontrolled pain and a mild confusional state (delirium).

Before planning an intervention the psychiatrist obtains a history of previous depressive episodes, family history of depression, concurrent life stresses, and the availability of social support. It is essential to distinguish between dementia and pseudodementia (depression) when the predominate presenting symptom is cognitive impairment. The depressed elderly cancer patient may be receiving commonly prescribed medications that can contribute to depressive symptoms either alone or through drug interactions, i.e., cimetidine, diazepam, guanethidine, narcotic analgesics, propranolol, methyldopa, *L*-dopa, and reserpine. Often the elderly take over-the-counter drugs in efforts at self-medication. The physician should inquire about the use of these drugs and about alcohol use. Some of the commonly used cancer chemotherapeutic agents can also cause depression including prednisone, decadron, procarbazine, vincristine, and vinblastine (Young, 1982). Evaluation of possible drug-induced depression should be completed before additional pharmacotherapy is prescribed for the elderly patient.

Treatment of the depressed older patient should combine short-term supportive psychotherapy with pharmacotherapy to control symptoms when appropriate. The elderly cancer patient may initially resist psychiatric consultation because such a consultation represents another social stigma, mental illness. Patient resistance diminishes when the psychiatrist's evaluation and treatment includes family or surrogate family such as close friends or companions and reviews the individual's life accomplishments as well as current distress.

The treatment of depression in the elderly with antidepressant medication has been reviewed by other authors (Salzman, 1984; Gerner, 1984). Tricyclic antidepressants have been the class of medications most commonly used. Nortriptyline and desipramine are usually better tolerated by the elderly because they are less likely to produce orthostatic hypotension at therapeutically equivalent doses than other tricyclics (e.g., amitriptyline, imipramine). Treatment is usually started with a low dose with dosage titrated slowly upward as tolerated.

A therapeutic daily dose of nortiptyline for elderly cancer patients may be as low as 30–40 mg. The tricyclics have a long half-life and hence the total daily dose is often taken at bedtime. The sedating effects are useful in the depressed patient with insomnia. The clinician should monitor blood levels of both nortriptyline and desipramine. Prior to starting antidepressants in the elderly, an electrocardiogram should be obtained.

Orthostatic hypotension is one of the most troublesome anticholinergic side effects of tricyclics in the elderly. Other anticholinergic side effects that may limit doses are delirium and cardiac arrhythmias (Friedel, 1983; Meyers & Mei-Tal, 1983; Stoudemire & Fogel, 1987). The elderly male with prostatic hypertrophy and urinary retention and patients of both sexes with constipation often have difficulty tolerating strongly anticholinergic drugs, as does the cancer patient who has obstructive symptoms associated with gastrointestinal or genitourinary surgery. Patients with stomatitis secondary to chemotherapy or radiotherapy likewise will benefit from the least anticholinergic drugs or from the benzodiazepine alprazolam.

Amitriptyline, imipramine and doxepin with a starting dose of 10–25 mg at bedtime are increasingly used as adjuvant analgesics in the management of pain in cancer patients (Foley, 1985). Elderly patients often benefit from these low doses without having troublesome side effects.

The new short-acting benzodiazepine, alprazolam, is of interest in older cancer patients. It has both anxiolytic and antidepressant properties and is being found to be useful in the treatment of depressed elderly patients (Ayd, 1984; Pitts et al., 1983; Rickels, 1985). Owing to its short half-life and absence of anticholinergic effects, it is well tolerated by the elderly.

The sympathomimetic stimulants (dextroamphetamine and methylphenidate) have been found to be useful for the treatment of depressive states in medically ill patients in whom tricyclic antidepressants are poorly tolerated or contraindicated (Kaufman & Murray, 1982; Woods, 1986). In the oncology setting dextroamphetamine has been found to improve both mood and appetite in patients who are in terminal stages of illness. A controlled trial of methylphenidate in patients with advanced cancer showed reduced narcotic consumption and improved activity and interest (Bruera, 1986). Amphetamines are useful to counter the sedating effects of narcotics in patients who require large amounts of analgesics. Methylphenidate may be preferable to dextroamphetamine in elderly patients because it has fewer troublesome side effects (Chiarella & Cole, 1987). The starting dose of dextroamphetamine in medically ill patients is 2.5–5 mg. given in the morning, and the starting dose of methylphenidate is 5–10 mg at 8 AM and noon.

MANAGEMENT OF DELIRIUM

Delirium, the second most common psychiatric diagnosis among hospitalized elderly cancer patients, is due both to the direct effects of cancer through structural damage by invasion or extension into the central nervous system, or more commonly to nonmetastatic involvement or metabolic encephalopathy. The cause of global cognitive impairment is often organ failure (liver, kidney, lung, thyroid, or adrenal gland); electrolyte imbalance (hypercalcemia, hyponatremia; vitamin deficiences [vitamin B^{12}]); drug effects (narcotic analgesics, chemotherapeutic agents, sedatives, hypnotics, and cumulative effects of medications with anticholinergic properties); sepsis; intravascular coagulation (often associated with lung cancer); and hormone-producing tumors (Posner, 1979; Lipowski, 1983).

Often failure of multiple organ systems contributes to the patient's confusion. Prompt recognition and treatment of delirium in the elderly cancer patient can reduce distress for both patient and family. Having recorded a "baseline" mental status examination makes it easier to identify the early symptoms of delirium in the elderly, such as personality changes of irritability, emotional lability, suspiciousness, or cognitive changes such as mild disorientation, recent memory impairment, and change in judgement.

The early symptoms of delirium are often misdiagnosed by the referring physician as depression (Levine et al., 1978; Massie & Holland, 1987b), the erroneous assumption is that the impact of the disease has finally caught up with the patient. Because elderly cancer patients are often reluctant to report mild mood disturbances or changes in thinking to physicians, delirium often progresses to late or more severe stages with symptoms of paranoid delusions or hallucinations before etiologic workup is started or treatment is instituted.

Careful evaluation of central nervous system dysfunction must be included in the medical and psychiatric evaluation of the elderly cancer patient. Several points should be kept in mind during the evaluation and treatment of delirium (Massie et al., 1983):

1. It is often necessary to treat a patient's agitated or disturbed behavior while simultaneously trying to determine its cause.

2. Careful serial review of mental status and medical and laboratory data must be undertaken; neurologic consultation should be obtained.

3. Patients with delirium benefit from short, frequent contacts with a supportive person, preferably a family member, who speaks quietly and reassuringly about the environment, correcting misinterpretations and assisting in the patient's orientation to objects and people around him or her. Permitting a family member to remain in the patient's hospital room at night and continuity in nursing staffing from shift to shift can help allay the patient's anxiety about surroundings.

4. When agitation is severe or the patient is delusional or hallucinating, one-to-one nursing observation is indicated. suicidal ideation and behavior may develop in response to frightening hallucinations or delusions or awareness of change in mental functioning.

5. A psychopharmacologic approach should be used with patients exhibiting agitation or disruptive behavior as a part of their delirium. In our experience, haloperidol is the most effective drug. Oral or intramuscular administration of 0.5–1.0 mg often reduces agitation without causing oversedation or hypotension in the elderly. Doses repeated at 30- to 60-minute intervals are titrated against behavior. Extrapyramidal effects of haloperiodol are more common in elderly patients and, if they occur, they should be treated early with antiparkinsonian medication.

COMPLIANCE WITH ACTIVE TREATMENT

It is essential that patients adhere to cancer treatment for best results. Haug (1979) reported that older patients are more likely to comply with therapeutic regimens than younger patients. Maisiak and colleagues (1983) found that elderly cancer patients missed clinic appointments because of lack of faith in treatment and confusing clinic settings. An important factor in helping older patients comply is the presence of supportive people who encourage the elderly to utilize available services (Lewis, 1983). Social isolation has been related to poorer resistance to illness in general (Berkman & Syne, 1979). Blazer (1982) found mortality rates varied with the number of living family members in the household. There is a great need for attention to support systems as part of the psychosocial care of older patients who must receive lengthy and arduous regimens of either chemotherapy and/or radiotherapy.

PSYCHOLOGIC ISSUES ASSOCIATED WITH PALLIATIVE CARE

For those elderly patients in whom curative treatment is not possible, assuring maximal comfort during stages of advanced disease is the goal. The psychiatric consultant is often called during this period to assist with: (1) management of behavior related to delirium; (2) evaluation and treatment of pain, depression, and anxiety; (3) evaluation of suicidal statements (which may be secondary to delirium or depression); (4) help in reducing staff conflicts regarding patient care; (5) evaluation of both patient and family conflict, which can arise from a prolonged and uncertain illness course; and (6) anticipatory bereavement counseling for family members.

In the terminal stages of cancer a decision to respect the patient's comfort usually precludes establishing a cause of delirium. The delirium of terminal illness is likely irreversible, and management is predicated on providing maximal psychologic support. As much as possible, pharmacologic management of delirium, pain, and anxiety should include symptom reduction without oversedation.

Patients, their families, and staff members at times suffer from the uncertainty of the course of cancer illness and its often-prolonged terminal phases. The psychiatric consultant may be called in to assist the family with the stress of long or repeated hospitalizations. Awaiting and anticipating how and when death will occur become major preoccupations for the family or spouse. Families often need help in deciding where terminal care should be given. If a decision is made for the elderly patient to die at home, family members should be taught about available home care programs and nursing support. However, both the elderly patient and the family need the continued follow-up and support given by the patient's primary physician if the patient chooses to die at home.

Anticipatory bereavement and bereavement counseling for elderly widows and widowers can provide support for the survivors of cancer patients and may reduce the frequency and morbidity of the range of illneses that occur more frequently in settings of loss and grief. A study of increased mortality following loss of a wife indicates vulnerability of men ages 55–75 (Helsing and Szklo, 1981).

SUMMARY

Cancer in the elderly has several psychologic risks. We have reviewed common issues in the elderly; delay with early symptoms, a greater tendency toward development of delirium, and the need for cautious use of psychotropic medications when treating depression. Management during active treatment and terminal care each pose challenging problems for the psychiatric consultant.

REFERENCES

Antonucci, T.C., Kahn, R.L., & Akiyama, H. (1988). Response to cancer symptoms by the elderly. In Yancik, R., & Yates, J. (Eds.), *Cancer in the elderly: Approaches to early detection and treatment.* New York: Springer.

Ayd, F.J. (1984). Psychopharmacology update: Alprazolam–anxiolytic and antidepressant. *Psychiatric Annals, 14*:393–395.

Berkman, L., & Syme, S. (1979). Social networks, host resistance and mortality: A nine year follow-up study of Alameda County residence. *American Journal of Epidemiology, 109*:186–204.

Blazer, D. (1982). Social support and mortality in an elderly community population. *American Journal of Epidemiology, 115*:684–694.

Bukberg, J., Penman, D., & Holland, J.C. (1984). Depression in hospitalized cancer patients. *Psychosomatic Medicine, 46*:199–212.

Bruera, E., MacDonald, N., Chadwick, S., & Brenneis, C. (1986). Double-blind cross-over study of methylphenidate with narcotics for the treatment of cancer pain. *Proceedings of the American Society of Clinical Oncology, 989*:253.

Chiarello, R.J., & Cole, J.O. (1987). The use of psychostimulants in general psychiatry. *Archives of General Psychiatry, 44*:286–295.

Cohen, H.J. (Ed.) (1987a). Cancer I: General aspects. *Clinics in Geriatric Medicine, 3*:419–586.

Cohen, H.J. (Ed.) (1987b). Cancer II: *Clinics in Geriatric Medicine, 3*:595–801.

Evans, D.L., McCartney, C.F., Nemeroff, C.B., et al. (1986). Depression in women treated for gynecological cancer: Clinical and neuroendocrine assessment, *American Journal of Psychiatry, 143*:447–452.

Foley, K.M. (1985). The treatment of cancer pain. *New England Journal of Medicine, 313*:84–95.

Friedel, R.O. (1983). Affective disorders in the geriatric patient. In Grinspoon, L. (Ed.), *Psychiatry update, Vol. 2.* Washington, D.C.: American Psychiatric Association Press.

Ganz, P.A., Schag, C.C., & Heinrick, R.L. (1985). The psychosocial impact of cancer on the elderly: A comparison with younger patients. *Journal of the American Geriatric Society, 33*:429–435.

Gerner, R.H. (1984). Antidepressant selection in the elderly. *Psychosomatics, 25*:528–535.

Haug, M. (1979). Doctor–patient relations and the older patients. *Journal of Gerontology, 34*:852–860.

Helsing, K.J., & Szklo, M. (1981). Mortality after bereavement. *American Journal of Epidemiology, 114*:41–52.

Holland, J.C., Hughes-Korzun, A.H., Tross, S., Silberfarb, P., Perry, M., Comis, R., et al. (1986). Comparative psychological disturbance in patients with pancreatic and gastric cancer. *American Journal of Psychiatry, 143*:641–643.

Holland, J.C., & Massie, M.J. (1987). Psychosocial aspects of cancer in the elderly. *Clinics in Geriatric Medicine, 3*:533–539.

Jaeger, H., Morrow, G.R., & Brescia, F. (1985). A survey of psychotropic drug utilization by patients with advanced neoplastic disease. *General Hospital Psychiatry, 7*:535–360.

Kaufmann, M.W., & Murray, G.B. (1982). The use of d-amphetamine in medically ill depressed patients. *Journal of Clinical Psychiatry, 43*:463–464.

Levine, P.M., Silberfarb, P.M., & Lipowski, Z.J. (1978). Mental disorders in cancer patients: A study of 100 psychiatric referrals. *Cancer, 42*:1385–1391.

Lewis, C., Linet, M., & Abeloff, M. (1983). Compliance with cancer therapy by patients and physicians. *American Journal of Internal Medicine, 74*:673–678.

Lipowski, Z.J. (1983). Transient cognitive disorders (delirium, acute confusional states) in the elderly. *American Journal of Psychiatry, 140*:1426–1436.

Maisiak, R., Gams, R., Lee, E., & Jones, B. (1983). The psychosocial support status of elderly cancer out-patients. *Progress in Clinical and Biological Research, 120*:395–403.

Massie, M.J., & Holland, J.C. (1987a). The cancer patient with pain: Psychiatric complications and their management. *Medical Clinics of North America, 71*:243–258.

Massie, M.J., & Holland, J.C. (1987b). Consultation and liaison issues in cancer care. *Psychiatric Medicine, 5*:343–359.

Massie, M.J., Holland, J.C., & Glass, E. (1983). Delirium in terminally ill cancer patients. *American Journal of Psychiatry, 140*:1048–1050.

Meyers, B.S., & Mei-tal, V. (1983). Psychiatric reactions during tricyclic treatment of the elderly reconsidered. *Journal of Clinical Psychopharmacology, 3*:2–6.

Pitts, W.M., Fann, W.E., Sajadi, C., & Snyder S. (1983). Alprazolam in older depressed inpatients. *Journal of Clinical Psychiatry, 44*:213–215.

Plumb, M.M., & Holland, J. (1977). Comparative studies of psychological function in patients with advanced cancer-I: Self-reported depressive symptoms. *Psychosomatic Medicine, 39*:264–276.

Plumb, M., & Holland, J.C. (1981). Comparative studies of psychological function in patients with advanced cancer-II: Interview rated current and past psychological symptoms. *Psychosomatic Medicine, 43*:243–254.

Popkin, M.K., MacKenzie, T.B., & Callies A.L. (1984). Psychiatric consultation to geriatric medically ill inpatients in a university hospital. *Archives of General Psychiatry, 41*:703–707.

Posner, J.B. (1979). Neurological complications of systemic cancer. *Medical Clinics of North America, 63*:783–800.

Rickels, K., Feighner, J.P., & Smith, W.T. (1985). Alprazolam, amitriptyline, doxepin, and placebo in the treatment of depression. *Archives of General Psychiatry, 42*:134–141.

Rimer, B., Jones, W.L., Wilson, C., Bennett, D., & Engstrom, P.F. (1983). Cancer and the elderly: A cancer control challenge. *Progress in Clinical and Biological Research, 130*:123–133.

Salzman, C. (1984). *Clinical geriatric psychopharmacology.* New York: McGraw-Hill.

Snider, E.L. (1980). Awareness and use of health services by the elderly: A Canadian study. *Medical Care, 28*:1177–1182.

Stoudemire A., & Fogel, B.S., (1987). Psychopharmacology in the medically ill. In Stoudemire, A., & Fogel, B. (Eds.) *Treatment of psychiatric disorders in medical–surgical patients.* Philadelphia: Grune & Stratton.

Woods, S.W., Tesar, G.E., Murray, G.B., & Cassem, N.H. (1986). Psychostimulant treatment of depressive disorders secondary to medical illness. *Journal of Clinical Psychiatry, 47*:12–15.

Young, D.F. (1982). Neurological complications of cancer chemotherapy. In Silverstein, A. (Ed.), *Neurological complications of therapy: Selected topics.* New York: Futura.

15

Geriatric Oncology: Challenges in Nursing Care

Deborah Welch-McCaffrey

In caring for the older cancer patient, major nursing responsibilities include the provision of support and education for both patient and family and ensuring optimum symptom management. Advocacy responsibilities encompass many nursing interventions with the elderly as well. Because nursing transcends all aspects of cancer care, so do nursing challenges. The American Nurses Association and the Oncology Nursing Society have developed Outcome Standards for Cancer Nursing Practice (ONS & ANA, 1987). These standards primarily reflect the high incidence problem areas of patients in any stage of disease, regardless of care setting. The clinical practice outcome standards address the areas of prevention and early detection, information, coping, comfort, nutrition, protective mechanisms, mobility, elimination, ventilation, and sexuality. This chapter will highlight five of these standards and identify specific implications for the nursing care of geriatric oncology patients. Recommendations for cancer nursing practice will be offered.

PREVENTION AND EARLY DETECTION

The elderly are the age group most vulnerable to develop cancer and should be targeted with the most intensive educational efforts to promote prevention and early detection behaviors (Stromborg, 1982). However, as a group they have received minimal intervention to encourage preventive self-care strategies. Reasons for this relate both to the potential consumer of the education and the health care providers offering the programs.

Programs on cancer prevention and early detection for the elderly may be underused due to the older person's perception that "it's too late, I can't do anything about my chances" or "even if it is diagnosed early, I'll die from it anyway." Hence, perceptions about one's vulnerability to develop cancer is a critical factor in the determination of an individual's readiness to hear about cancer prevention and early detection options. The concept of "cancerophobia" must be acknowledged as a real and important entity forming the basis of the perception about cancer. As the elderly perceive cancer to be in epidemic proportions around them within their network of family and friends, one can see why this fatalistic attitude about cancer is so apparent.

This sense that "it's too late" may be a factor in the orientation of health professionals to the educational needs of the elderly with respect to prevention and early detection. The fact that there are so few programs oriented specifically to the elderly indicates a similar fatalistic perception on the part of many providers of the education.

Transportation is another key issue because available programs are often not brought to the elderly, rather, the elderly are expected to come to the program with multiple problems associated with such. A label of disinterest or noncompliance may then not reflect the true reason for missed attendance.

Options for nursing intervention in the realm of cancer prevention and early detection are plentiful. Older Americans exhibit fewer early cancer detection behaviors than any other age groups, and nurses as educators can make a significant impact on this reality (Celentano et al., 1982; Weinrach & Nussbaum, 1984). In one study of 84 elderly cancer patients, nearly three-fourths of the sample reported that they had greater comprehension from teaching when performed by nurses rather than by physicians (Heinrich et al., 1984). Major goals in the realm of prevention and early detection include assisting the elderly to recognize significant personal risk factors for cancer's development, identifying a plan for seeking health care assistance when an alteration in health status occurs, and teaching appropriate cancer self-detection measures. Some specific recommendations include the following:

1. Assess potential barriers to initial instruction and implementation of preventive and self-detection practices, i.e., transportation problems to attend class or individual appointment; visual acuity impairment as it effects reading; negative perceptions promoting avoidance.

2. Whenever possible, integrate a behavioral check into the teaching program, i.e., observe patient doing a hemoccult testing, performing breast self-examination [BSE].

3. Encourage a mobile, individual approach rather than an institutional, group

approach, i.e., consider a mobile screening van to reach the elderly; acknowledge the therapeutic value of the individual versus group approach.

4. Customize programs to the specific needs of the elderly, particularly BSE education, i.e., anticipate selected performance obstacles such as alterations in vision, range of motion, and peripheral sensation; expect some aversion regarding the performance of BSE; utilize teaching tools that address physiologic changes in elderly breasts rather than models and illustrations oriented to the younger female (Welch-McCaffrey & Dodge, 1988b).

PROVIDING INFORMATION

The standard of providing the elderly with information about cancer and its treatment to facilitate self-care, participation in therapy, and optimal functioning, is complicated by many potential barriers within the elderly age group (Welch-McCaffrey, 1986). Neurosensory impairment, misperception, and participation preferences are several of those barriers that require deliberative assessment and intervention as informational needs are considered.

Some normative neurosensory aspects of aging have implications for planning educational endeavors for the elderly. These include decreased pupil size, changes in the lens, decreased color discrimination, presbycusis and decreased acuity of peripheral sensory nerve receptors. Some additional cancer considerations include potential central nervous system (CNS) and/or spinal cord involvement by a tumor, and concurrent therapy with busulfan, steroids, cisplatin and vinca alkaloids, which may selectively cause or exacerbate some of the above-mentioned neuro-sensory changes with age (Welch-McCaffrey, 1986).

Cancer patients in general are strongly influenced by a lack of or incomplete knowledge regarding the disease (Wilson et al., 1984; Weinrich and Weinrich, 1986). However, the elderly are particularly influenced by the accumulation of years of misconceptions and by information gathered from an extensive lay referral system. This, coupled with a fatalistic attitude, makes educational intervention within the elderly often difficult.

Eagerness to participate in care may not be evident with many elderly patients. Noninvolvement characterized by a lack of assertiveness in asking questions about one's cancer as well as deferring decision-making to the physician and health care team often is closely tied to cultural expectations and a cohort effect. This noninvolvement is evidenced in the fact that the elderly in general know less about their disease process and use of medications than do younger patients (Klein et al., 1982). Suggestions for dealing with barriers that affect the provision of information for the elderly include the following:

1. In anticipating altered perception with age, consider using short sentences, and large, bold print whenever possible; assess hearing impairment initially;

supplement verbal messages with hand gestures and written information; allow extra time for patient responses.

2. Thoroughly assess expectations from treatment based on the patient's past experiences; then clarify the difference or uniqueness of the patient's situation, ideally with a family member in attendance.

3. Respect the individual patient's desire for participation in his or her care and the elderly's common difficulty in using the word "cancer," and discomfort with communicating problems with physicians.

4. Acknowledge a general discomfort on the part of the elderly with airing questions in group settings.

5. Anticipate worry over unanswered questions and hence the need to reinforce teaching begun by the physician (Rimer et al., 1983).

COPING

The stresses associated with a cancer diagnosis in the elderly can emanate from a wide spectrum of physical, psychologic, and spiritual etiologies. Again, misperceptions about cancer are a major factor influencing coping strategies. Stereotyping the elderly by health professionals is common when psychosocial responses in geriatric oncology are addressed.

Jennings and Muhlenkamp (1981) noted that oncology nurses considered older cancer patients less depressed, anxious, and hostile than what the patients themselves reported. Assumptions often prevail when depression and confusion are problematic symptoms. However, recent studies have suggested that psychosocial distress as a result of a cancer diagnosis in the elderly may be less intense than that in younger age groups.

Cassileth et al. (1984) reported that age appeared to offer a diagnosis-independent advantage in that better mental health scores were found with the older chronically ill patients studied. Ganz et al. (1985) found that the elderly male cancer patients whom they studied generally experienced less psychosocial disruption from cancer than did younger individuals. Both groups of researchers concluded that the experience of developing coping skills to manage stress over the years most likely was responsible for the lower level of psychosocial distress among the elderly.

In evaluating depression as a correlate of coping in female cancer patients, Lansky et al. (1985) found that the prevalence of depression was within the range seen in the general population and that elderly female cancer patients had no higher incidence of a major depressive disorder. The most significant indicator of depression in an elderly cancer patient is not a diagnosis of cancer, but rather a premorbid history of depression.

There is psychopharmacologic evidence suggesting that depression in older age is associated with alterations in the synthesis, storage, release, and utilization of chemical neurotransmitters (Lipton, 1976). The typical burdens of the elderly must also be considered in the evaluation of depression in old age. These burdens include physical impairment, illness, bereavement, loneliness, boredom, poverty, and lack of independence (Lipton, 1980). Hence, physiologic and psychosocial factors may interplay in the causation of depression in the elderly. Cancer-related variables become factors to consider as well. Neurologic involvement by tumor and fluid and electrolyte imbalance may cause neuropsychiatric symptoms (Welch-McCaffrey, 1985a). Cancer of the pancreas, a common malignancy in old age, has been noted to present with depression as an early symptom (Douglas et al., 1977; Joffe et al., 1986). Multiple losses (both personal and social) become profound factors for the elderly, particularly when the loss is that of a spouse. Murphy (1985) found that the absence of a significant relationship involving the reciprocity of warmth and understanding promotes depressive responses in the elderly.

Confusion in the older cancer patient is not an automatic correlate to the disease or its treatment (Welch-McCaffrey & Dodge, 1988a). However, to many physicians and nurses the clinical appearance of confusion in the elderly is perceived as an expected occurrence. Hence, the aggressive workup of a confusional state in the elderly is often neglected. Most confusional states are both acute and reversible in the elderly cancer patient. (Welch-McCaffrey & Dodge, 1988b).

Drug-related causes often evolve from polytherapy, particularly drugs with central anticholinergic effects, antipsychotics, antihistamines, and antispasmodics. As the common sequelae of pain, emesis, obstruction, and anxiety are treated in the elderly cancer patient, potential etiologies of confusion abound. Other causes of confusion such as infection, dehydration, ischemia, and metabolic imbalances must also be considered in the evaluation of confusion in the elderly cancer patient. Suggestions for emotional support to enhance coping in the elderly patient with cancer include the following:

1. Assess coping requirements the same way for any age group (Table 15.1). Make no assumptions about the appropriateness of a given response without validation from the patient and family. Plan supportive interventions around an individualized psychosocial assessment.
2. Look for multiple, significant losses or the recent loss of a spouse to enhance depression and complicate coping. Unresolved losses from years past and a premorbid history of depression are high-risk factors as well.
3. When confusion is a clinical problem determine if the confusion is new or a gradual worsening of an insidious problem. This information provides substance for the differential diagnosis of an acute versus chronic confusional state.

TABLE 15.1 Psychosocial Assessment of the Cancer Patient by the Nurse

Category	Knowledge Goal	Sample Questions
Previous or standard style of coping with crisis	What should I expect regarding communication?	What were some major setbacks you've had in the past? How did you react when they occurred? What help did you get through that difficult time?
Past experiences with cancer	What assumptions, misconceptions are present?	Has anyone close to you had cancer? How did he/she fare? What have you read or heard about cancer?
Transmission of information	What and how was the patient told about the cancer?	What is your perception of where you stand with your cancer? In what manner were you told? Do you feel hopeful? How much do you want to know about your cancer?
Availability of support	Who is helping the patient deal with the cancer?	Who is your main support? Are they nearby? Do they want to help? How is the main support doing? How much do you talk about the cancer?
Current stressors	Where should I place my priorities?	What is your main concern now? What is the main factor interfering with your ability to get on with your life? What can the nurses do to help you cope with your cancer?

Adapted from Knobf MK, Fischer D, Welch-McCaffrey D 1984: *Cancer Chemotherapy: Treatment and Care*, Chicago: Yearbook Medical Publishers, with permission.

COMFORT

Cancer is a disease immediately associated with an alteration in comfort. However, the incidence of significant pain in the general population of cancer patients is less than 50%. Because most elderly are dealing with other chronic illnesses concurrently with cancer, the distress caused by nonmalignant conditions must be determined in the evaluation of discomfort. Arthritis, neuralgia, angina, and peptic ulcer disease are just a few possible nonmalignant sources of physical distress to consider.

When the elderly cancer patient does have a problem with cancer-related pain, pharmacologic treatment may be hampered by age-related alterations in the synthesis and metabolism of drugs and the interaction of multiple prescribed drugs. However, there is no evidence that pain threshold or pain tolerance is significantly different among the elderly with intact mental function than in other age groups (Long, 1985). When narcotics are required to treat cancer-related pain, longer-acting drugs such as methadone or the sustained-release morphine compounds often work well with the elderly owing to the decreased demand for repeated pill-taking throughout the day. It seems appropriate at this time to elaborate briefly on the issue of compliance with drug regimens because this clinical problem affects not only pain management but also the overall success with symptom management in the promotion of comfort throughout the course of cancer.

To date, no studies have addressed the issue of medication noncompliance in the elderly cancer patient population. However, in the general aged population it is estimated that one-half of the elderly do not comply with their prescribed drug regimens. Some manifestations of medication noncompliance include the following:

- Failure to fill prescriptions;
- Filling the prescription but failing to take the medication;
- Taking only a portion of the medication;
- Failure to follow the frequency or dose instructions;
- Sharing medications;
- Using over-the-counter medications as a substitute for prescribed drugs;
- Putting all of one's daily medications in one container and taking them randomly throughout the day (Buckalew & Sallis, 1986; Welch-McCaffrey, 1986).

Compliance is often inversely related to the number of prescription medications (Darnell et al., 1986). When more than four drugs are prescribed for the patient, at least one will be mishandled. Hence, it is interesting to note that at least 25% of all elderly discharged from a hospital will have six or more prescriptions that require self-administration (Smith, 1979). The cancer experience, then, induces a potential high-risk situation for the elderly when antiemetics, analgesics, oral chemotherapy, and sedatives are prescribed in addition to the drugs ordered for the patient's other concurrent chronic illnesses.

Sleep disturbances may be a particularly troublesome deterrent to psychobiologic comfort. The presence of pain, anxiety, and changes in orientation associated with hospitalization may exacerbate existing sleep problems. Colling (1983) cited frequent complaints by the elderly in relation to sleep:

- More frequent awakening during the night;
- Increase in total time awake;
- Longer time in bed before the onset of sleep;
- Subjective expression of poor sleep;
- Early morning awakening.

Monitoring continuous infusions of chemotherapy-uncontrolled bouts of diarrhea for lower pelvic irradiation, protracted emesis, and pain are some examples of cancer-related variables that can interfere with an elderly patients' pattern of sleep.

In working with elderly cancer patients and their families to promote comfort, goals include encouraging the patient and family to report alterations in comfort level and identifying measures that enhance comfort. Some suggestions for meeting these goals include the following:

1. Identify the etiology of the patient's pain(s) and consider nonmalignant as well as malignant sources.

2. Consider the use of longer-acting drugs to treat pain when planning a medication regimen.

3. To enhance compliance promote the use of various reminder tools; written instruction should supplement verbal teaching; follow-up phone contact and home care support should be coordinated; and review current medication schedule and adapt accordingly to decrease requirements to take medications constantly throughout the day (Welch-McCaffrey, 1985b).

4. Acknowledge alteration in sleep as a major potential cause of symptom distress and intervene accordingly, also acknowledging the need for nap time with age (Hayter, 1983).

MOBILITY

Because mobility is a critical element in longevity and quality of life, alterations in mobility must be assessed in an ongoing fashion as should potential causes of an impairment in mobility. In the cancer experience decreased mobility may be caused by the cancer itself or by complications of the disease and its treatment.

The problem of bone metastases creates many real and potential threats to optimum mobility. Bone involvement by cancer is the third most common site of metastatic implantation. More than 80% of all patients who develop bone metastases have tumors originating in the breast, prostate, or lung cancers, malignancies occurring frequently in the elderly (Welch-McCaffrey, 1988). Bones most frequently affected by metastases include the pelvis, ribs, femur, and vertebral bodies.

The problem of spinal cord compression as a result of bone metastases is yet another major consideration in altered mobility. Lung and breast cancer, lymphomas, and cancers of unknown primaries account for one-half of this oncologic emergency.

Primary nursing has an important role in the early diagnosis of spinal cord compression because changes in gait and bowel and bladder function may be early symptoms of ensuing compression that can be assessed by nurses over time (Welch, 1980).

Problems in gait can also be attributed to the neurotoxic effects of the vinca alkaloids. Stumbling, loss of balance, loss of sensation, or numbness and tingling in the foot and toes are all symptoms of this chemotherapeutic toxicity. An assessment of this problem can be done by asking the patient to walk on his or her heels. The inability to do so often points to peripheral neurotoxicity. Certainly, dyspnea, nutritional compromise, weakness, and fatigue, common correlates of both cancer and its treatment, increase the likelihood of impaired mobility.

The tendency of older persons to fall and injure themselves is so common that it is considered almost an inevitable part of aging (Craven & Bruno, 1986). However, falls in the elderly patient with cancer must be minimized owing to the multiple potential complications that may result. In particular, falls that happen concurrently with bone marrow depression and bone metastases increase the likelihood of bleeding, thrombosis, infection, and fracture, in addition to compromising the patient's quality of life and overall rehabilitative process. Hernandez and Miller (1986) outlined risk factors in the profile of the elderly patient most likely to fall. These factors are listed in Table 15.2 with the cancer implications noted.

Robinson and Conrad (1986) stated that the word "accident" in discussing falls is inappropriate in that it connotes evidence of random events in the causation of falls. The authors advise the use of the term "nonintentional injury," with its implications of preventive interventions. Regardless of terminology, mobility status should be included in the overall evaluation of rehabilitation needs of cancer patients, and in particular, the older cancer patient (Schag et al., 1983).

Nursing interventions associated with altered mobility encompass both therapeutic and preventive strategies. Some of these include the following:

1. Assess cancer-related causes for impaired mobility and plan prophylactic interventions.
2. Evaluate postural competence and environmental demand with individual geriatric oncology patients.
3. Implement a protocol to prevent falls for high-risk patients.
4. Utilize physical therapy services during prolonged periods of immobilization to increase strength and range of motion.
5. Assess potential hazards to mobility at home before discharge.

CONCLUSION

In addressing the current or potential geriatric oncology population, many education-intensive programs are needed. However, as Rimer (1983) noted, educating

TABLE 15.2 Risk Factors for Falls and Their Cancer Implications

General risk factor	Cancer implication
History of falls	Assess premorbid history
Postural hypotension	Increase time in bed
Sensorimotor deficits	Peripheral neuropathy from vinca alkaloid therapy
	Steroid-related cataracts
	Cisplatin-related ototoxicity
	Brain metastases
Gait instability	Weakness/cachexia
	Peripheral neurotoxicity
	Spinal, pelvic, or lower extremity bone metastases
Confusion	Polytherapy, particularly with drugs having central anticholinergic effects
Incontinence/urgency	Bladder outlet obstruction
	Prostatic hypertrophy
Cardiovascular disease	Assess concurrent nonmalignant disease
	Cardiotoxicity from anthracycline antibiotic chemotherapeutic agents
	Pericarditis
Neurologic disease affecting movement or judgment	Brain metastases
Orthopedic disorders or devices affecting balance	Bone metastases surgical therapy
Medications affecting blood pressure or level of consciousness	Analgesics, antiemetics, antianxiety agents, diuretics to treat symptom distress
Agitation, increased anxiety, emotional ability	Uncontrolled pain, stress of initial or recurrent diagnosis

Adapted from Hernandez, M. & Miller, J. (1986). How to reduce falls. *Geriatric Nursing*, 7:97–102.

the lay community without educating the professional community would produce negligible outcomes. It is hoped that this chapter has identified some implications for care of the elderly cancer patients and has encouraged further interest and investigation into this field.

One of the greatest disservices to the elderly with cancer is the immediate attribution of troublesome signs and symptoms to a given cause without aggressive workup of the problem's etiology. Figure 15.1 summarizes some of the common problems of old age and their potential cancer implications. It is time that we acknowledge the special needs of geriatric oncology patients much like we acknowledge the special needs of children with cancer. The fact that one-half of all cancers are diagnosed in the older age group mandates a close scrutiny of problems and care requirements which has not been performed to date. Because chronologic

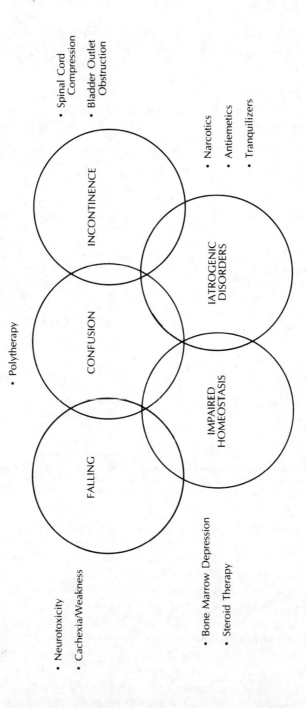

FIGURE 15.1. Morbidity-associated old age syndromes with references to cancer. Adapted from: R. Cape, 1978.

age is the single greatest risk factor for cancer's development, we cannot ignore the importance of the specialty of geriatric oncology.

REFERENCES

American Nurses Association & the Oncology Nursing Society. (1987). Standards of oncology nursing practice. Kansas City: Author.

Buckalew, L.W., & Sallis, R.E. (1986). Patient compliance and medication perception. *Journal of Clinical Psychology, 42:*49–53.

Cape, R. (1978). Aging: Its complex management. New York: Harper and Row.

Cassileth, B., Lusk, E.J., Strousse, T.B., Miller, D.S., Broan, L.L., Cross, P.A., et al. (1984). Psychosocial status in chronic illness: A comparative analysis of six diagnostic groups. *New England Journal of Medicine,, 311:*506–511.

Celentano, D., Shapiro, S. & Weisman, C. (1982). Cancer preventive screening behavior among elderly women. *Preventive Medicine, 11:*454–463.

Colling, J. (1983). Sleep disturbances in aging: A theoretic and empiric analysis. *Advances in Nursing Science, 6:*36–44.

Craven, R., & Bruno, P. (1986). Teach the elderly to prevent falls. *Journal of Gerontological Nursing, 12:*27–33.

Darnell, J.C., et al. (1986). Medication use by ambulatory elderly: An in-house survey. *Journal of the American Geriatrics Society, 34:*1–4.

Douglass, H.O., Karakousis, C.P., & Nava, H. (1977). Guide to the diagnosis of pancreatic cancer. *Hospital Medicine, 13:*6–13.

Ganz, P., Schag, C., & Heinrich, R. (1985). The psychosocial impact of cancer in the elderly: A comparison with younger patients. *Journal of the American Geriatrics Society, 33:*429–435.

Hayter, J. (1983). Sleep behaviors of older persons. *Nursing Research, 32:*242–246.

Heinrich, R., Schag, C., & Ganz, P. (1984). Living with cancer: The cancer inventory of problem situations. *Journal of Clinical Psychology, 40:*972–980.

Hernandez, M., & Miller, J. (1986). How to reduce falls. *Geriatric Nursing, 7:*97–102.

Jennings, B., & Muhlenkamp, A. (1981). Systematic misperception: Oncology patients' self-reported affective states and their caregivers' perceptions. *Cancer Nursing, 4:*485–489.

Joffe, R., et al. (1986). Depression and carcinoma of the pancreas. *General Hospital Psychiatry, 8:*241–245.

Klein, L., et al. (1982). Aging and its relationship to health knowledge and medication compliance. *Gerontologist, 22:*384–387.

Lansky, S., et al. (1985). Absence of major depressive disorder in female cancer patients. *Journal of Clinical Oncology, 3:*1553–1560.

Lipton, M. (1976). Age differentiation in depression: Biochemical aspects. *Journal of Gerontology, 31:*293–299.

Lipton, M. (1980). Pharmacotherapy of depression in the elderly. *Psychosomatics, 21:*816–824.

Long, D. (1986). Management of pain in the elderly. In Andres, R., Bierman, E.L., & Hazzard W.R. (Eds.), *Prinicples of geriatric medicine,* (pp. 199–208). New York: McGraw Hill.

Murphy, E. (1985). The impact of depression in old age on close social relationships. *American Journal of Psychiatry, 142:*323–327.

Rimer, B., Jones, W., Wilson, C., Bennett, D., & Engstrom, P. (1983). Planning a cancer control program for older citizens. *Gerontologist, 23:*384–389.

Robinson, B.E., & Conrad, C. (1986). Falls and falling. In Ham, R.J. (Ed.), *Geriatric medicine annual*. Oradell, NJ: Medical Economics.

Schag, C., Heinrich, R., & Ganz, P. (1983). Cancer inventory of problem situations: An instrument for assessing cancer patients' rehabilitation needs. *Journal of Psychosocial Oncology, 1*:11–24.

Smith, C.R. (1979). Use of drugs in the aged. *Johns Hopkins Medical Journal, 145*:61–64.

Stromborg, M. (1982). Early detection of cancer in the elderly: Problems and solutions. *International Journal of Nursing Studies, 19*:139–156.

Weinrich, S., & Nussbaum, J. (1984). Cancer in the elderly: Early detection. *Cancer Nursing, 7*:475–482.

Weinrich, S. & Weinrich, M. (1986). Cancer knowledge among elderly individuals. *Cancer Nursing, 9*:301–307.

Welch, D. (1980). Spinal metastases from carcinoma of the breast. *Nurse Practitioner, 5*:8, 10.

Welch-McCaffrey, D. (1985a). Coping with cancer: the elderly patient receiving chemotherapy. In *Nursing Considerations in Geriatric Oncology*. Adria Labs: Columbus, OH.

Welch-McCaffrey, D. (1985b). Medication use in the elderly cancer patient. *Oncology Nursing Forum, 12*:89.

Welch-McCaffrey, D. (1986). To teach or not to teach? Overcoming barriers to patient eduction in geriatric oncology. *Oncology Nursing Forum, 13*:25–31.

Welch-McCaffrey, D. (1988). Metastatic bone cancer. *Cancer Nursing, 11*:103–111.

Welch-McCaffrey, D., & Dodge, J. (1988a). Acute confusional states in elderly cancer patients. *Seminars in Oncology Nursing, 4*:208–216.

Welch-McCaffrey, D. & Dodge, J. (1988b). BSE for elderly women: considerations in program planning. *Oncology Nurisng Forum, 15*:811–814.

Wilson, C., Rimer, B.K., Bennett, D.J., Engstrom, P.F., Kane-Williams, E., & White, J. (1984). Educating the older cancer patient: Obstacles and opportunities. *Health Education Quarterly, 10*:76–87.

Index